Dr. ROMI
HUP. D.
3400 S
PHILA, PA 19104

(PAge 139)
292
148

JONATHAN E. RHOADS, M.D.

JONATHAN E.

QUAKER SENSE AND SENSIBILITY IN THE WORLD OF SURGERY

JOHN L. ROMBEAU, M.D.
DONNA MULDOON

HANLEY & BELFUS, INC. *Philadelphia 1997*

RHOADS, M.D.

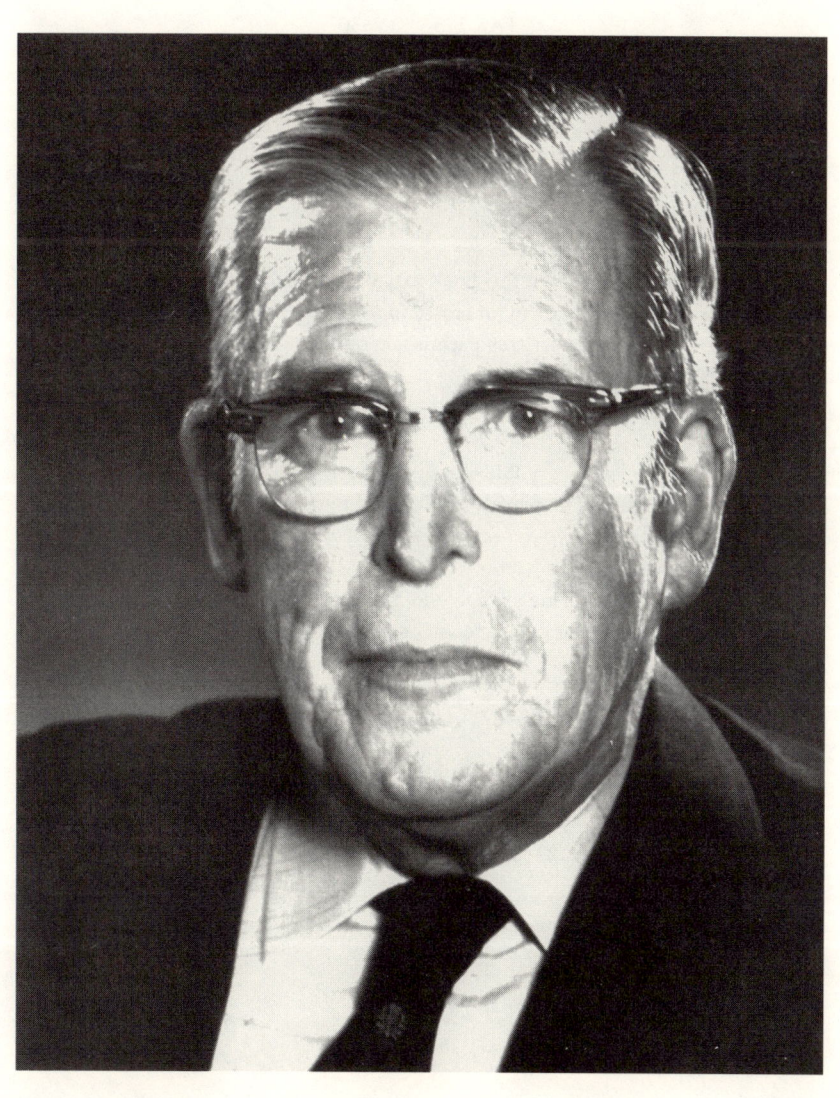

HANLEY & BELFUS, INC.
Medical Publishers
210 South 13th Street
Philadelphia, PA 19107

215-546-7293; 800-962-1892
FAX 215-790-9330
INTERNET http://www.hanleyandbelfus.com

Copyright © 1997 by Hanley & Belfus, Inc.

All rights reserved. No part of this book may be reproduced, reused, republished, or transmitted in any form, or stored in a data base or retrieval system, without written permission of the publisher.

ISBN 1-56053-252-1
Library of Congress Catalog card number 97-71848

Hanley & Belfus books are available for special promotions and premiums. For details, contact the publisher.

DESIGNED BY ADRIANNE ONDERDONK DUDDEN

Printed in the United States of America

1   3   5   7   9   10   8   6   4   2

CONTENTS

Preface vii
Foreword ix

INTRODUCTION
They Came to Do Good and Did Well 1

ONE
Friends for Life 7

TWO
Swimming the Bosporus 45

THREE
Can We Give Him Back His $18? 65

FOUR
Mr. Pim Passes By 101

FIVE
The Battle of Spruce Street 121

SIX
The Chief, the Cow, and the Cortisone 147

SEVEN
Thought for Food 175

EIGHT
A Happy Faculty 215

NINE
I Wonder Where That Plane Is Going? 229

TEN
Wise Counselor, Firm Friend 249

Acknowledgments 272
Endnotes 273
Selected Bibliography 290
Index 293

PREFACE

John L. Rombeau, M.D.
Donna Muldoon

Jonathan E. Rhoads is an amazing enigma. How was one surgeon able to accomplish so much in clinical care, research and teaching, reach the pinnacle of American surgery, and still be devoted to his family, friends and community? What role did his Quaker upbringing play in those achievements? How has he remained an active contributor to society at the age of 90? Those are just a few of the questions we pondered in 1992 when we began researching this book. Throughout the preparation, our goals were steadfast: namely, to portray the humanistic and scholarly qualities—with an emphasis on the former—that distinguish this unique person. This book is not intended to be a definitive scientific biography. By design, and with the hope that the readership will extend beyond academic surgeons, no attempt was made (with the exception of the discovery of intravenous feeding) to critique the 350 scientific publications of Dr. Rhoads. For this information, the reader is referred to *Jonathan E. Rhoads—Eightieth Birthday Symposium*, edited by Clyde F. Barker and John M. Daly and published by J.B. Lippincott in 1989.

Many methods were used to obtain information for this authorized biography. Extensive interviews with Dr. Rhoads were conducted and transcribed. We interviewed more than 40 individuals, including family, close friends, and colleagues. Letters were received from 109 former surgical residents and many others. Telephone interviews were conducted with those unable to be interviewed in person. The response was overwhelming. Regrettably, page limitations prevent the inclusion of comments from every contributor. The reader is referred to the Acknowledgments for a complete list of contributors. Site visits were made to the many schools and homes that figure so prominently in this book. Archival information from Germantown Friends School, Westtown School, Haverford College, The Johns Hopkins Medical School, the College of Physicians of Philadelphia and the University of Pennsylvania were especially contributory. Excerpts were selected from

66 of Dr. Rhoads' talks. Approximately 100 scientific publications were reviewed, particularly those relating to nutrition research.

It is impossible to adequately acknowledge every contributor to this book. We are indebted to Maureen Rombeau and Anita Moorer for their editorial assistance and detailed reviews of the manuscripts. The historic information provided by David Y. Cooper was extremely helpful for the chapter on nutrition research. Robin Noel's preparation of the photographs and Adrianne Onderdonk Dudden's elegant cover and text design grace the book. The expertise of Linda Belfus at Hanley & Belfus publishers was invaluable. Finally, and most importantly, this book would not have been possible without the encouragement and generous support of Clyde F. Barker, M.D., John Rhea Barton Professor and Chairman, Department of Surgery, University of Pennsylvania.

We hope this book will provide at least a modicum of insight into the reasons this enormously gifted individual made a difference in our world. Moreover, it is our hope that Jonathan Rhoads' distinguished surgical acumen and his graceful *Quaker Sense and Sensibility* will continue to inspire the young surgeons of today and beyond.

FOREWORD
Clyde F. Barker, M.D.

For the last seven decades, Jonathan Rhoads has served the University of Pennsylvania as faculty member, provost, department chairman and its ambassador to the worlds of medicine and science. While chairman of surgery, he guided his department to a preeminent position in U.S. surgery. From his full-time faculty (which never exceeded 20 in number), eight members became chairmen of medical school departments. Of the residents he trained during his 13 years as program director, 62 have become faculty members in 34 different medical schools, 28 as full professors and 12 as chairmen of their own departments. This biography provides considerable insight into how this remarkable individual inspired his trainees and colleagues to excel in academic medicine.

The remarkable breadth of Rhoads' contributions has been facilitated by the coincidence that his long career coincided with what might be called the renaissance period in surgery. The biography will be an important source for historians since few of the advances made in the entire field of medicine during Rhoads' long career escaped his attention and he had an important influence on many of them. He was among the first to use antibiotics for surgical problems, to use vitamin K to stop bleeding, and coumadin to stop clotting. He pioneered the use of intubation to treat intestinal obstruction. He probably performed the world's first peritoneal dialysis for renal failure and was one of the first to employ hemodialysis. He was one of the earliest to base the treatment of shock and burns on scientific studies. For decades Dr. Rhoads has been a world expert on malnutrition and the surgical treatment of cancer, areas familiar to both authors—John Rombeau, an acclaimed surgical nutritionist at the University of Pennsylvania, and Donna Muldoon, former Managing Editor to Dr. Rhoads for the journal *Cancer*. Dr. Rombeau is an ideal narrator of the story of the landmark development of total intravenous nutrition by Rhoads and his associates, one of the greatest advances of 20th century medicine, and Ms. Muldoon successfully captures important insights into the soul and mettle of Jonathan Rhoads' life beyond medical academia.

As chairman of surgery at a major university, Dr. Rhoads saw to it that his faculty pioneered programs in the emerging fields of open heart surgery, vascular surgery and transplantation. In a day when even the triple threat man appears to be extinct, it is safe to predict that we are unlikely to see the likes of this career again.

The book is fascinating because it provides so much new information about Dr. Rhoads' multi-dimensionalism. It details his experience as a scholar, athlete, editor, scientist, teacher, administrator, statesman, reconteur and driver of fast automobiles. The book abounds with personal anecdotes. As a youth and an adult, he has been fascinated with world travel. His adventures in Europe while on college vacation included swimming the Bosporus. Last year he flew over Mt. Everest in a small plane, one of the last travel experiences to elude him. The book also emphasizes Dr. Rhoads' physical stature, energy and stamina. The records show that before he reached his full height he was the tallest member of his college freshman class. This giant of a man has always seemed larger than life size. His personal impact on those of us who grew up under his wings seemed in part to derive from his sheer physical size.

Another important dimension known best to his surgical colleagues is his ability to cut and sew. Not all famous surgeons are great operating surgeons, but Dr. Rhoads was truly a surgeon's surgeon. Chosen to perform a major operation on his famous chief, I.S. Ravdin, less than a year after he finished his residency, Dr. Rhoads was still operating 50 years later, only recently electing to give it up while his skills were intact and much in demand.

Time, sometimes referred to as the fifth dimension, is crucial to the legend of Jonathan Rhoads. His father was an intern at the Hospital of the University of Pennsylvania when this oldest of U.S. university hospitals opened its doors 123 years ago. Jonathan Rhoads became a HUP intern 65 years ago and has been here ever since. Thus, his active career in medicine spans more than half of HUP's existence and the last two-thirds of the 20th century.

Present time continues to be an important part of Rhoads' mystique. In his case the University of Pennsylvania waived its rule that faculty members assume emeritus status at age 70. He remains an active professor of surgery at age 90. In fact the 1990s have been one of his best decades. During this decade he has added many major awards to a list of 30, which includes the Philadelphia Award (emblematic of the city's first citizen) and the Benjamin Franklin medal, the highest award of the American Philosophical Society, and in the spring of 1997 the prestigious Cosmos Club Award. He continues to travel the world to attend meetings, to lecture, and to write and publish papers, some 390 so far. Another important part of this decade is Dr. Rhoads' new and wonderful marriage, which is described with great charm. Kitty, like his first wife Terry, was a pediatrician. She is also the widow of David Goddard, who succeeded Rhoads as provost of our university. This provoked the comment by one wag that he only marries pediatricians and she only marries provosts. Kitty is Jonathan's distant cousin, but he says with a twinkle in his eye they're not concerned over consanguinity.

Finally, what can be said of Dr. Rhoads' importance to his university in time future? In leaving the University of Pennsylvania a century ago, William Osler delivered the famous address "Equanimitas." He said, "It is not the pride and pomp and circumstance of an institution which bring honor, nor its wealth nor the number of its schools." Instead, he said, "The greatest possession of any University is its great names . . . such names amongst . . . [Penn's] . . . founders as Morgan, Shippen, Rush and . . . their successors Wistar, Physick, Barton and Wood." Penn's history in the last 100 years allows the addition of other famous names to Osler's list, including Osler himself, the Peppers, A.N. Richards, and I.S. Ravdin. No such list would be complete without the name of Jonathan Rhoads. Penn is fortunate to have him in person as he begins his tenth decade. Generations from now I feel quite sure that Dr. Rhoads' name will remain secure in the annals of our university and those of American medicine. This book tells us why, and the story makes great reading.

Clyde F. Barker, M.D.
John Rhea Barton Professor
of Surgery
Chairman, Department
of Surgery
University of Pennsylvania
School of Medicine
Philadelphia, Pennsylvania

There is an aphorism attributed to President Hutchins of the University of Chicago: "Whenever I get the urge to exercise, I lie down until it wears off." We have a saying in our family: "Whenever I get the urge to lie down, I think of Jonathan Rhoads and get up."

Robert Austrian[1]

INTRODUCTION

THEY CAME TO DO GOOD AND DID WELL
THE RHOADS LEGACY

On May 16th, Jonathan Rhoads drove to the Hospital of the University of Pennsylvania to attend the Thursday morning Morbidity and Mortality Conference at 7:00 a.m. By 10:30 he was downtown at the annual meeting of Vishay Technologies. At 12:00 he drove across town for the American Philosophical Society Committee on Meetings. By 4:00 p.m. he was back at the hospital to attend the Schmidt Richards Lecture and dinner program. The next day, he and his wife flew to Rome to attend a joint meeting of the American Philosophical Society and the Academia Nazionale dei Lincei. They, along with other members of the American Philosophical Society, attended a reception at the American Embassy in Rome and later met with Pope John Paul at the Vatican. The next day Rhoads and his wife flew to Sicily to go sightseeing. Leaving Palermo, they flew back to Rome and on to New York. The year is 1996 and Jonathan Rhoads is 89 years old.

Anyone who knows Dr. Rhoads will not be surprised by this revelation. His days and nights continue to be filled with scientific, financial, educational, and religious meetings. He continues to participate actively in the scientific sessions of nearly all of the major surgical societies in the United States and abroad.

The influence of the Quaker ethos on the personality and mind of Jonathan Rhoads cannot be underestimated. Educated at the Germantown

1

Friends School, The Westtown School, Haverford College, and Johns Hopkins Medical School (all Quaker affiliated or initiated institutions), and the son of a physician who was also an active Quaker "minister," Jonathan Rhoads' early life was bathed in Quaker theory and practice, with little or no deviation from the ways of that distinctive society.

To most American minds, the word *Quaker* conjures up the name of an oatmeal cereal or a can of motor oil. The Quaker name is no doubt affixed to these products for a very good reason: Quakers are known to be industrious, honest, and direct in their dealings with people. Founded by George Fox, the Religious Society of Friends dates its existence to 1652 in the Lake District of England.[2] Quakers, or Friends as they are properly called, first came to this country in 1656. Persecuted in England and banned from universities, Friends became successful in those areas to which they were confined: trade, industry, and medicine. Their success is attributed to those values which Friends hold dear: industriousness, honesty, frugality, kindness, and gentleness in their dealings with people. Indeed, the Society of Friends, like a number of other minority groups, has contributed to the professions out of proportion to its numerical strength. While idleness is considered a vice to be avoided, Friends believe that "work should be approached not with frenzied striving for unattainable goals, but with deliberate calm."[3]

The Quaker religion is based on "testimonies" or doctrines which inform the ethical, moral, intellectual, and physical being. Howard Brinton, a Quaker historian, divides these into primary, secondary, and tertiary classes.[4] Included in the primary class is the belief that all men and women are equal before God; thus, no intermediary is needed, such as a minister or priest. Friends communicate directly with God within the confines of what they call the "meeting for worship," which is conducted in silence. If a Friend is so moved by what Fox calls the "inner light" during a meeting, he or she will stand up and deliver a short homily or commentary. It is not unusual for a meeting to go on in total silence. The meeting for worship and the meeting for business are included in the secondary class: the meeting for worship is the religious counterpart of the meeting for business.[5] The tertiary doctrines are defined by the values of community, pacifism, equality, and simplicity.

The relationships which are formed within this framework of Quaker doctrines are transferred to the outside world and become a way of life and thinking.[6] Indeed, his daughter-in-law, Julia, observes of Dr. Rhoads' religion:

In a way it's an identity rather than a religion. But it has informed his ethics. It has been clearly a rock for his whole sense of community.[7]

The Quaker meeting is a kind of "laboratory or training ground for a desired social order."[8] The mind and personality of Jonathan Rhoads, having been nurtured in this unique "laboratory," epitomizes in so many ways the sense and sensibility for which Quakers are so well known.

If Jonathan Rhoads is the embodiment of the Quaker way of life and thought, he is also considered by colleagues and friends the quintessential surgeon. Yet, it would seem that the ethos of those who inhabit surgery's high-tech, ego-driven environment is, in many ways, the very antithesis of that of the Quaker community. A former surgical resident of Dr. Rhoads relates her first meeting with him:

At times Dr. Rhoads was referred to as "the Sphinx" during the years I was a medical student, intern and resident. Early in my senior year of medical school, I paid the perfunctory visit of an aspiring surgeon to the Chief of Surgery, Dr. Rhoads. As always, he was courteous and guardedly encouraging to me as a female interested in surgery. During the course of the meeting he said, "Barbara, you have the personality of a surgeon." I was encouraged by this positive statement from him. Only later as I reflected upon his words, I was uncertain whether this was a compliment or an insult. All of my classmates knew that surgeons were "SOBs."[9]

The words *operating theater* call forth the drama, sterility, and detachment dominating that arena into which human beings are cast when matters of life and death are at stake. In this authoritarian, hierarchical system, the senior surgeon is the director in a drama which involves a supporting cast of residents, interns, nurses, and technicians, all of whom perform specifically delineated roles within the confines of the operating room (theater). The surgeon's world is defined by "event" rather than "process."[10] A decision is often made and acted upon in a specific period of time, with no turning back—unlike internal medicine, where time and medicine are the prescribed methods of action for less acute problems. This is a task-oriented profession requiring great mental and physical stamina. It is a world dominated by the intensity and immediacy of life-and-death decisions requiring a certain kind of personality and temperament. More than any other medical specialties, men who choose surgery as their specialization (it is still a male-dominated profession) are very often the sons of physicians.[11] A surgeon describes the typical person who goes into surgery:

I think we do believe that there is distinct characterization of the surgeon which sets us apart and makes us immediately recognizable, a cutting personality, so to speak. But the reason for that belief is part of what we are, an ego-centered group, made possible by our high prestige and status in the community. Everyone's not alike, of course, but enough of us are. We're aggressive, hard-driving elitists. We've become hardened through responsibility and task orientation which require emotional detachment, obsessive-compulsiveness, and high physical stamina. . . . We can get pretty temperamental if something gets in the way.[12]

In 1955, Dr. Rhoads wrote an essay on Quaker tenets and their relationship to the medical profession. He begins by qualifying his observations:

There are within the 160,000 members of the Society of Friends such differences in practice and precept and among the 200,000 physicians and surgeons in the United States such divergent philosophy and practice that any attempt to compare the two may indeed be unwise.[13]

He points out that the philosophy of Quakers, in many ways, parallels that of the medical profession:

The author believes that the religious philosophy of the Society of Friends is amazingly parallel to much that leaders of the medical profession have stood for from Hippocrates in ancient times to Osler and the best of the contemporary medical statesmen.[14]

It was Osler who rated equanimity as the most important quality in a physician. Certainly, many of Rhoads' colleagues have commented on his equanimity in and out of the operating room. In concluding his essay, Rhoads observes:

In thus reviewing consonances and dissonances between the religious philosophy of the Society of Friends and the principles and aims of the medical profession, one is nearly forced to conclude that the consonances far outweigh the dissonances, perhaps especially in this country where class distinctions are relatively amorphous; that the profession of medicine is almost an ideal medium of expression for Friends having the usual educational prerequisites, except insofar as it may involve military duties.[15]

What is the Rhoads legacy? In the area of research, it is the discovery of intravenous feeding. His loyalty and service to his community and its educational institutions is another. Whether as Provost of the University of Pennsylvania, or in his role as a board member of Haverford College, Bryn Mawr College, the Westtown School, Germantown Friends School, or the Philadelphia Board of Education, he has left his unique mark.

Equally important, and perhaps more lasting, is the example he set for the young men and women who trained under him. Bill Curreri, on the occasion of Rhoads' 80th birthday, observed:

I cannot help thinking how much pride Dr. Rhoads must have in the attendance today of all the professors and all of the chairmen he trained who are not only passing on the surgical principles he taught but also passing on the principles of education and research that he considers so important. This applies not only to the present generation but to several generations of surgeons to come, all of whom in a sense will have enjoyed the benefit of his wise counsel.[16]

Victor Hanson, commenting on the imprimatur Rhoads left on the Department of Surgery at Penn, adds:

His kindness and compassion while guiding a huge and complex organization of ambitious talent to achieve excellence was truly remarkable.[17]

Finally, no discussion of the Rhoads legacy would be complete without mentioning Dr. Rhoads' uncanny ability to achieve consensus in the many meetings he has attended. Quakers place great value on reaching consensus. Douglas Steere, a Quaker scholar, defines the qualities Friends look to in the clerk, the major official of the Friends business meeting:

He or she is a good listener, has a clear mind that can handle issues, has the gift of preparing a written minute that can succinctly sum up the sense of the meeting. . . . A good clerk is a person who refuses to be hurried and can weary out dissension with a patience borne of the confidence that there is a way through.[18]

This ability or talent is sorely needed in a world which has become increasingly impatient and contentious.

The Quaker aphorism, "They came to do good and did well," applies not only to Jonathan Rhoads but also to most of his close associates, colleagues, and friends. As he enriched the lives of these people, they enriched his. He surrounds himself with individuals of tremendous intellectual and financial accomplishment who share his traits of kindness, gentleness, and innate wisdom. The story of Jonathan Rhoads, then, is also the story of the great institutions he has attended and the remarkable people who have played an important role in his life.

Whatever atmosphere men are brought up in persists—their first impressions largely determine what they revere and love—or hate

O.W. Holmes, Jr.[1]

ONE

FRIENDS FOR LIFE
THE EARLY YEARS AND WESTTOWN

It was into an active, happy family that Dr. Edward Rhoads delivered his second son, Jonathan Evans Rhoads, at 8:00 a.m. on May 9, 1907. Named after his grandfather, his arrival was especially welcome since a first son, Edward Garrett, had died from pneumonia at 5 months of age. Indeed, 6 of his 12 male cousins died before the age of 23. Jonathan weighed a healthy 8 pounds, 2 ounces, and he was the last of 4 children. His sisters, Ruth, Esther, and Caroline, were 13, 11, and 7 years old.

His parents were both members of the Religious Society of Friends. His father, Edward Garrett Rhoads, was born on February 18, 1863, in Marple, Delaware County, Pennsylvania, where his ancestors lived since 1702. He was the third of 6 children born to Jonathan Evans Rhoads and Rebecca Garrett Rhoads. The Rhoads and Garrett forebears came to America from Lincolnshire, England, and Wales, respectively. Presumably, these Quakers came to America for a combination of reasons: adverse governmental regulations, religious persecution in Great Britain, and economic opportunity. In the family tradition, Jonathan Rhoads farmed and tanned leather and, at times, dug up stone in nearby Darby Creek from which scythe stones were made. He was a very religious man who also enjoyed travel, as revealed in a letter he wrote to Samuel Morris in 1891:

I have long had an appreciation of a call to religious service along the Pacific Coast of our country and the lands beyond the great ocean.[2]

His calling was realized in 1892 when he traveled to Australia and Japan to spread the Quaker message. It was during this trip that he met Robert Louis Stevenson and tried to convince him to become a pacifist.[3]

7

He was a recorded minister in the Quaker Meeting. While Quakers do not believe in intermediaries in their religious meetings, certain members who are gifted speakers are acknowledged with the title "recorded minister." In the custom of the Society of Friends, Jonathan Rhoads used the singular form of address "thee" and "thou" rather than the plural "you." His grandson and namesake continued to use this form of address with Rhoads' sister Caroline until her death in 1995. Another Quaker custom was to refer to the days of the week as First Day (Sunday), Second Day (Monday), and so forth rather than the pagan names of Sunday, Monday, and so on.

Because Friends are conscientious objectors, Rhoads was not involved in the Civil War, which was being fought in nearby Gettysburg. It is known that he visited local prisons and workhouses to deliver his religious message, and at one point he helped a local Negro orphanage with its financial affairs. He was socially active in the community and brought to the attention of the local government the need for various reforms. While work and religion were serious pursuits, Jonathan Rhoads did have a droll sense of humor, as evidenced in a story passed down through the family:

When he was farming, before he moved to Wilmington [Delaware], he was planting wheat in the field, and the farmers in that area had certain theories about the phase of the moon in which you should plant wheat and when you should not. So one of his neighbors saw him out planting wheat at the time you were not supposed to plant wheat and said that his crop would never be any good because it was the wrong phase of the moon. Jonathan responded that he was planting his wheat on the earth not on the moon![4]

Rhoads' grandfather was a very hospitable person, profoundly interested in his growing family, and he told them engaging stories of his foreign travels that always contained lessons as well.[5] He especially enjoyed reading the Bible at family gatherings.

With the impact of the Industrial Revolution, Jonathan Rhoads moved his business to Wilmington, Delaware, and changed the focus of the company to the manufacture of leather industrial belts, although they continued to make leather harnesses, saddles, shoes, and shoe laces. Admiral Richard Byrd gave his personal endorsement to the Rhoads company for the leather shoelaces he wore on his trip to the North Pole.[6] Rhoads brought his five sons into the business and changed the name to J.E. Rhoads and Sons in 1887. At one point, J.E. Rhoads and Sons had branches in Atlanta, New York, Philadelphia, and Cleveland. Later on, the company moved to Newark, Delaware, and until 1995 it was considered to be one of the oldest businesses in continuous operation in the United States.

Young Jonathan's memory of his grandfather is limited in that he was only 7 years old when his grandfather died in 1914. He was told that when his grandfather came to visit his namesake, the little boy was making porcine noises, and he said: "Thee little piggie thee!"[7]

Young Jonathan's grandmother, Rebecca Garrett Rhoads, was born in Philadelphia in a home near Fourth Street below Market, where her father had a business. Similar to the Rhoads, the Garretts had an interesting heritage. Rebecca's great great grandfather, Phillip Garrett, was a clockmaker and was said to be responsible for taking care of George Washington's clocks when he was in Philadelphia as President of the United States.[8] Later, the family moved to a larger home near Vine Street in Philadelphia, where her family lived until they moved to Germantown, on the outskirts of Philadelphia. Rebecca was sent to the Westtown Boarding School, in Chester County west of Philadelphia, for a year or two until graduation. As a child she preferred outdoor sports. She lived in a very large household with her six siblings, two aunts, an uncle, and a hired helper. After she married Jonathan Rhoads, she spent most of her time looking after her own large family and running a busy household. It was once rumored that "she debated her husband as to who was the head of the household. Finally she admitted that he was the head, but that she was the neck who turned the head!"[9] Caroline Rhoads remembered that her grandmother was kind and sensitive to children.

Why Jonathan and Rebecca's son Edward decided to become a doctor is not entirely clear. It is known that he gave serious thought to becoming a missionary. Writing to his daughter Esther, he tells her:

I used to think of missionary work as a desirable life in my younger days and I am glad for thee to have this taste of it, partly because of the association it brings with active Christian workers.[10]

It is probable, however, that he decided to follow in the footsteps of his Uncle James, who graduated from the Medical School of the University of Pennsylvania in 1851 and began practice in Germantown shortly thereafter. Subsequently, James gave up his medical practice, became deeply interested in education, and in time served as the first president of Bryn Mawr College.

Edward Rhoads attended the Westtown School as his father and mother had before him. After he graduated in 1881, he was appointed as an assistant teacher there and served in that capacity from 1881 to 1882 and then again for a period of time in 1883. Additionally, he served as president of the Westtown Alumni Association from 1881 to 1882. When Edward Rhoads entered the Medical School of the University of Pennsylvania in 1882, he was 6 feet 2 inches, had very broad shoulders, and sported a mustache and goatee. He had dark hair and blue eyes and spoke very slowly and softly. An imposing figure, he inspired confidence in those around him. Medical education at that time consisted of a three-year course and required no undergraduate college. Very little is known about his experience in medical school and, for that matter, his experience as an intern and house officer. His son recalls one experience his father related to him:

My father was very concerned about honesty in medicine. When he was a young house officer he helped operate on a man with cancer and the patient later asked him about prognosis and after telling him, the man went out and committed suicide. He didn't like to lie and probably passed on bad news by various circumlocutions.[11]

At the end of three years, medical students at the University of Pennsylvania were required to take examinations and write a thesis. Edward Rhoads' 67-page thesis, entitled "Epidemic Cholera," was thoughtfully and thoroughly researched. He concluded his thesis with the recognition that the future of medicine lay in prevention. On the basis of high scores in the examinations (he received grades of 99$\frac{3}{5}$ in his final exams), and his excellent thesis, Edward graduated from the Medical School of the University of Pennsylvania in 1885 at the age of 22. By this time he was living in Germantown at 5353 Greene Street, near his Uncle James' practice and the home of his aunts. Following graduation he won one of the four openings for internship at the Hospital of the University of Pennsylvania in West Philadelphia. Following his intern year he was appointed chief resident at America's first hospital, Pennsylvania Hospital at Eighth and Spruce Streets in Philadelphia. By 1887 Edward Rhoads had set up practice in Germantown, then a suburb of Philadelphia.

Edward Rhoads was shy, although not in his medical practice or at Quaker Meeting. A man of tremendous energy and bearing, he established a large medical practice, was very active in the Germantown Friends' Meeting and Philadelphia Yearly Meeting. On most Sundays he visited the quieter meetings whose members enjoyed the words of a recorded minister. He was very bright and well informed on most subjects. His daughter Caroline remembers that her mother could never make him save money (and she had to sequester it away), as he often gave it to the needy and to various missionary causes. She describes her father:

Father had a very good grasp of the English language and he was quite the Quaker minister. He loved to go to conferences in Northfield, Massachusetts. He went around and visited different meetings and particularly small meetings where there was very little speaking. He was a popular doctor and people were very fond of him. Father could tell wonderful stories. He could tell it right so that the point came through all of the time. He was a very religious man and it came through in the way he lived, and he was very kind and generous. He was in a way more quiet and a little bit shy at times, not where it concerned his competence but just in general social relations.[12]

His son, Jonathan, adds:

I thought him a very bright man and very well informed person, not just about medicine which he didn't talk about much in family dinners but on subjects in general. I think he would have been quite current on what has come out on health care programs and he had a keen interest in the single tax. . . . I think that perhaps my dominant impression of my father was a combination of intelligence and conscientiousness. But he was a good conversationalist.[13]

Edward Rhoads, like many of the Quakers of his day, was a conscientious objector. Of the American Quaker Meetings during World War I, the Philadelphia Orthodox took the strongest anti-war stand.[14] Too young for the Civil War and too old for World War I, Edward was not subject to the draft, when many young Quaker men were imprisoned for their beliefs. During his leisure time he visited these confined friends and worked for their release. If not successful in that endeavor, he at least helped to improve their conditions.

Edward Rhoads and Margaret Ely Paxson, whom he would marry, had many opportunities to become acquainted. Both attended the Westtown School during the same period, and both had relatives in Germantown whom they frequently visited. Moreover, Edward's Uncle James was married to one of Margaret's aunts. Edward Rhoads made special trips to Maple Grove in New Hope, Pennsylvania (30 miles northeast of Philadelphia), to visit the Paxson girls. These trips undoubtedly enhanced the friendship with Margaret, and the couple married in nearby Lahaska, Bucks County, on November 16, 1892.

Margaret Ely Paxson was born on December 21, 1863, to Oliver Paxson and Ruth Anna Ely on the farm named Maple Grove. Maple Grove was composed of two farms, one of about 60 acres and the other originally three times that size. Her father ran the farm and performed duties similar to those of a modern-day notary public. The house is still standing and continues to be occupied by the Rhoads family. The New Hope Historical Association noted that it is a home of some historical importance:

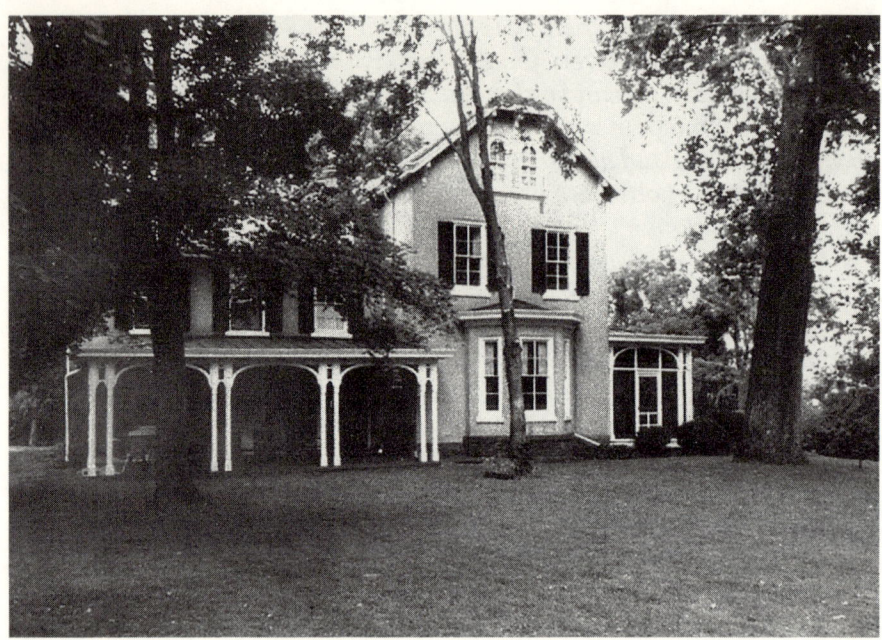

Maple Grove, New Hope, Pennsylvania.

The original house stands since 1775 or 1776 on land purchased by Oliver Paxson from Coryell in 1770. The east end of the house was rebuilt in 1850. The farm once extended to the Delaware River and it is said that Washington's officers used the original house in 1775 and 1776. The parlours were last decorated in the 1880's and are typical of the period. Nine generations, descendants of Thomas Paxson, have enjoyed this home, which contains furniture, china, silver and treasures from foreign travel of most of these generations.[15]

Margaret was the second of four children. Her youngest sister, Caroline, was a member of the first class to graduate from the Bryn Mawr College. Margaret was educated at home and then was sent to Westtown School, from which she graduated in 1883. Although she did not go to college, she was an avid reader and was artistically inclined. There were two unhappy events in her childhood: her mother died from uterine cancer when she was only 4 years old, and her father died when she was 13. As the result of these traumatic experiences, she strongly disliked funerals for the rest of her life.[16] She and her siblings were raised by a kind and sensitive widow whom her father married shortly after the death of her mother. Margaret's uncle, Richard Ely, who lived nearby, was their appointed guardian and looked after Maple Grove.

Margaret was 5 feet 7 inches, with a trim figure and brown hair and green eyes. She probably suffered from polio at some point, as one of her hands was weak, which made writing a bit difficult. She loved horseback riding, tennis, gardening, and ornithology. She was a strong believer in travel and the importance of science. In addition to raising four children and tending to the needs of many visiting relatives and missionaries, Margaret was active in the Germantown Meeting, School Committee, and the Women's Foreign Missionary Association. John Webster, a schoolmate of Jonathan's, remembers her as an "enthusiastic, ebullient person, friendly, straightforward . . . a torpedo of energy, very active and quick talking."[17] Caroline describes her mother:

My mother was a very open person. . . . She was very adaptable. . . . She could get along with anybody and she was a friendly, outgoing person and had a great many friends. . . . She was exceedingly tactful without you ever thinking of her being tactful. She was very intuitive. . . . She could go into any situation and seem to be at home.[18]

Caroline tells another story of her mother revealing her kindness to others:

I remember I had a friend with awful, I call it acne, that may not be the correct term, but I could hardly bear to get near her. And I remember Mother just taking her in her arms and giving her a big kiss. I said to my mother, "How could you bear to kiss her?" because her face was so broken out, and Mother said, "Oh she needed it so badly!" And she was that way with people.[19]

She was above all else, according to her son Jonathan, "a resilient person and regardless of what happened her response was always quick."[20] He never saw her despondent or depressed. With regard to her views on discipline, Caroline remembers her mother "was a very human person and she didn't think you had to be restrained a whole lot to be good."[21] Jonathan underscores this view of his mother and her outlook concerning her children:

She was not, I don't think, a very rigorous disciplinarian. And she had a conviction that you couldn't shake. She thought you were going to be all right even when there was ample evidence to the contrary. . . . She had a great conviction that her children would turn out all right. Her faith in her children often seemed to me completely blind, and as the grandchildren came along, she showed similar and equal interest and devotion to them. She was, I would say, a happy person, sort of innately happy. . . . She didn't brood over things very much and I think she had a happy life.[22]

He adds:

When she and my father became engaged, my grandfather remarked that "'Margaret is so transparent." She didn't have any [hidden] side to her or didn't try to secret herself in any way. . . . She did a great deal of reading, particularly biographies. . . . Her favorite poet was Longfellow and she was fond of quoting his statement made early in life that he didn't know what he was going to do but he was going to excel in it, or words to that effect. But I think she had sort of a native business sense. She had an instinct about things. . . . She didn't marshall a lot of facts as a rule to support an argument and carry it on in a logical way. She sort of went from where she was to where she thought she ought to be . . .[23]

Rhoads' mother, Margaret, was the business person in the family and took wise advice from her Uncle Richard in managing the finances of her family, her husband's practice, and the farm.

Prior to her marriage, Margaret kept herself busy with the demanding chores of running a farm. Edward and Margaret complemented each other, and their daughter Caroline never recalls an argument between them. By all accounts, their marriage was a happy one. They settled in Germantown but kept the property of Maple Grove as their summer home.

Germantown was a community composed primarily of German immigrants, although it also included a sizable Quaker population. Philip Benjamin, in his book, *Philadelphia Quakers in the Industrial Age*, describes Germantown in the late 1800s:

Germantown with its own Orthodox and Hicksite Meetings was a sophisticated settlement. Rural oriented, conservative Friends felt estranged from its residents. When Joseph Elkinton planned a religious meeting there in 1894, Jonathan Rhoads warned him that "the rich and cultivated residents of that place" required wisdom and learning in a preacher before they accepted him.[24]

Benjamin further relates the reason Friends were attracted to Germantown:

Combining elite status, the atmosphere of an old rural town, and proximity to the business center of Philadelphia, Germantown attracted many Friends in the new century.[25]

The Germantown home at 159 West Coulter Street, where the family spent much of the winter, was large enough to accommodate the medical office of Edward Rhoads, a growing family, and, at times, many visiting missionaries and relatives.

The first child born to the couple was a girl, Ruth, in 1894. It was a difficult birth, and the child sustained some neurologic damage so that she had difficulty talking. She had low resistance to infections and suffered many illnesses over the course of her life. According to Caroline, her sister Ruth was "quite intellectual and very sweet looking."[26] She was sent to the Westtown School for a period in 1914, but was frequently ill and finished high school at Germantown Friends School. She went on to Bryn Mawr College, where they planned to apportion her work over 5 years rather than 4 because of her decreased energy and frequent illnesses. She managed to finish 4 years, but once again her studies were interrupted because of poor health. She never finished her fifth year at Bryn Mawr but continued to attend social affairs at the college and made many friends there. After college she worked for the Society of Organized Charity for several years but never became a social worker in the professional sense.[27]

Margaret Rhoads, Ruth Ely Rhoads, Caroline Paxson Rhoads, Edward G. Rhoads, and Esther Biddle Rhoads in 1902.

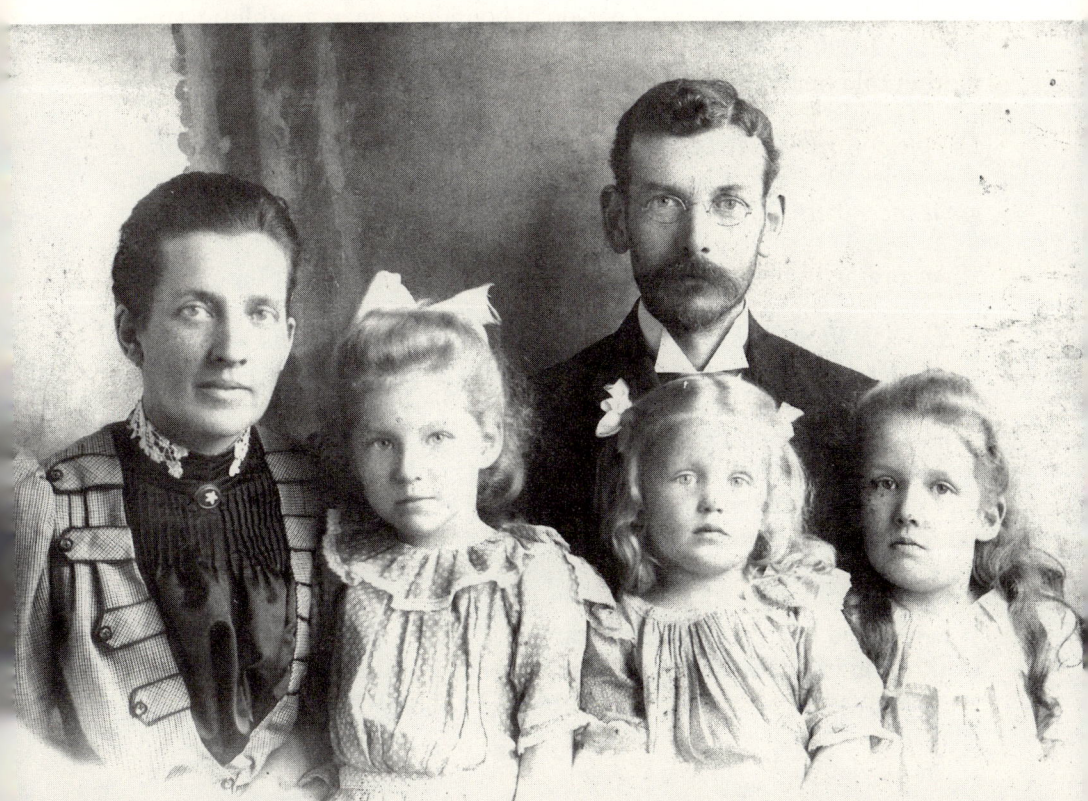

In addition to working in her father's office, she worked on a part-time basis in the Friends Free Library, which was part of the Germantown Friends School. She was admired for her work there, and as Caroline recalls:

If anybody in the Friends Library wanted something looked up they went to Ruth, not the head librarian. She enjoyed her work there very, very much.[28]

She played a pivotal role in her father's office and in the home, as her mother wrote:

Ruth does all of father's accounts extremely well at work and she is also a very good housekeeper. Her judgment is good and she has more decisions now. She remembers things and keeps us all jogged up so we quite depend on her.[29]

In her later years she spent her leisure time reading a good deal, helping out with the family, and traveling. She passed away in 1967 after a prolonged illness.

The second sibling, born in 1896, was another daughter, Esther. Esther was, by everyone's account, a person of boundless energy, athletic, smart, and headstrong. She left her imprint on others very early on, as her mother told her:

I so often think what David Forsythe told Aunt Margaret Rhoads about thee when thee went into kindergarten: "Thee has a very independent great niece here."[30]

According to her sister Caroline:

Esther was like mother in that she couldn't spell . . . but she was the one that later went on and did quite a bit of writing. She hated all English work as a girl. I guess she was quick enough so that she was very good at mathematics and I guess was quick enough so that she could kind of toss aside what she didn't care about and concentrate on what she did care about. But she made good friends at Westtown and was much more athletic than I. Quite well coordinated, she played hockey and had a good time.[31]

Esther had a large and varied stamp collection and would spend hours working on it. She was very outgoing, sociable, and energetic. Her boundless energy is revealed in a diary entry in 1914, in which she wrote:

I have played 38 games of tennis today, winning 18.[32]

She attended the Germantown Friends School where, according to her brother, "she proved to be a particular irritant to one of the math teachers."[33] She was not considered the academic but was particularly talented in the sciences. Later in high school, Esther decided that she wanted to study physics, so she transferred to the Westtown School in her junior year and graduated in 1914. The following fall, Esther attended Drexel University, where she majored in domestic science. She graduated from the program two years later.

Why Esther decided to become a Quaker missionary in Japan is not entirely clear. She did share her father's deep religious beliefs, and they would attend various Friends conferences and religious meetings together. Esther's early interest in Japan was spawned, perhaps, when her grandfather recounted his visits to that country to spread the Quaker message. Most likely, her parents also influenced her decision to become a missionary. They were very active in the Mission Board of the Philadelphia Yearly Meeting, whose chief interest was the work in Japan. Edward Rhoads was the Board's vice chairman, and his wife was its secretary. The Binfords and the Bowles, Quaker missionaries in Japan, visited the Rhoads family whenever they were in the United States. There was a children's missionary society which was an outgrowth of the ladies' missionary society of which her mother was a member. The stories the missionaries would

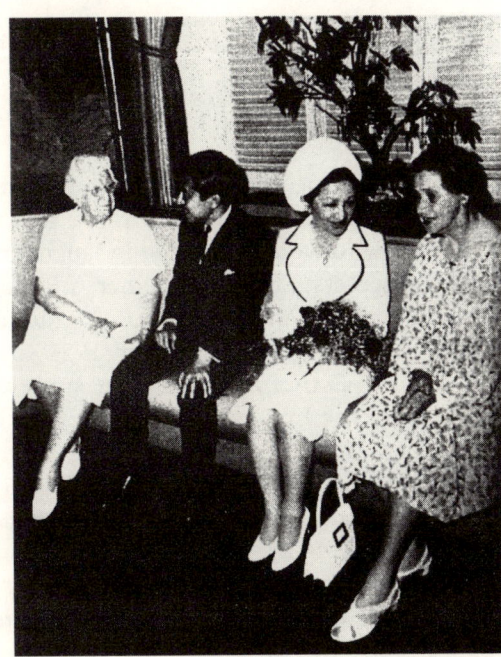

Esther Rhoads, Crown Prince Akihito, Princess of Japan, and Elizabeth Gray Vining.

tell probably fascinated the adventurous Esther. In addition, she came into contact, through her father, with the leading Japanese educator of the time, Inazo Nitobe. It was Nitobe who thought that the greatest contribution the Friends could make to Japan was in the area of education for girls.[34] To this end, a Friends Girls School was established by Quakers in 1887. In 1911 the school was recognized by the Japanese government as one of the best schools in Tokyo. At age 21 years, Esther left San Francisco on the *S.S. Korea Maru* for Japan in August 1917 and arrived in September.

Many years later, Esther shared her early experiences with her nephew's wife Julia, as Julia relates:

She shared once how difficult it was when she first got to Japan when she was teaching in the school. She had grown up in a whole milieu that valued a woman in a rather extraordinary way that the rest of society had not caught up with, even here in America. By the time she got to the school in Japan, she just had a clear sense that a woman was to be valued as an individual and to go as far as they could intellectually and in terms of achievement. It was a world without walls as far as she was concerned. I guess it was a woman who was running the school, the person who was her first supervisor, [who] had to take her aside and counsel her about the role she expected [of] her students, as young women coming in to their own in Japan, that they could not expect of themselves and their life in Japan what she was putting forward to them. It was not compatible with their role in society. They could not be what she was expecting of them. She had to turn that loose and learn more about the culture that she was to grow so close to. Evidently, that was a very painful and a very hard step for her.[35]

She spent one year there and returned to attend Earlham College in Richmond, Indiana. Earlham was a favorite Quaker college of the missionaries who were interested in Japan, and so it was a place sympathetic to her interests. She received her A.B. degree from Earlham in 1921 and returned to Japan shortly after graduation. She then attended the Japanese Language School from 1921 to 1924. Elizabeth Gray Vining, a colleague of Esther's who later became the first of the Quaker missionaries to tutor the Imperial family, wrote of Esther:

Esther Biddle Rhoads though only 27 in 1924 was already a leader in the school and the Institute. She'd first gone to Japan in 1917 and then returned to the mission in Tokyo with a life long commitment. She was a lovely woman with wavy brown hair, strong and enthusiastic and dedicated from childhood to working in Japan. . . . She taught English, Cooking and the Bible.[36]

The family wrote to Esther sometimes twice a day. Early letters reveal that her mother, Margaret, had very definite ideas about how her daughter should comport herself, especially concerning the matter of marriage if it arose:

You will be in very close quarters but thee will have time to look after thy "darling sin" of leaving things around. If thee could correct this great fault thee would be nearly perfect. So correct it for the bliss of thy future husband may depend on it, but be sure thee comes back to America to get him and also take him from our walk of life. After the glamour of first love has worn off and you settle down to the humdrum of life, it is fortunate not to be annoyed by mannerisms and ideals of another grade of society. I am presupposing that you would be attracted on congeniality of religious thought and tastes.[37]

Her brother Jonathan remembers her as "a vigorous person":

She went at everything pretty much. I think she played hockey and I expect basketball and so forth. Never seemed to get tired. At a later time there was a brand of overalls that would advertise that it would not rip, tear or wear out. We used to say that Esther would not rip, tear or wear out.[38]

Julia Rhoads describes Esther:

Such a powerful woman, powerful in the sense of her own sense of herself and mission that she had had. . . . I don't think I have known too many who have been clear about their role in life, what they wanted to do and what they hoped to accomplish, and yet at the same time she was so self-effacing. . . . She did not call attention to herself. . . . She didn't need to. She was just one of those people who would think, kind of like Jonathan, who had an extraordinary comfort with themselves. . . . They didn't need to make an impression on anyone because there was this sense of comfort and integrity that was very very strong.[39]

By 1926, Esther had a Master's degree in religious education from Columbia Teachers College in New York. She returned home on furlough in the spring of 1940, before Japan entered the war, and applied for a passport to go back. The U.S. State Department, perhaps anticipating imminent hostility, would not authorize her return to Japan. Esther was in the United States when Pearl Harbor was attacked, and she promptly got involved in looking after people of Japanese descent on the West Coast, who were U.S. citizens displaced by government fiat. From 1942 to 1945 she worked out of the American Friends Service Committee

Office in Pasadena, California, and dealt largely with interred Japanese-Americans. Later, she was able to get some of the young people out of the camps for educational opportunities in the East.

In June 1945, Esther and J.P. Elkinton, a fellow Quaker, went to Washington, D.C., to represent the Philadelphia Yearly Meeting to express their concern for peace and condemn the bombing of Japan. The missionary groups who had been in Japan were anxious to go back to see what they could do to help. General MacArthur, then in charge of occupied Japan, envisioned many problems if the missionary groups returned to look after people to the exclusion of those with non-Christian beliefs. MacArthur decided that the Christian missionaries could only distribute relief supplies through the Japanese Ministry of Welfare. He proposed that the missionary groups send a few delegates to represent them. They collectively formed an organization called Licensed Agencies for Relief in Asia, subsequently known as LARA. Because of her leadership qualities and her knowledge of Japan, Esther was permitted to return as a representative of LARA. In that role she visited 28 cities which had been bombed. Because she was working under the aegis of the U.S. military, Esther was given a rank which corresponded to Lieutenant Colonel.[40]

Esther returned to the Friends school in Tokyo, which had largely been destroyed during the war. The teachers carried on with their classes under the most difficult of circumstances. These concerns led Esther to serve as an intermediary for Friends in the United States who raised money for the restoration of the school. Esther proved to be a very astute business woman and garnered the trust and admiration of all who came in contact with her.

During the military occupation of Japan, MacArthur decided very early on not to try the Emperor as a war criminal. He recognized that the emperor was a religious entity, revered and worshiped by many Japanese, and not solely a governmental person. It became known that he wanted an American tutor for his son, and his thoughts turned to the Quakers because they had not joined in the attack or in the war. Initially, Esther was approached to fill this position. As she was already busy with her tremendous responsibilities in LARA and the reconstruction of the Friends School in Tokyo, she recommended Elizabeth Gray Vining, a Quaker and Bryn Mawr graduate for the position. Vining agreed to come to Japan and tutor the crown prince and other members of the Imperial family. She remained in that position for three years and then returned to the United States. It was at this point that Esther was called upon to replace her as the tutor to the crown prince. She became well known to the Imperial family and was invited to go duck hunting with them. She would go to the Palace to teach her lessons but would also invite them to the school so they could see how Americans worked and lived.[41] Esther became principal of the school in 1949 and was appointed Chairman of the Board of Trustees in 1955.

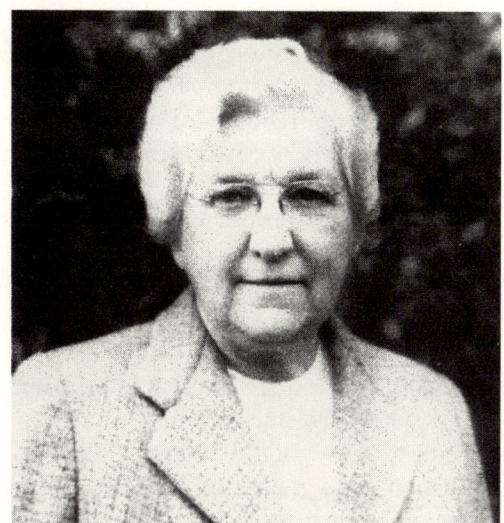

Esther Rhoads at 65 – retirement from Tokyo Girls School.

After 40 years of service, Esther retired in 1960. Emperor Hirohito awarded her the Fourth Order of the Sacred Treasure in 1952, and upon her retirement she received the Third Order, rarely given to a woman. The Japanese Red Cross gave her its highest decoration, and the Tokyo government presented her with the "keys to the city." Her life is recounted in a book, *Footprints of a Quaker: Esther Biddle Rhoads*, which remains to be translated from Japanese to English.

Esther returned to Germantown and lived with her sisters Ruth and Caroline. However, her retirement was short lived—less than four months after retirement, she went to Tunisia to aid refugees from the Algerian war. Frustrated with the impossible conditions and lack of resources there, she returned home a year later.

She became increasingly active with the Friends Services Committee, the Philadelphia Yearly Meeting, and the Germantown Meeting. Similar to her father and grandfather, Esther was formally recognized as a recorded minister by the Meeting. So fond was the Japanese Emperor of Esther and Mrs. Vining, that he interrupted a trip to Brazil to visit them in Philadelphia in 1978. Later, she received honorary degrees from Haverford College, Earlham College, and Drexel University in recognition of her lifetime devotion to the welfare of humanity. On February 4, 1979, Esther Rhoads passed away in her sleep at the age of 82. Although she was not alive to share in the event, the Friends School of Tokyo celebrated its 100th anniversary in 1987.

Caroline, the third daughter of Edward and Margaret Rhoads, was born on her father's birthday, February 18, 1900. Caroline, Jonathan's youngest sister, was a tall, statuesque girl with a lovely complexion and a shy disposition compared with her other siblings. She describes her childhood as quite happy, although she expressed disappointment that her mother, who was very outgoing, did not teach her more of the social graces.[42] She had great powers of concentration and loved to read. As Jonathan tells it:

My mother left her at home studying and asked her to cover the telephone, and my mother came back after a period of time and the phone was ringing off the hook and Caroline was deep in her book and not hearing it at all.[43]

Caroline attended the Germantown Friends School until the 10th grade, when she transferred to the Westtown School. She was by all accounts a very good student. She was happy with her experience at Westtown, and graduated in 1917. The family decided to send her to Mt. Holyoke College in Massachusetts because of their great admiration for the school's Quaker founder, Maryanne Wooley. Mt. Holyoke proved to be both stimulating and broadening. Her mother urged her to major in science. To partially satisfy her mother's interest in science and her own love for history, Caroline majored in economics. She graduated from college in 1921 and secured a teaching job at the Wilmington Friends School in Delaware. She subsequently accepted a position at the Moorestown Friends School in New Jersey, where she taught for 3 years. Caroline secured a teaching position at Girard College, a private school for orphaned boys in Philadelphia. She received a Master's Degree in Education from Columbia University and taught fifth grade until she retired in 1965. Caroline was considered to be a very successful teacher.

Like the other members of her family, she was an avid traveler. In her early 20s she took an extended tour of the Mediterranean, visited historic sites, rode a camel, saw the pyramids, took a boat along the Nile and visited the Holy Land. In later years she visited the Scandinavian countries and, in 1959, with her sister Ruth, visited Esther in Japan.[44] Caroline divided her time between 43 West Walnut Lane, in Germantown, and New Hope. Later in life, she moved to a Quaker retirement home in Germantown. Her love of reading helped make her a superb Scrabble player well into her early 90s. She loved her nieces and nephews and played an integral role in their upbringing. She took care of her mother and sister Ruth during their long illnesses. Caroline passed away in 1995 at the age of 95.

Jonathan was the second but only surviving son and last child of Edward and Margaret Rhoads. In the early 1900s, many changes occurred in Philadelphia and throughout the world. In the first decade of his life, advances in transportation, communication, and mass population movements

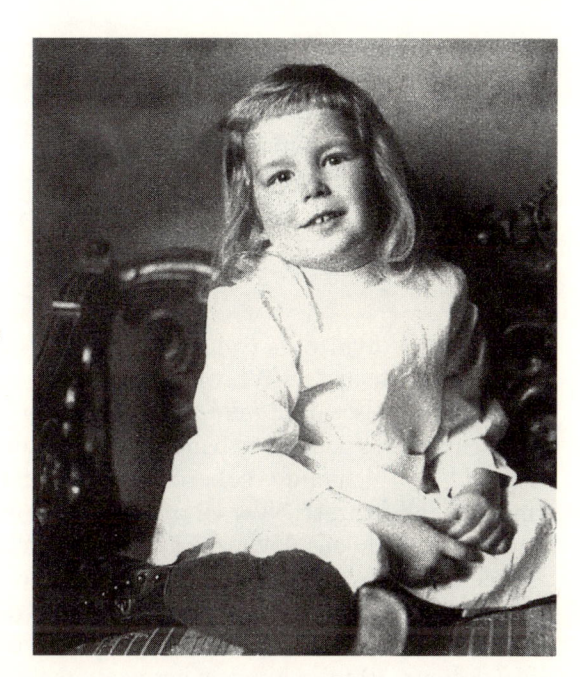

Jonathan Evans Rhoads at the age of 3—1910.

created an awareness of an interdependent world. Emigration soared in the first decade of the 20th century: nearly 9 million people immigrated to the United States. "Heavier than air flights" had begun in 1903 with the Wright brothers, and by 1910, automobiles were being mass produced. Locally, a wide channel was developed in the Delaware River, enabling Philadelphia to compete with the world's great seaports. The first airplane flight from New York to Philadelphia was sponsored by the New York Times and the Philadelphia Public Ledger. Radio transmission of human speech advanced rapidly. Telegraphic transmission of photos was lending immediacy to news reports. Phonographs made for quick international exposure to many types of music. Newsreels first appeared in 1909. The Rhoads family lived very well by most standards of the day. Edward Rhoads bought his first car in 1898, a three wheeler, but had so much trouble with it that he went back to using horses.

Writing to Esther in 1909, Margaret Rhoads reports on the activity of her 2-year-old son, Jonathan:

Jonathan showed me a great amount of scribbling on the wallpaper in the dining room and said, "mine!" so I had to remonstrate with him for marking the wallpaper, but it was so honest of him to own up to it.[45]

It is most likely that Jonathan at the age of 2, was proud of his handiwork, rather than exhibiting an early example of his scrupulous honesty. He was a handsome chubby little baby with big blue eyes, long flowing hair, and a wonderful smile. She writes again to Esther in that same year, expressing great pride in her little boy:

We went in the auto to Aunt Tatt's where we left it and walked up the Wissahickon [Creek, near Germantown] and back to the auto. Papa bought Jon a cute little cart which was easily carried in the auto and then trundled him along. He is perfectly splendid. He can even say "New Hope."[46]

The family divided its time between their summer home, Maple Grove, and their home at 159 West Coulter Street in Germantown. Typically, Margaret Rhoads would take the children to New Hope at the beginning of the summer, and her husband would remain behind with the domestic help and would spend weekends with the family at Maple Grove. The trip back and forth to New Hope was arduous. The York Road was a toll road. Edward Rhoads devised a system whereby he would exit York Road and reenter it beyond the various toll gates to reduce the cost to 75 cents. This was quite expensive, as most doctors received a dollar for an outpatient visit. For many years Margaret drove a horse-drawn carriage for the 7–8-hour, 30-mile journey between New Hope and Germantown.[47]

The Rhoadses spent their leisure time visiting friends and relatives, canoeing, swimming, and playing board games with the children. They tended to the farm animals, including chickens, horses, pigs, and cows. They tried to raise turkeys, but the birds would often stray to adjoining farms. The children were as much a product of country life as city life. There were a good many chores for them to do at New Hope. He helped feed the animals and gathered eggs from the hen house. His biggest job on the farm was harvesting bundles of hay to be stored in the barn. Jonathan spent one or two summers riding around the neighborhood and taking care of the family horse. He was given riding lessons in Germantown several times a week. Maple Grove was beautiful and the family loved being there—Margaret writes to Esther in 1909:

It is delightful to be home. Everything is in beautiful order. The grass is very green and shrubbery fine and peas and peaches in the distance. People drop in to see us. It is delightful to live in so much love.[48]

They grew currants, gooseberries, and blackberries and had beds of mint and horseradish. While corn, lettuce, cabbage, kale, parsnip, and turnips were cultivated, asparagus and tomatoes were especially abundant. The cows were milked, and cottage cheese was made in the summers. Jonathan's mother made jellies, and she worked tirelessly canning and putting up fruit and vegetables, which the family would live on for the entire year. Margaret writes:

I packed 40-odd jars of canned fruit this a.m. and, consequently, my arms ache! and besides Mary and I did up to 7 qt. jars of tomatoes and 6 pint jars of peaches.[49]

In the fall the family retained a farmer who would ship a market basket containing a couple of chickens, eggs, and garden truck to the family in Germantown. Jonathan met the train at Wayne Junction station, picked up the produce, and went about the neighborhood selling some of the surplus food from the summer.

The Rhoads children grew up in an atmosphere dominated by the Quaker values of economy, simplicity in dress, conservative lifestyle, and honesty and forthrightness in their dealings with others. This was a very religious family: the Bible was read to the children every morning. Edward Rhoads, like his father before him, took this religious moment to teach the children the geography of the Holy Land. He pulled out maps and showed them the sites of the various Bible stories he read to them. The family not only attended Germantown Meeting but would often visit other nearby meetings.

Jonathan skipped kindergarten and, at the age of 6, entered the first grade in nearby Germantown Friends School—the same school his sisters attended and where his father was the school physician. Assessing his early childhood, Rhoads says:

Well I'm not sure that I enjoyed my boyhood but I had to go through it.... I found it a little hard to get used to being away from home and I muddled through first and second grade.[50]

Founded in 1845, Germantown Friends School, like other Quaker schools, only admitted the children of Quakers. Many of Jonathan's classmates and their parents were patients of his father. The Friends Library, adjacent to the school, carried only nonfiction works since Friends believed that works of fiction were unnecessary and a waste of time. Science was always strongly emphasized as a subject for Friends to study and discuss. A determined mother wrote to Esther of her precocious 10-year-old son:

I am reading to Jonathan when he retires, "Old, Old Tales from an Old Old Book" by Nora Archibald Smith. They are Old Testament tales. Some of those old characteristics I would not want to take an examination upon myself. Jon said if I was going to read him that kind of a book he would as leave have the Bible! I did not know what to say for if I read him pages and pages—say of Joshua, he would not know as much of that judge as one short chapter in this book. I admire his sentiment and think I will get the characters and stories in his head and then read the original by degrees.[51]

One of his fellow students remembers that Jonathan was quiet, retiring, and modest to a degree, but was also considered the brightest member of the class and known to have a good sense of humor. In general, he did not like athletics, as he was too big for his age, ungainly, and uncoordinated. Dorothy Brooks was his sixth grade teacher whom he remembers fondly. In addition to being very nice to the young Rhoads she recommended him for promotion from the sixth to the eighth grade. His sister Caroline tutored him through the summer, and their efforts proved to be successful, as Jonathan skipped seventh grade in 1919 and entered the eighth grade at the age of 12.

Germantown Friends, in addition to being an outstanding school, was also innovative in that foreign languages were taught as early as the fifth grade. Jonathan took both French and Latin, and while he didn't enjoy them very much, he excelled in both. He attributed much of his talent to the enthusiasm of his Latin teacher, Miss Zebly, whom he recalls had a rather compelling personality.[52] A survey of his school records at Germantown Friends School revealed that he received high credits in mathematics, Latin, French, science, and geography. He distinguished himself by having been on the honor roll every marking period during the school year 1918–19. He remembers that he did not enjoy English very much, and it is the only subject in which he did not receive high credit, although he performed reasonably well. He did not, by his own account, have a large number of friends at school.[53]

His sister Caroline, who was seven years older, would often look after her younger brother. He was a good child and would never cross the street without permission. He rode his bicycle quite a lot, and he once peddled his bike to Northeast Philadelphia, 12 miles away, to watch the construction of the Sears Roebuck building.

Two historic events influenced the United States and the Germantown community during this period: the great influenza epidemic and World War I. The first wave of influenza struck in 1918 and is estimated to have killed 548,000 people in the United States and 20 million worldwide.[54] Schools and churches were closed. Jonathan's father was very busy during this period, seeing as many as 50 patients in one day because so many people were ill with influenza. As nursing care became scarce, his father would enlist neighbors and healthy patients to care for the sick. A great many people succumbed to the disease, as there were no antibiotics and other therapies at the time. To his father's credit, he lost only one patient to influenza.[55]

World War I particularly affected the Rhoads family because of their place of residence and religious beliefs. They lived in what was predominantly a German community. There was a rapid buildup of animus, both nationally and from neighboring communities, against the Germans. The German Hospital in the city was renamed Lankenau. A movement to rename Germantown emerged, but this was eventually defeated. There was a great worry about indigenous German spies, and anyone who had a German name or accent was suspect.[56] Additionally, the Quakers' noncombatant views were not well received by the U.S. judiciary. A good many Quakers who were conscientious objectors were interred at Camp Meade, Maryland. As a young boy, Jonathan remembered the announcement of armistice:

There was an announcement on the 9th of November that an armistice had been signed and there was a tremendous celebration. I think classes were discontinued and people were just so happy about it and then it turned out that it hadn't been signed, but it was signed two days later. It was celebrated again, but the first celebration was more enthusiastic.[57]

Following the war, Quaker groups organized and left to do relief work in France, Germany, and Russia. His mother writes to Esther:

Everything is about disarmament now days. The President issued an order for two minutes of prayer everywhere at just after 12 p.m. tomorrow, the anniversary of the Armistice day, a general holiday. To read the papers and hear people talk, one would think the world was for disarmament and peace. After a while the war element will make itself known, but I hope it will be overruled.[58]

In 1915 the family went on a western trip to the World's Fair in San Francisco. Since it was during wartime, friends and relatives advised against the trip. However, Margaret Rhoads had been planning the trip for years and finally persuaded her husband to go. The trip was a wonderful experience for the family, and it was expanded to 6 weeks so they could see Niagara Falls. They went out by the Canadian Pacific Railroad, traversing the lower part of Canada, through Detroit and over to Chicago. They changed to the S.O.O. Line and went up to Medicine Hat, Alberta. The Canadian Rockies, Banff, and Lake Louise were highlights en route to Vancouver, where they took a boat to Victoria and to Seattle, where some relatives lived. The family journeyed down past Mt. Rainier and Mt. Hood to San Francisco and stayed there about a week at a hotel which was right on the fairgrounds. They continued southward through Santa Cruz, Santa Barbara, and Los Angeles. Esther, writing to her Aunt Hetty, describes some fun on the beach at Jonathan's expense:

We had dinner at Santa Cruz and went down to the beach where Jonathan and Caroline and I with 20 other ladies went wading. Jonathan got to giggling when a wave up to knees began to draw the sand out from under his feet and down he went right over backwards and we all just stood and laughed so that he was thoroughly soaked before we could pick him up. He played in the hot sun on the sand and I think will be none the worse for his dip in the Pacific.[59]

The family even managed to cruise on one of the glass-bottomed boats at Catalina Island. After a detour to San Diego to see the zoo, they traveled across the desert, to the Royal Gorge, Colorado Springs, and the Garden of the Gods near Pike's Peak. The family returned home via Denver, where the train diverged to accommodate riders with New York or Philadelphia as their final destination. Prior to leaving for Philadelphia, Edward Rhoads was terrified when he could not find Jonathan, fearing that he had been shipped off to New York. After much searching, the young and curious Jonathan was found and the reunited family returned home to their very busy lives in Germantown and New Hope.[60]

During the summer of 1920, Jonathan's father, mother, and Esther traveled to England for a Friends' conference, and then Esther and Dr. Rhoads journeyed to Dresden, in southern Germany, to visit Friends who were doing relief work. Jonathan spent the summer picnicking, biking and hiking around New Hope under the watchful eyes of sisters Caroline and Ruth.

For the first 19 years of his life, Jonathan watched his father's medical practice grow, and then drop off after Edward Rhoads became ill. As his father's office was in the house, Jonathan saw firsthand what it was like to be a doctor and the many demands it made on his father and the family. As a boy, he often thought that he did not want to be a doctor since he was not able to spend the time with his father as the other boys his age could with their fathers. Jonathan writes of his father's practice:

My father was in general practice, yet that term does not convey today the professional and indeed the social position that it did then. He did a large volume of obstetrics, including the more difficult deliveries that necessitated hospitalization. He did everything in pediatrics, non-operative nose and throat work, infectious disease, heart disease, allergy, some neurology, rheumatology, psychiatry in a common sense kind of way, and other parts of internal medicine including diabetes. . . . He also did fractures before x-ray, and minor surgery, such as the suture of lacerations and drainage of superficial abscesses.

I think the thing that brings out the difference between his practice and what you think of general practice today is that if he had a difficult problem and sought a consultant, he wouldn't seek one from the medical school, he would draw on a fellow practitioner in the community.[61]

While there was no talk of medicine at the dinner table, his father would take him on home visits to see his patients. He spent a good deal more time on house calls than on office visits. There were regular office hours, but he would leave at around 10 a.m. and make house calls for 2 or 3 hours before coming back for lunch and then going out again in the afternoon. Not many patients had automobiles, and it was very inconvenient to go to the doctor's office. Additionally, most of the automobiles were open cars, and a person would get a good deal of exposure in the winter. His practice was very busy, and the office was never left without making his itinerary known. When Edward Rhoads left in the morning, he would leave a little outline of where he would probably go so that if an emergency arose, the family could call one of those houses on his list.[62]

Another incident that stands out in Rhoads' memory of his father's practice was when he was sent with a horse and buggy to meet the then-famous surgeon, Francis Stewart, of Jefferson Medical School at the train station. Stewart was summoned to repair a Colles' fracture Rhoads' father had sustained from the kick of a model-T Ford when he was cranking it—not an uncommon occurrence in those days.[63]

Jonathan's talents and abilities were evident by his early teens. The summer he was 14, his father's cousin, Alfred, arranged for him to go to their place in the Berkshires, where he got him a job on an adjacent farm. At the end of the summer his father wrote to Esther:

Alfred says they have enjoyed Jonathan much and remarked on his interest in mechanical things.[64]

His interest in "mechanical things" was spurred on by an uncle who sold hardware and would often give different tools to Jonathan for Christmas. Presumably, Jonathan inherited these qualities from his father who was quite skilled with his hands, as he was required to make splints out of wood. Jonathan made a variety of things with his tools. Later he became interested in automobiles, as nearly all boys do, and put new piston rings in the family auto. One summer, he remodeled the pantry into a kitchenette.

With Caroline away in her senior year at Mt. Holyoke and Esther in Japan, the family decided to move to a somewhat smaller home in Germantown at 108 Queen Lane. The family had employed servants throughout his sisters' childhood, including a man who took care of the horses and served as chauffeur when the family had cars. Later, the Rhoadses retained a husband and wife who lived in the house and took care of the cooking and yard work. As a result of the Immigration Law of 1921, inexpensive help became less and less available so that by the time the family moved to 108 Queen Lane, they were largely without servants, although they employed a maid when they were at New Hope. Edward Rhoads writes to Esther of the move and of the family's lovely summer at Maple Grove:

The new house is being painted and papered and electrified and plumbed, even tho' we have not yet received the deed. . . . We certainly have had a nice summer here. The garden is yielding tomatoes and lima beans in plenty. There is corn in the orchard. Eggplants have done well and squash and cabbage and lettuce are still to be had. . . . I have specially enjoyed Solebury First Day School this summer and the meetings have seemed to me more vital than they used to and the Friends have been very cordial. . . . Jonathan is putting Jumbo through some of his stunts. He is to go to the back farm when we go to be the watch dog for the McDowells on loan. I should have liked to have him with us in Germantown but mother seems to think it would add to her cares and I want to avoid that in every possible way.[65]

While both the Rhoads and Paxson families had traditionally attended the Westtown School, families in Germantown Meeting encouraged their members to send their children to Germantown Friends School. By the end of his freshman year in high school, Jonathan decided to transfer to the Westtown School:

I just thought that I needed sort of a fresh start and I had an uncle by marriage who was married to my mother's oldest sister. His name was Robert Mickle. An engineer by training, he graduated from Cornell. He had gone to Westtown and urged me strongly to go to Westtown. He said, "You will find that the friends that you make at Westtown will be your friends the rest of your life."[66]

The Westtown School, situated on 600 acres in Chester County, Pennsylvania (20 miles southwest of Philadelphia), was founded in 1799 by the Philadelphia Yearly Meeting of the Religious Society of Friends, which continues to oversee school policy and activities. From the beginning, Westtown was coeducational. Many of its founders were descendants of the Philadelphia upper class in the 19th and 20th centuries. Westtown was considered by many to be the Groton of Philadelphia Quakerism. Digby Baltzell, in his book, *Puritan Boston and Quaker Philadelphia*, describes the school:

Philadelphia Quakerism has a far older boarding school tradition, which dates to the founding of the Westtown School in 1799. Quakers after all have always wanted to guard their children from dangers of secular city life.[67]

Jonathan Rhoads was the fourth generation in his family to attend Westtown. Indeed, the Westtown catalog lists 98 members of the Rhoads family. His own great grandfather, Joseph, was the first Rhoads to come to Westtown, entering in 1800.[68]

Jonathan Rhoads entered the sophomore class of Westtown School in the fall of 1921. His application reveals that he was 5 feet 9 inches tall and weighed 130 pounds. His health was described by his father as good, with previous childhood diseases listed as chickenpox and measles. Occasional bouts of tonsillitis and an average tendency toward colds was noted. Commenting on his early adjustment to Westtown, Rhoads has said:

While my work at Germantown Friends had been satisfactory, though never outstanding, my social adjustment was distinctly below par and this continued during the 10th grade at Westtown. However in the 11th and 12th grades, I gained much better acceptance from my classmates and was elected to various school offices which provided additional opportunity for self expression.[69]

Westtown was a rather austere place and had strict hours when students had to be in the building. The school maintained the Quaker standard of simplicity in dress and speech. The student body was more mixed than Germantown Friends and consisted of the children of farmers in addition to those from the city. Like Germantown Friends in an earlier era, only children whose parents were both members of Orthodox Meetings were admitted. Classes followed a routine, predictable schedule until 2 p.m., when all students were required to spend an hour outdoors. Sports were important to students and Jonathan, while not particularly athletic, tried out for soccer. Students could, instead of spending their spare time with sports, chop wood for $2 a cord. While Jonathan recalled that he had difficulty adjusting to his first year at Westtown, this is not confirmed in a letter his father wrote to Esther:

We have good accounts from Caroline and Jonathan. Both seem happy. I think Jonathan is taking hold well in his studies and we were pleased to hear that he had gone out for soccer and was on the second team although he did not feel sure that he could stay there, but he appears to have gone in with the determination to do the proper thing in athletics as well as in his studies.[70]

At Westtown, students had monthly dining room place assignments. Normally, there were 8 students from different classes and one teacher at each table. Indeed, Jonathan's letters to Esther as early as his sophomore year are full of humorous evaluations of his dining companions:

J. Parker Hull—most foul but a talker
Rebecca Parker—housekeeper the old fashioned type
Eileen Brinton—a senior and fair talker
Hugh Russel—very good for Eileen's talking ability
Ralph Cope—22—knows his habits
David Pennoch—an awful rep for a temper
Amy Sharpless—24![71]

He writes of his roommate, Stanley Moore, from Guilford College, North Carolina:

He is rather worldly, very amusing and quite fond of shiking![72]

Shiking was a local term for when a student left the premises of Westtown without permission. His mother writes to Esther:

Then J. and I went canoeing, and he scandalized me by telling me a boy advised being very good until you got a [good] reputation and then shiking so as not to be found out. I have written him at length on the advantage of a truthful, honest and fair character. Also I hope he will get on Student Council some day.[73]

Jonathan's hobbies at this time were chess, collecting stamps, riding his bicycle, reading Poe and Dickens, and exploring the Wissahickon Creek when he was home from Westtown. There was much reading aloud. As a whole, the Quaker community was opposed to drama, light reading, fiction, and music; however, the family attended orchestra concerts. They did not attend movies, although students would often talk about them.

Within the school, there was avid interest in world and local events. Jonathan Rhoads belonged to three organizations in his first year at Westtown: the Brightonian Literary Society (membership prepared freshman and sophomore boys for participation in the Parliamentary Society), the Rustic Club (an all male club which encouraged interest in agriculture), and the Societas Latina or Latin Club. He was interested in radio and built a small, one-tube set, and he soon became president of the radio club.

He also was frequently ill during his first year at Westtown. In her letters to Esther, Margaret Rhoads reports Jonathan's illnesses with some regularity and remarks on the difficulty of raising boys:

J continues to have colds when I phoned him and he sounded so hoarse and coughed too much. I hurried out on a 1:00 o'clock train to find him cheerful and bright and afraid to come home on account of making up lessons. . . . Boys are hard for me to understand. They are entirely satisfied with a room and no embellishments. No cushions. No rug. No bed cover, no pictures or pennants.[74]

And again:

Jonathan is home on grades and he has such a bad cold, laryngitis, that we will keep him home a day or two. Boys don't have any sense, run about without enough clothes and do all sorts of reckless things.[75]

Jonathan seemed mildly amused with his mother's concerns when he writes to Esther:

I hope that thee and Peg are well. I have been staying at home since Thanksgiving with a cold which I have had for some weeks. It doesn't bother me much except for a while it made me awfully hoarse and then it began to make me deaf so that I couldn't hear Pa's watch more than an inch or so from my ear. This got the family excited (thee has doubtless heard the story many times over in Ma's letters) and they kept me home although I had not any ear ache during this cold merely during another one previous to this. I feigned a protest but it has given me a chance to get acquainted with the new house.[76]

Looking forward to summer, he writes to Esther about his prospects for a job:

I'm awfully hard up for a job this coming summer (could thee furnish me with sufficient scandal to write stories up for the Country Gentleman and so forth).[77]

The school year ended uneventfully, and Jonathan returned to New Hope for the summer.

Levis Phipps, the son of a local Quaker farmer, was assigned as Jonathan's roommate in his junior year. That, however, would change with the arrival of a new friend, John Webster, from Frankford, Pennsylvania, in the fall of 1922. Webster remembers the day they first met:

I went to Westtown as a junior. They called it first class. I met Jonathan and we liked each other right away and he proposed that we be assigned

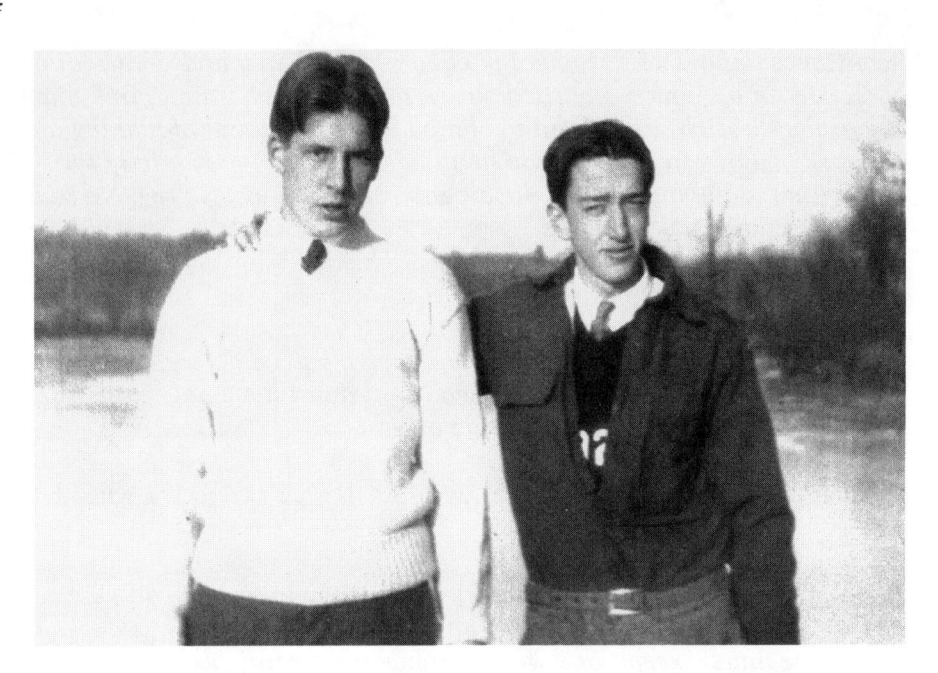

Jonathan Rhoads (left) and John Webster (right) on the ice skating pond at Westtown School – 1924.

as roommates. I can just see him standing there, he and I in a certain location but how to do it, because I had been assigned a roommate and didn't know anybody else so he said we have to make sure that Levis Phipps had to be changed because you can't just change the roommates when you were assigned. So he thought of ways of creating an atmosphere of "dirty tricks." He fixed Levis' bed . . . so that when Phipps sat on it, it fell to the floor. So Phipps knew he had friends there but also some enemies . . . so sure enough, Phipps asked to have his room changed.[78]

John Webster, later to become one of Rhoads' closest friends and a lifelong confidante, was a year and a half older than Jonathan. He was tall and thin, wore glasses, and like many of the other Westtonian boys, parted his hair in the middle. He had come from the Frankford Friends School. His father, an engineer and city surveyor, was instrumental in designing the layout of Roosevelt Boulevard, a major thoroughfare in Philadelphia.[79] Webster appealed to the humorous side of Rhoads and vice versa. He was fun loving and enjoyed a good time, but was also a serious student. Their backgrounds were somewhat similar in that their parents were professional and well-educated people and solid Orthodox Quakers. Rhoads remembers his first impressions of Webster:

John was a person who could talk to almost anybody. He interested them and he was interested in them. He said that you didn't have to like everything about a person in order to derive something worthwhile out of your association with them.[80]

Webster distinguished himself in and out of the classroom. He was a skilled debater and a very talented athlete. He was President of the prestigious Literary Union, editor-in-chief of the yearbook committee and manager of the track team. Webster describes his life as Rhoads' roommate:

Now as a roommate, for two years, he was as you would expect an excellent scholar. I was above average too, so we were well suited. But he was fun loving. We had earthy bull sessions, yet we balanced that off with systematic reading of the Bible every night although we chuckled over it off and on . . . did it any way all the way through the New Testament. . . . And even though we were desirable students we broke the rules occasionally.[81]

Webster remembers that Rhoads gave him good advice from time to time. He discouraged him from bragging or showing off because he had broken records in track.

By the fall of his junior year, Rhoads' mother writes, "Jonathan has grown like a weed."[82] He continued to excel in Latin, math, and chemistry. Webster remembers one night when Jonathan became so engrossed in his Latin lesson that he forgot to eat dinner. Webster recalled that they shared a life-long ambition of earning $5000 a year. They had a pact that the first one who earned a thousand dollars a month would have to buy the other a three-fingered steak at the Bellevue Hotel. Webster ended up buying the dinner.[83]

Later, when Webster and Doris Blackburn (another Westtonian) married, Rhoads was the best man. Following graduation from Penn State, John Webster worked for Sears and then became interested in banking. He got a master's degree from Rutgers and eventually headed the trust division of the Provident Bank of Philadelphia.

Jonathan Rhoads never forgot his friend's birthday. He would visit Webster at his office in Center City, and the two would celebrate Webster's birthday with banana splits. So wed was Rhoads to this ritual, that one year, during a severe snow storm, Rhoads and Webster went across the street to a local drug store and ordered their banana splits. The soda jerk informed them that he had no bananas. Dr. Rhoads walked out, went to a local grocer, and purchased two bananas. Returning to the drug store, he gave the clerk the bananas and said, "Now we want our banana splits!"[84] The friendship that developed at Westtown lasted for 70 years until Webster's death in 1992.

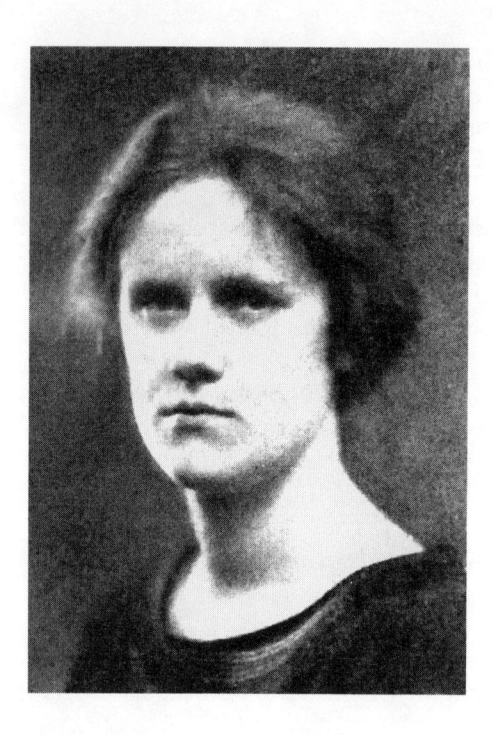

Helen Bell, a classmate of Jonathan Rhoads at Westtown.

Rhoads recalls his increasing social maturity:

The second year I became more interested in the other people around the class. I got to know more people. I found that if I could tell funny stories that I got along better. I didn't have any great supply of these but usually one could come up with something that would make people laugh. I got acquainted with more of the girls in the class. There was Helen Bell who was a crackerjack student.[85]

Helen Bell was from New York City and the only child of William and Susan Bell, both graduates of Westtown. Indeed the family's connections to Westtown go back to her great-grandparents on both sides. This was a Quaker family distinguished for its contributions to education.[86] A lawyer by training, her father was president of American Cyanamid and a trustee of the Duke Foundation. Rhoads admired him for his success in life and the way he used it. He was an avid yachtsman. He impressed Jonathan with his detailed knowledge of Dumas and other authors. Rhoads, Bell, Webster, and another classmate, Ted Hetzel, were invited to spend weekends on Long Island on the Bell yacht. As Webster tells it:

We had two big house parties in New York. This is because Helen Bell was very wealthy. . . . Her father was millionaire many times over and she was the only child and was like all of us friendly with Jonathan. We were treated royally. One time we spent the day on the yacht that was used to sail to Spain. We were given a chance to steer the thing, jump overboard and swim around. We had fabulous meals and tickets for Cyrano de Bergerac and we were driven around in two big Locomobiles, which were the biggest cars of that day. This was quite mind boggling for a 17-year-old![87]

It was evident to everyone early on that Helen Bell was one of the brightest, if not the brightest, student in the 1924 class at Westtown. Her record was marked by just about every distinction a school can bestow on one of its own. Her yearbook notes some of her qualities and accomplishments:

All "A's" is her favorite pastime. She can debate like Webster, read books like Master Carroll and write like Shakespeare. Still, Helen has a keen sense of humor, as her best friends know.[88]

Bell was one of two seniors to be admitted to the Cum Laude Society, which was the Westtown equivalent of Phi Beta Kappa in college. After graduation from Westtown, Helen Bell went on to Vassar College, where she roomed with Terry Folin, later to become the wife of Jonathan Rhoads. Later, Bell taught at the Westtown School for 4 years and then married a fellow teacher, Alan Hole. The couple had three children who also attended Westtown. In 1942, Helen (Bell) Hole wrote a history of the Westtown School, *Westtown Through the Years*. In a foreword, Carroll Brown, then the principal, describes her:

A deeply concerned Friend to whom the Quaker tradition is a precious possession, she has added to these qualifications a richness of culture unusual in any circle. A sense of humor, a sense of proportion and a sense of requirements of her public, and considerable experience of non-Quaker European and American life have precisely fitted her for this task.[89]

Helen Bell and her husband moved to Indiana, where they joined the faculty of Earlham College. Like her life-long friend Jonathan Rhoads, she too served as a provost. The two friends kept in touch over the years and faithfully attended Westtown class reunions. Helen Bell passed away at age 77 in 1983.

Theodore Hetzel, another of Rhoads' close friends at Westtown, was a very handsome, "well put together" fellow.[90] While he was the son of a

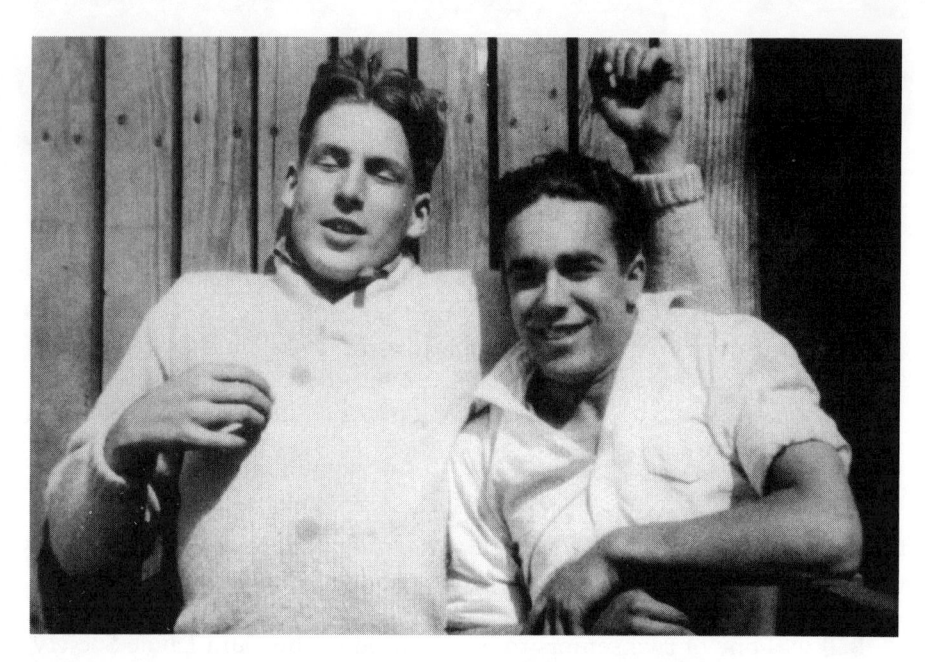

Ted Hetzel (right), one of Rhoads' close friends at Westtown (1923).

birthright Quaker (his mother), his father, under the friendly persuasion of Edward Rhoads, became a convinced Friend. Ted and his sister were delivered by Edward Rhoads. Hetzel's father, who was also someone the young Rhoads admired, was an engineer for the Link Belt Company. He retired early, but as Rhoads says, "was a genius and a thoughtful man; he did not aspire to great wealth and there wasn't anything he couldn't do."[91] Like Bell, Ted Hetzel had one of the longest and most distinguished entries in the yearbook of 1924.

Unlike Webster and Rhoads, Hetzel was not one to joke around. He was very mechanically inclined and a leader in the many organizations to which he belonged. He was an expert figure skater (as was Rebecca Wills, his future wife). He was an excellent photographer at an early age and a proficient violinist. He was president of the class of 1924. Ted possessed many of the same remarkable qualities as his father. After graduation Hetzel joined Rhoads and a few other Westtonians at Haverford College. At Haverford he majored in Engineering and German and graduated with many honors. He went on to get a Ph.D. in Engineering at Penn State. Hetzel secured a teaching position at Haverford College, where he remained for the rest of his professional life. The Hetzels had six children and named their last son, who later became a doctor, after Jonathan Rhoads.[92] They were active in the American Indian rights movement and spent many summers working on reservations throughout the United States. Ted was honored by native Americans for his distinguished work with their community. Ted Hetzel and his wife Becky remained close friends with Jonathan Rhoads all of his life. Ted died in 1990 at the age of 84. His wife Becky lives at Crosslands, a Quaker retirement community.

By his junior year Jonathan and his close friends were dubbed the "whiz kids" by their fellow classmates. They were at the top of their class academically and had many intellectual interests outside of school. Webster recalls that Rhoads encouraged them to attend the Academy of Music and to listen to Gilbert and Sullivan and Mozart.[93] They skated a good deal in the winter, as there was a large pond on the school grounds. They belonged to the Natural History Club, which was one of the few coeducational clubs. Rhoads later noted that they studied nature, but it was mostly human nature they were interested in.[94] They belonged to the honorary societies, language, parliamentary, and debating clubs. Rhoads' ability to steer and conduct meetings was evident early on in his membership in the Parliamentary Club. *Roberts' Rules of Order* was drummed into every Westtonian, and Rhoads and Hetzel became experts at it. A fellow classmate, Francis Harvey, recalls his experience with these fellows:

I knew Jonathan as a super brain. We had a parliamentary society after the House of Representatives and I was the Speaker of the House. Jonathan and his buddy Ted Hetzel would drive me nuts with parliamentary rules and filibustering. He made me learn the Roberts' Rules of Order *so that later in life I knew what I was doing when I got to be moderator of a Baptist church and also in politics.*[95]

Time and again, Jonathan's classmates were impressed with his ability as a quick study, in Latin and chemistry especially:

I remember Jonathan when he sat next to me in Latin class. He had no time for homework because he was studying chemistry by himself in order to pass the college board test, so that he translated Virgil when he first saw it in class. He got an A and no doubt in chemistry too.[96]

Another classmate remembers a facet of his personality that many have come to recognize as a life-long trait:

I remember Jonathan as a very wholesome nice looking young man— often smiling, a very bright, astute student. Sitting at his desk at the aisle next to mine I would so often see his hand raised, so eager to give the correct answer. My respect for him was enormous not because I realized he was gifted but in answering problems I had failed, he would do it in a loving non-judgmental attitude, nothing smug or egotistical about Jonathan.[97]

Becky Hetzel assesses his personality:

He's very quiet but he has limitless qualities. He was certainly extraordinarily bright and ... I remember in Latin class at Westtown we were all struggling to get our sight reading in good shape so that we could make a good translation in class. Jonathan somehow or another could read it at sight in class and didn't seem to have to do it beforehand. He was slow but he got it. ... He was very quiet ... and I think that you made an approach to him rather than his approaching you. I do remember that he was growing so fast that when we were about 15 his blue serge suit was short in the arms and short in the legs. And he was fun...everybody liked him and of course everybody realized how bright he could be without making much of an effort.[98]

Besides an improvement in his social life in the junior year, Jonathan continued to excel in his studies. His grades that year reflect his keen interest and natural talent in chemistry and math. A survey of his conduct record during these years reveals a young man who seems to have had occasional problems with neatness, punctuality, and thoroughness in school work. It was noted that he was industrious and courteous, paid attention in class, and had a fine attitude toward the best interests of the school. Neatness appeared to be a particular problem, as his mother writes to Esther:

Jonathan met me at Browning, King and Co. and it is well we planned to meet there for he was a wreck. Pants torn, mended with adhesive plaster, shoes muddy and cap over his eyes. Jonnie says I looked like a sight as I wore that stiff brown hat which is not as becoming to me as it is to thee. When I go to Westtown, I wear my best.[99]

In another letter to Esther she says:

Jonathan gives me continual worriment because of his lack of self assertion in dress and general independence. ... It is such an emancipation to think and act for yourself provided you don't hurt anyone else.[100]

Jonathan spent the summer following his junior year at the Brown's camp in Indian Lake in the Adirondacks. The camp was named after Thomas Brown, who had been head master of the Westtown School. It was founded and run by Westtown people, "on Westtown ideals in a wilderness setting."[101] It was not a camp for children but mostly for the faculty without families who vacationed there for a few weeks during the summer. Four or five Westtown boys were recruited to help out at the Backlog Camp. Along with Jonathan, Ing Richardson, Hewlings Cooper, and Francis Harvey were chosen to go to Backlog. Work at the camp consisted of carrying wood to the various tents for camp fires and accompanying campers on day trips and overnight trips around the territory. It was here that Jonathan became interested in Brown's daughter Alice, who was equally interested in him. Rhoads and his fellow Westtonians worked long and hard. For 2½ months, they were paid $50 plus rail fare from Philadelphia to Indian Lake, New York.

Ing Richardson remembers him as a hard worker and one who would not indulge in the usual adventures of young men who were growing bored with life at camp:

The camp was . . . accessible only by water from the town which was 12 miles away. We knew that T.K. Brown did have a model-T Ford which was hidden in the woods at the nearest road some 2 miles away. Late in the summer, the temptation to get to town for an ice cream became overpowering. One of us proposed "borrowing the vehicle." He said he knew how to drive a model-T and also how to jump the ignition without a key. Three of us readily agreed to go but Jonathan thought twice. He said, "Look you guys, I like ice cream and I would love to go but I have to make this job last for a lot of summers." . . . The trip was a success, we thought. But Jonathan's intuition paid off. He alone was invited back the following summer.[102]

In September 1923, Jonathan's senior year at Westtown, Margaret Rhoads was worried about her daughter Esther, who had had a major abdominal operation a few months before. She decided to travel to Japan to reassure herself that Esther was all right. Shortly after her arrival in Japan, the news that a tremendous earthquake had destroyed the city of Tokyo, the site of the Friends School where Esther worked and lived nearby, reached the family. Edward Rhoads anxiously wrote to his wife and daughter after hearing the news:

We have been very anxious, of course, since the news of the earthquake reached us. I happened to buy a final Evening Ledger *on the 1st and saw the report in that, since which time we have scanned many papers which have been full of reports and rumors. We have been comforted by the hope that you had not changed your plans and were therefore probably in Kanazawa, which a London report said was not damaged. . . . Caroline saw the papers on the second day and returned by rail from*

> *Boston . . . and tonight Jonathan arrived from camp, looking well and measuring 6 ft. 2¾ in his shoes and weighing 163½ lbs.*[103]

Still not hearing of the fate of his wife and daughter, he writes again on the ninth of September:

> *We wonder a great deal about what mother and thee may be doing in this time of trouble in Japan. The newspapers devote a great deal of space to the earthquake and there are a good many people waiting for news from friends in Japan.*[104]

On September 14th, Edward Rhoads finally received word that his wife and daughter were safe:

> *We and others are very thankful for Mother's cable from Kanazawa, for it is the only direct word we have had from any of the mission group.*[105]

By the time he was a senior at the Westtown School, Jonathan gained much greater acceptance from his classmates and was elected to various school offices, which provided additional opportunities for self-expression. He belonged to 13 organizations or societies and was president of three. In addition, he served as a scribe for the Philadelphia Yearly Meeting and was associate editor of the yearbook.

Election to the prestigious Triangle, the boys honorary society, was considered to be the highest achievement at Westtown. The society was founded to promote interest in school activities, to reward good conduct and all-around ability. Qualifications for membership were good scholarship, leadership, athletic ability, and loyalty to the best interests of the school. Jonathan, up to this time, met all of the requirements save one: participation in athletics. By his senior year he was well over 6 feet tall, was "gangly," and at times was teased by his fellow schoolmates regarding his athletic abilities. He solved this, Webster said, by quietly going off and teaching himself to figure skate, making the third rank, "not a distinction to be taken lightly."[106] It was also during this period that Rhoads mastered the Westtown method of walking on ice, something he reused 71 years later during the famous ice blizzard of 1994 in Philadelphia. In addition to figure skating, Rhoads took up pole vaulting. As a result, he was elected to the Triangle, which he still considers one of his major achievements at Westtown.

During Rhoads' senior year in 1924, changes, albeit slowly, began to occur at Westtown. There was an increase in fiction in the library, joint cheering at interclass games was allowed, and group singing was finally approved.[107]

College board exams in the 1920s were administered serially: i.e., one could take some each year for three years close to the time that a student had completed the work. A student in the senior class complained to Rhoads that he found the physics exam particularly difficult. On looking at some of the questions and answers, Jonathan thought that it didn't look particularly hard and entered into a wager with the senior that he would be able to pass the exam even though he had not taken the physics course. The exams were not closely monitored at the time, and Rhoads was able to take the examination without the permission of the head master, George Jones. His mother writes to Esther:

Jonathan is tremendous! He wanted to try physics in college board exams though he had not had it in class, so not finding George Jones to ask permission he plunged in and got a 98! The 2 boys who were prepared for the exam got in the 50's. It is a howling joke, anyway it will raise the average of WBS in physics.[108]

The headmaster was both surprised and pleased at his accomplishment.

A considerable part of the senior year was devoted to planning his future. Jonathan's mother writes to Esther about his immediate plans:

Jonathan came home before dinner and will return before supper 1st day. He is thinking about next year. Our large ideas of having him in college 6 years dwindle and he thinks he is [too] young for a scientific school. He and John Furnas and Webster think they would like to teach!! a year. Did such an idea ever occur to thee? We expect to pay much attention this fall to the subject of what is best for him to do. He is a fine fellow. Funny how he and Caroline can analyze themselves and the situation and just miss making a tearing success. . . . Probably they will develop late.[109]

By the end of his senior year, Jonathan Rhoads and Ted Hetzel decided to go to Haverford College, John Webster was accepted at the University of Pennsylvania (later transferring to Penn State), and Helen Bell was accepted at Vassar. Just about all of the members of the Westtown class went on to college. Rhoads graduated from Westtown feeling a good deal part of the group and particularly one of its abler students.

The summer following graduation, Jonathan was scheduled to return to Backlog Camp. Once again his health was compromised by the whooping cough so that he ended up spending the summer convalescing at New Hope. By August his Mother reports to Esther:

I put my traveling money into gasoline so to give Jonathan a good time. He has been contented externally and patient but we have got our

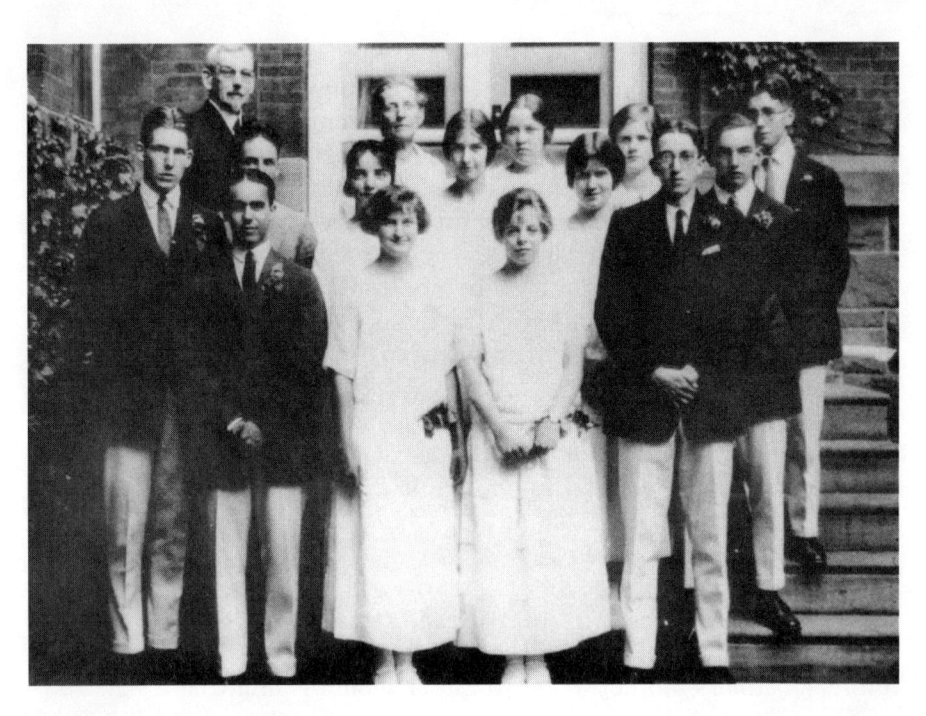

Jonathan Rhoads (far left), his mother and father (back row), and his classmates at graduation from Westtown School in 1924.

entertainment from being together until now. He has lots to read—he has received many books and bought some with the money from his peace prize.[110]

Once again the family spent a lovely summer at Maple Grove. Jonathan Rhoads, now 17 years old, left the sheltered life of Quaker Westtown and entered Haverford College, with its broadening influences, in the fall of 1924.

Jonathan has been off on a trip—his kind—preserve me!
                                                    Margaret Rhoads[1]

TWO

SWIMMING THE BOSPORUS

HAVERFORD COLLEGE

With the encouragement of Stanley Yarnall, the principal of Germantown Friends School and his father's cousin, Jonathan Rhoads applied to Haverford College in the spring of 1924. Surprisingly, it was the only school to which he applied. His experience with Quaker education thus far had been very positive, and Haverford, with its fine academic tradition and small size, appealed to him. In addition, its proximity to home was of some importance because of his concern over his father's declining health. In the end, Rhoads concluded that Haverford and he were a "good fit." Based on his high score on the college board examinations, Jonathan Rhoads won one of the four prized Corporation Scholarships to Haverford College.[2]

Rhoads and his fellow classmates Ted Hetzel, Ing Richardson, Dick Lane, John Furnas, and Dick Wistar entered all-male Haverford College along with 46 others in the fall of 1924. Haverford, located 9 miles west of Philadelphia on the idyllic Main Line, is the oldest Quaker college in the United States. Founded in October 1833 by the Guerneyite branch of the Quakers, Haverford was transformed, under the masterful leadership of Isaac Sharpless, from a sheltered Quaker school to an academically respectable institution by the early 1900s.[3]

In 1924 Haverford College had a student population of 220 with a faculty of 25, most of whom resided on campus. The library contained 85,000 books, and the physical facilities included 20 buildings, an acre of land per student, and 5 athletic fields (including cricket, baseball, American rugby, and association football). There were also 7 tennis courts, a running track, and a skating pond. Offering 100 courses, 4 Corporation Scholarships and among its graduates an impressive 7 Rhodes scholars, to many the Haverford College of 1924 seemed on keel with its stated aims:

To encourage the growth, among a limited number of young men, of vigorous bodies, scholarly minds, strong characters and a real religious experience.[4]

While only 16.4% of the student body were members of the Religious Society of Friends, vestiges of the college's Quaker origins were still evident in the 1920s (although the custom of addressing others using "thee" and "thou," common at Westtown and in the Rhoads home, was not used at Haverford). All students were required to attend fifth day (Thursday) Meeting for Worship. Attendance at Collection (the Quaker equivalent of assembly) was also required 4 times a week.[5] However, commenting on the Quaker notion of social service and his days at Haverford, former dean William Cadbury noted:

I entered here in 1927. Sure we went to Meeting as a matter of course. We went to Collection 4 times a week, but as far as the social message of Friends is concerned, a young man didn't pay any attention to social messages. We were quite isolated from the rest of the world. . . . This kind of thing that we talk about as the Quaker tradition today simply wasn't in the cards then.[6]

Indeed, *The New Yorker* magazine was much in evidence at Meeting. In its irreverent treatment of college days at Haverford, the yearbook staff posed the question: "Can you suggest the text of a speech to enliven Meeting?" to which they replied, "O sleep, it is a blessed thing!"[7]

While the Westtown school adhered to the witness on equality of men and women, Haverford did not. Robert Stevens, former president of Haverford College, points out that many Friends in the late 1800s thought higher education played a negative role in the upbringing of women:

Despite the witness on equality, many shared the view of the Friend which wrote in 1899 about the dangerous effect intellectual ambition could have on women. It made them cold, unloved, and unhelpful instead of joyous, affectionate and unselfish. Many Friends thought that higher education for men was a bad thing; they thought that it was even worse for women.[8]

The quiet and dignified atmosphere of the Westtown School and the repose of the Rhoads' home were in stark contrast to the distinctly boisterous male environment at Haverford. Freshmen were suddenly thrust into a campus where food fights, water fights, and bed dumpings were commonplace. One snowball fight became so fierce that all 208 windows of Roberts Hall were broken. As one of the few women employed at Haverford, a former librarian recalls the undergraduate response to her and the few other females who would occasionally appear on the quadrangle between the dormitories:

When male students spotted a woman, they would hang out of Barclay and Lloyd windows and yell fire, fire to bring other fellows to the window. We'd hot foot it out of there.[9]

Because there were no fraternities, freshmen had to endure the mild equivalent of a Haverford hazing, usually at the hands of the sophomores. Freshmen were called *rhinies* (Greek for little worm) and were required to wear a green beanie with a yellow button, name tag, black bow tie, black socks with garters, and a clean, stiff collar to dinner and meeting. Knickers were strictly forbidden. Freshmen were required to rise when spoken to, keep their hands out of their pockets, have their galoshes fully buckled, and tip their hats to their professors and seniors. Worse, freshmen were dragged out of bed in the middle of the night and pelted with rotten eggs and tomatoes.[10]

First-year students were measured for body height, weight, chest expansion, lung capacity, and hand-grip strength. The results, along with those of freshmen at other U.S. colleges, were reported in the *Haverford News*. Freshman Haverfordians compared very favorably to their fellow collegians: while the average body weight of freshmen in the United States was 136.5 pounds, Haverford freshmen weighed in at a robust 145 pounds. They exceeded other freshmen in height by 2 inches (the tallest in the class of 1928 was Jonathan Rhoads, measuring 74.4 inches); in chest expansion by one-half inch; lung capacity by 15 cubic inches; and hand-grip strength by 8 pounds. These findings were especially interesting because the Haverford freshmen were younger by 1 year than their peers.[11] They were politically conservative and largely Republican, favoring Coolidge over La Follette and Davis in the freshman straw poll.[12]

Jonathan moved into Barclay Hall in the fall of 1924 and roomed with Chester Olinger, a fellow from a Pennsylvania Dutch farming family. As early as October of his freshman year, Rhoads expressed his disappointment with college life:

Life here is rather disheartening as your efforts seem to count for very little. I am not surprised that Haverford has a reputation for fellows having too good a time for it is supremely situated for that.[13]

Required courses in the first year were English composition and literature, two foreign languages (of which Latin or Greek had to be one), mathematics, and physical education. In addition to these, Jonathan Rhoads elected to take courses in German, algebra and quadratics, ancient history, and biology. His considerable talent in mathematics was clear. Having received grades in the high 90s, he won the college math prize for that year.

While the year for Jonathan was marked by periods of disappointment and pessimism, his sense of adventure and sly humor are evident when he writes to Esther in October 1924:

In the meantime, I am working up a naughty little scheme with brother Hetzel et al. to get a second hand Ford and drive up to the Cornell game at night, stop at Syracuse to see Cooper, a Westtown fellow who roomed with Hetzel last year. We figure on about 5 fellows getting a $75.00 car and selling it soon after the game for about $50.00 since the college authorities "cease to be responsible for our moral and scholastic welfare if we have a car at college." I trust whoever drives the car will not deviate from the straight and narrow path for there is likely to be a ditch of death on either side. Even the Devil can quote scripture to his own purpose. So I have been taking no thought for the morrow. I hope this will not be the occasion for any depression on account of the waywardness of the younger generation.[14]

The "naughty little scheme" came to fruition one Friday night in November 1924. Five fellows—Dick Lane, Ted Hetzel, Johnnie Webster, Ing Richardson, and Jonathan Rhoads—bought the car for $50, each contributing $10, and named it Becky after Hetzel's girlfriend. Jonathan's father contributed a battery, and the group took off for Ithaca, New York by 8:00 p.m. that evening. The trip was not without its problems, as Ing Richardson recalls many years later:

On the way up and back we had several flat tires, each requiring a tube, patch and rubber cement. We kept the jack at a fixed height until we found that Rhoads could lift any wheel high enough to slip it under. We were ill prepared for New York state in November in a car with no curtains. We stuffed newspapers under our clothes to keep from freezing. By the time we reached Cornell at noon on Saturday, we found the game having been moved up to the morning was already over and Haverford had lost. The trip back was a repeat performance of the trip up. In the early hours of Sunday morning near Scranton, we had more flat tires, right rear and front left. A screwdriver was used for the tire iron but slipped to make a third puncture.

It was on this trip that we came to appreciate the considerable mechanical talents of Jonathan. The early Ford was equipped with "spark

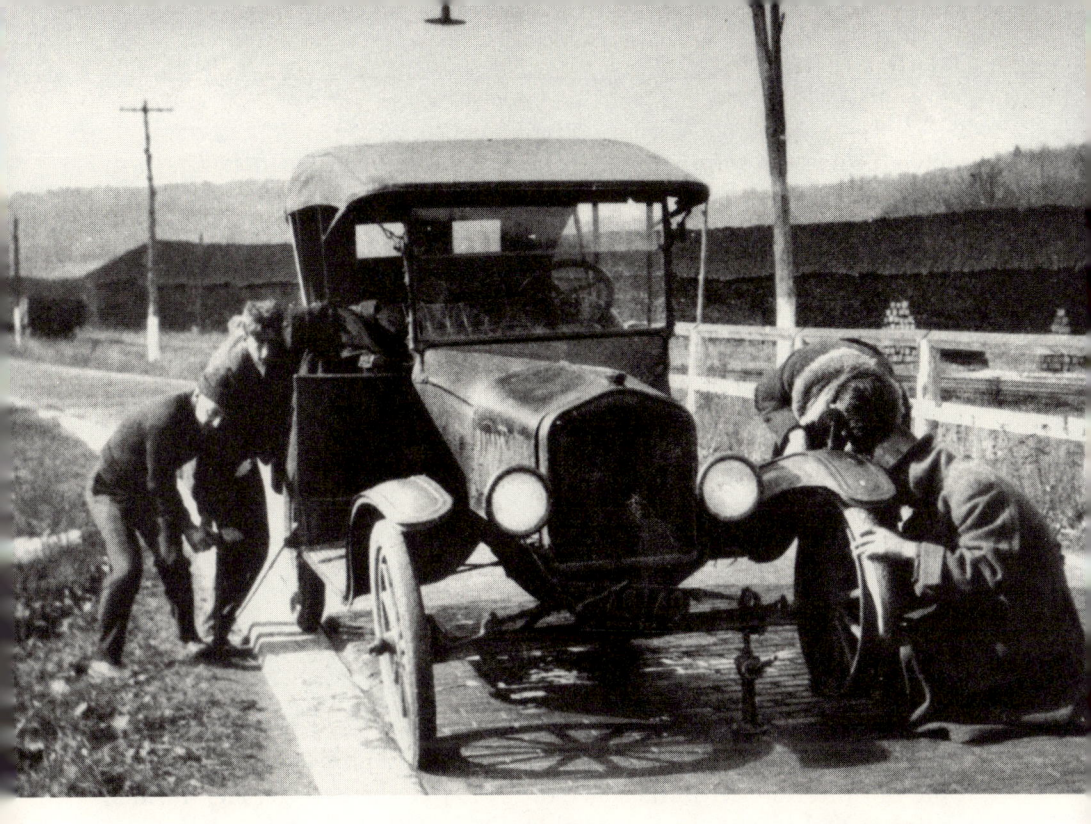

The return trip from the Haverford-Cornell Soccer game in 1924: John Webster (left rear), Dick Lane (left front), Ing Richardson (right rear), and Jonathan Rhoads (right front).

coils" in a wooden box just inside the hood on the right and were a very essential part of the ignition. In addition to all of our other troubles, the engine began to miss. It was Jonathan who diagnosed the problem—faulty spark coils. We found that by jiggling one of the contacts the engine would return to normal. So mile after mile, lying on the fender and running board, Jonathan jiggled the contact of the defective coil. As we drove through Stroudsburg, the ignition returned to normal. As a reward Jonathan got the best seat in the car, the warm seat in the center of the back seat.[15]

Before rolling into Haverford, they stopped by the Rhoads' home. Reporting the incident to Esther, his mother writes:

Jonathan came in and if we had not so many others we would have taken in his 4 friends (6th day, 8 p.m.) . . . [when they] arrived here 12:30 bleary-eyed and red. We put J on the lounge in front of the fire after the other friends left which they promptly did after dinner, then he went to bed and looked quite natural the next morning. He had that old leather lined overcoat of father's. What the other fellows did I don't know for J was cold enough after two nights riding. They were such perfect dunces.

They could have slept at Cornell and started out decently first day morning. . . . Now they are going to sell the car.[16]

Well into the second half of his freshman year, Rhoads once again expresses his disenchantment with college life:

The world we live in moves on with much of the tediousness of a drunk trying to get home. I'm not so very enthusiastic about college life and while perhaps I have not had enough of it to judge, still I don't feel that I am getting quite what I had hoped out of it. Perhaps my hopes were too indefinite to be realized.[17]

His father reports much the same to Esther:

Jonathan does not expect to come this weekend or next. He seems to be in a good many things at Haverford, though he talks rather pessimistically about his life there.[18]

While it would seem Jonathan was disappointed in Haverford College, it did not interfere with his sense of loyalty to the college. His mother, writing to Esther, noted what would become a life long trait in her son:

He brought his roommate home with him. He is short, slender, low forehead, nice eyes from near Reading, doesn't use his napkin but I guess he is a steady sort. . . . At least he does not get the bounce, which he says several boys have had for drinking. Jonathan is too dignified or too loyal to the college and had not told us the gossip.[19]

Despite his disappointments Jonathan was very active as a reporter for the *Haverford News*, and he sold advertising for the *Haverfordian*, the literary magazine, and became acquainted with the aspiring mystery writer, John Dixon Carr. Recognizing that he was not talented in football after trying it for a while, he turned to track and field and specialized in the pole vault. He was also very active with the chess team, 1924 being the year that an arranged radio chess match between Haverford and Oxford University took place, the first of its kind in the country. The 1924–25 pages of the *Haverford News* reflect the common interests of college students of the day (and now): sports, guest lecturers, college rules, social events, and club activities.[20] As the articles were unsigned, it is not clear which contributions were Rhoads'. He often said that his experience with the school newspaper subsequently helped his scientific writing.

Although his health was improved over what it was at Westtown, Jonathan began to experience severe bouts of acne, which afflicted him for many years. Once a week he would travel into Philadelphia, to 38th and Chestnut Streets, to the office of Dr. John Stokes. He recalls these visits:

His idea was that if you not only drained these pustules but if you cut the rim around the blackhead, it might go away. I had about 70 of them one morning, and I got dizzy going out. I don't think he used any anesthesia. He had an x-ray tube in his office and would spray the face, back and front with x-rays.[21]

And he writes in 1924:

My honorable parents are having a doctor work on my face. He makes from a dozen to 20 holes in my epidermis, has me eat about half a scanty meal and drink medicines and apply smelly lotions and hair tonics and absorb greasy salves through an epidermis already slippery . . . came away from a special session with the Honorable John Stokes M.D. with x-rays all over my countenance and sunburn clear down to my waist.[22]

Later, in the same letter, he humorously comments on the counsel of family members:

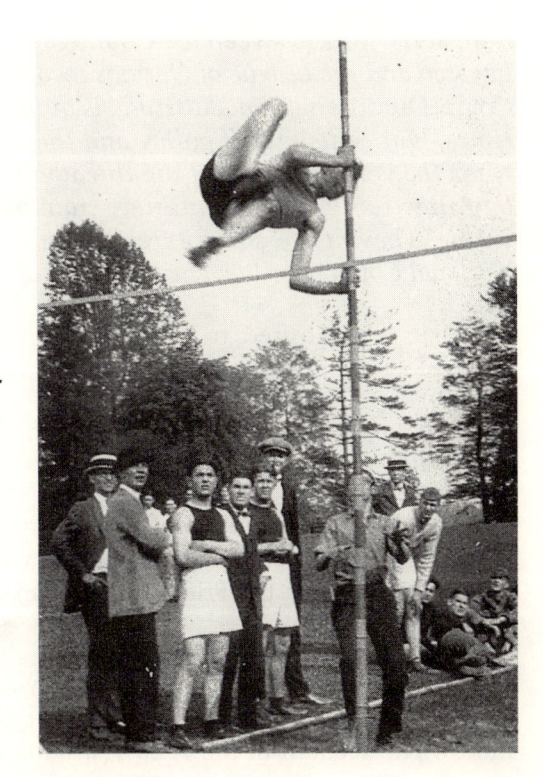

Jonathan Rhoads as a pole vaulter at Haverford College.

I had a couple of valuable documents from my parents today. Pa wants me to rub Doctor Stokes' salve in harder; Ma wants to see me study harder; now if cousin Madgie would send me a moral treatise my salvation would be complete, physical mental and spiritual![22]

Family life during his first year at college continued to be very active and busy. Visiting relatives and missionaries populated the Rhoads' household on a regular basis. Ongoing committee work and attendance at Quaker meetings punctuated the days, nights, and weekends of the family. Lectures and cultural events also played a significant role in their lives. They attended lectures on prison reform, Friends' International work, and travel in the Swiss Alps. Reading letters, books and magazines silently and aloud were other favorite activities. They subscribed to *Harper's*, *National Geographic*, and *The Literary Digest*, but not the Sunday paper, since reading comics was held in low esteem. A man of wide interests, his father read books by Jack London, devotional classics such as *The Life of Christ and the Saints*, *The Imitation of Christ*, *The Life of Saint Francis*, and treatises on psychology and economics. Politics were also of interest to Edward Rhoads, one of the few Democrats in largely Republican Germantown. He writes to Esther in the summer of 1924:

I am sorry for the sweep for Coolidge and would like to see the tariff lowered and the League of Nations recognized and the U.S. in the World Court. Our international attitude is quite depressing to my spirits sometimes. Our selfish tariff policy and the arrogance of our position as regards the yellow races and the threatening militaristic tendency shown by Army training camps, military training in schools, etc., all seem very wrong. They are to some extent counterbalanced by the work of the National Council for Prevention of War and other similar organizations.[23]

Music was limited to listening to the Victrola, and dancing was frowned upon. Jonathan's mother writes to Esther:

Can you have the Minuet or the Beautiful Blue Danube or are they too suggestive of dancing?[24]

While Esther remained in Japan, Caroline taught at one of the local Quaker schools, and Ruth continued to assist her father in the office and serve as librarian at the Friends Library in Germantown.

For Jonathan and his classmates the year ended with the annual cake rush, which marked the end of the rivalry between freshmen and sophomores. The account in the 1928 *Yearbook* describes the battle:

Having previously hidden several cakes in the gym when the set day came, it devolved upon us to prevent discovery. To several lodged in the attic Dempsey tried to apply chlorine from below but to his dismay that gas turned out to be heavier than air, and he was not seen again for several days. Sulphur fumes had a peculiar effect on Fox who passed out and crashed through the ceiling into Pop's (the coach) room. . . . The struggle was halted and called a tie about the middle of the afternoon by the Student Council for fear of greater damage.[25]

Jonathan's role in this was to climb a tree and pass food and drink to the freshmen who were in the rafters. Many years later one of the sophomores reminded Rhoads that it was he who tried to knock him out of the tree, noting that he was glad his efforts were unsuccessful.[26]

In the summer of 1925 Jonathan landed a job delivering ice cream for the Abbotts Company. The hours were grueling: he worked 7 days a week and had to rise at 3:30 a.m. to get to work by 5. After a few days a cousin offered him a "more attractive" job in nearby Chester, Pennsylvania, with the Philadelphia Quartz Company, which made silicates into a substance used for softening water. After accepting the job, he moved to Chester, where he lived at a boarding house with a fellow Westtonian, Rogers Heess. The eight-hour day was, for the most part, spent labeling cans of doucil (water softener) that were to be shipped out. Halfway through the summer Rhoads was rewarded with a 10% raise and put in charge of a crew. His tenure with the company lasted 10 weeks. Enamored with all forms of transportation, Rhoads persuaded the streetcar motorman to let him run the streetcar one morning.

The summer concluded with what would become a Rhoadsian trademark: traveling to a dizzying number of places in a short period of time. Jonathan began the trip by taking a trolley west on the Baltimore Pike to Media, Pennsylvania, then bumming a ride to Baltimore, followed by several different means of transportation to Washington. From there, he got a ride to Leesburg, Virginia, where he joined up with a fellow Westtonian, John Furnas. The next morning they left Leesburg and journeyed north through the Susquehanna Valley, slept in cornfields, and finally reached LaPorte, Pennsylvania, where another fellow Westtonian lived. Meeting with John Webster, who joined them in LaPorte, they bummed rides as far east as Doylestown, where Jonathan called his father at 10:30 at night to come get them. They arrived at home in Germantown at 1:00 a.m. Jonathan arose at 5:00 a.m. the next morning in order to get the 5:38 train to New York to meet his sister Caroline, who was arriving by boat from Europe.

Family letters to Esther early in 1925 disclose the declining health of their father. While he remained active with Quaker Meeting and committee work, Edward Rhoads retired from his medical practice in March

1925, when they sold 108 Queen Lane and made Maple Grove their permanent home.

Toward the end of that summer Edward Rhoads' health grew worse. He gave up Quaker meeting and committee work, staying for the most part in bed and only occasionally coming downstairs. Realizing that they would not be able to tolerate another harsh winter at New Hope, Edward and Margaret Rhoads decided to move to the warmer south to Fairhope, Alabama for 6 months.

Located on Mobile Bay, Fairhope was a 4000-acre experimental community established by the followers of Henry George, a land reformer, economist, and journalist who believed the principal cause of human inequality was the possession of land. He was also a great promoter of the single tax. The popularity of George's theories was buttressed by its humanitarian and religious appeal and society's deep discontent following the Great Depression of 1873–78.[27] Edward Rhoads was quite interested in George's theories and attended some of his lectures. By 1925 the community of Fairhope had been in existence for 29 years.

The decision to go to Fairhope came as a surprise to Jonathan, as he writes in 1925:

It certainly does seem exciting to think of the family tooting off to Alabama. When I decided to go to Haverford I rather regretted that I wasn't going to college a little farther from home, but it seems as though home was going to move away instead.[28]

On the basis of his freshman grades Jonathan secured another Corporation Scholarship for his sophomore year. Because of his keen interest and talent in the sciences, he declared a double major in mathematics and chemistry. He continued to work on the *Haverford News* and was appointed city editor for the year. He served on student council and gave talks on the accurate determination of atomic weights and the extraction of sugar from beets to the chemistry club. The *Haverford News* reported on a chess match in which he participated:

He has been displaying a steamy brand of chess in league competition and with some assistance in the way of victories from other members of the team should take the remaining matches. Rhoads has secured several draws.[29]

While life at school early in the sophomore year was generally uneventful, his father and mother were preparing for their trip to Fairhope. Living arrangements were hard to obtain in Fairhope, but by November the rental of a home was confirmed. Jonathan's father had become increasingly pessimistic about his fate, and his enthusiasm for the trip south had diminished somewhat. Plans went ahead, however, and on Monday, November 16, 1925—Edward and Margaret's 34th wedding anniversary—they left by train from North Philadelphia station. Staying overnight in Washington, D.C., they arrived three days later in Fairhope. Edward was exhausted and his health steadily declined.

The atmosphere at Fairhope was different from that of Germantown and New Hope. There were very few visitors, little activity, and no telephone. While such a change was immediately welcome, it must have seemed strange to experience such a radical departure in lifestyle with little or no family and friends surrounding them. They planned to stay until late March or April and then return to Maple Grove. With his father's health failing precipitously, his mother was totally devoted to the care of her husband. In addition to his sister Ruth, a nurse was retained to help care for him. By Christmas Edward Rhoads was totally bed-ridden. He experienced many bouts of "oppression," swollen legs, and cold feet and hands. His wife wrote to Esther:

I did not give up before Christmas. Father would rather go than be an invalid. He has always worked to the limit and nothing else satisfies him.[30]

Jonathan and Caroline visited Fairhope during the Christmas recess, having borrowed money from various relatives to travel by train. Esther, still in Japan, was expected to come home the summer of 1926, and the entire family was excited by this prospect. Edward Rhoads hoped he would still be alive to see his daughter one last time. But as his wife wrote to Esther:

Father said to send love to thee and said he supposed that he would never see Esther again.[31]

On the morning of January 24, Edward took his breakfast, and not long after he passed away. He was 63 years old.

Exhausted emotionally and physically with the ordeal of the past few months, Ruth and Margaret Rhoads remained behind in Fairhope until April of that year and did not attend his funeral in Germantown. Margaret writes to Esther:

It has relieved us of a tremendous strain not going to Germantown and having to greet all the relatives. I do hope that Jonathan and Caroline will not be over done. . . . I think it would have finished me to have gone North.[32]

Caroline believed that her mother did not attend the funeral because of her despondent state and hatred of funerals.

A close relative accompanied the casket from Fairhope to Germantown by train. As beloved and popular a doctor as was Edward Rhoads, his funeral was greatly attended, and it was held in the Germantown Friends Meeting House on Coulter Street. Caroline recalls that day:

Mother had always protected us from funerals. So I had prior little experience going to funerals and father's funeral was huge. There were men, all doctors, smelling of ether, all standing around the back door and the part where the family sat there was still some space but nobody wanted to go up in there.[33]

Jonathan did not remember the smell of ether dominating the room, but he recalls:

They arranged with Kirk and Nice [funeral directors] to meet the train and take the body out to his Aunts', my great Aunts' at 5353 Greene Street, which was opposite of the Friends Meeting and the Friends graveyard. He was buried there after the service at the Meeting. It was a big room [meeting house] and it was really very full because most of his patients were still living at the time he retired. There were a great many people who were connected with the Meeting who weren't patients necessarily. I remember that one of the talks by a woman named Esther Morton Smith. . . . She spoke very warmly of him. So then they assembled my cousins as pallbearers.[34]

Caroline returned to her teaching and Jonathan returned to finish his sophomore year at Haverford. The death of his father was quite a blow to him, and his grades suffered, though not to a considerable degree. Spring came and he secured his first letter in pole vaulting, no easy task for a person with his build. A classmate who watched him practice on the track relates:

I remember when we were on the track team I would go round and round the track seeing Jonathan's determination and perseverance at the pole vault. He did not have the build for vaulting; he got up there through sheer willpower.[35]

Margaret and Ruth returned to Maple Grove in April. Esther, having gotten a furlough earlier because of her father's death, returned to the United States in late spring. Jonathan and Esther then took a train to Fairhope to bring back the Ford which had been purchased for the family's use. On the way back they traveled along the Gulf coast from Mobile to New Orleans, then up the Mississippi River to Baton Rouge, on to Vicksburg, Memphis, Cairo (Illinois), into St. Louis, and then on to Iowa, where they had previously signed up for a Friends' youth conference. Esther returned home by train, and Jonathan drove back with the car and spent the rest of the summer at New Hope.

Rhoads moved from Barclay Hall to Lloyd Hall in his junior year. His mother and sisters rented an apartment at 147 West School House Lane, in Germantown, for the winter. Rhoads was not awarded a Corporation Scholarship for the year, so his mother sold small lots of Maple Grove to cover the $675 tuition and board. He took the required courses of Biblical literature and psychology, in addition to solid geometry, physical chemistry, and molecular physics. Having lost in his bid for editorship of the school paper, Rhoads resigned from the news but was recognized for his service with a gold key watch charm. He continued to be involved in pole vaulting, chess, and a new interest, the Curriculum Committee.

Undergraduates at Haverford, like undergraduates of today, were frequently dissatisfied with the curriculum and formed a committee to advance their ideas before the faculty. Rhoads and classmate Ed Hollander took the lead in pointing out the inadequacies of the psychology and education courses. The *Haverford News* reported that Rhoads spoke at length on the need for more education courses to meet the more stringent requirements for teaching in Pennsylvania.[36] Dissatisfied with the course in psychology, which emphasized the special senses (sight, hearing) and ignored Freudian theory, Hollander and Rhoads, along with a few other students, hired a female psychologist who taught what was referred to then as "experimental psychology." The required college entrance board exams also came under attack, although not by Rhoads. Haverford was one of only 4 colleges in the country which required the entrance exams at the time.[37]

Having sprained his ankle during track practice, Rhoads did not participate in the pole vault during the track meet at Union College on May 27, but attended nevertheless, because he was vying for the position as manager of the track team. It was during that meet that Rhoads and his teammates heard the news of Lindbergh's flight across the Atlantic. Will Rogers, writing in 1927, said that the news of Lindbergh's feat was second only to that of World War I.[38]

As the academic year came to an end, plans for his first trip to Europe started to take shape. It was a trip notable for its varied transportation: large and small boats, trains, airplanes, cars, bicycles, walking, and swimming.

The trip was conceived by Ted Hetzel, who spoke fluent German and was studying to become an engineer. Hetzel had become an agent for the Holland American Steamship Company and had recently read a book about sailing through Europe's many waterways. The idea intrigued Rhoads, so the two combined their funds—about $200—went to New York, and purchased a Johnson outboard motor, weighing 70 pounds, for their trip. They originally planned to sail from New York to Cherbourg but switched their destination to Rotterdam, since it was thought that they could more easily buy a row boat there. The trip across the Atlantic took 10 days. After arriving at Rotterdam, they discovered that most of the boats were too large for their purposes. The pair was sent by one of the boat sellers to a private rowing club where, they were told, they might find a boat more suitable for their needs. Lugging the 70-pound outboard motor and their luggage, they traveled several miles and finally found a more appropriate boat:

The boat was a long, sleek (open) boat with two rowing seats in it, it had a square back and we had that reinforced with an extra board and hung the outboard on it.[39]

Using tarpaulins and rain coats to protect them from the inclement weather, Jonathan and Ted proceeded through the canals of Holland near Utrecht. Then taking the Lek, one of the mouths of the Rhine, they crossed the border of Germany to Duisburg and Dusseldorf and then traveled south to Köln. Pressing on to Bonn, they moored the boat and took a train back to Köln to see the opera, *Die Meistersinger*. Returning to Bonn, they traveled up the Rhine and Main Rivers to Wurzburg, where they encountered trouble with the motor. They found that the bevel gears were beginning to wear out, so they returned to Dusseldorf and anchored the boat at a rowing club while Hetzel telegraphed Southbend, Indiana, for new bevels. During their stay they discovered that the canal they had planned to cross had 107 locks and cost 1.6 marks for each lock. Confronted with this formidable expense, they abandoned their trip by boat and decided to finish the trip by train.

They moved on to Nuremburg and then to Munich, where they stayed 3 or 4 days. They visited the English Gardens and the Deutsches Museum, savoring the good German beer along the way. Leaving Munich, Rhoads and Hetzel journeyed to Innsbruck and planned to hike through the Brenner Pass. From there they traveled to Venice, Trieste, Salzburg, and Vienna and took a train to Budapest.

It was in Budapest that Rhoads and Hetzel had their first ride in an airplane. Touring by plane was unusual then and not very safe. It was a mail plane, small and all metal, and the pair were stuck in the back with the cargo with no parachutes and were told by the pilot that the plane rarely landed where it was supposed to. In addition, the plane's exhaust leaked into the cabin, making their first aviation experience not particularly pleasant—but at least they could say that they had flown in an airplane.

They landed near Belgrade, took the Orient Express to Bulgaria, and then moved on to Constantinople (now Istanbul), where they spent a few days, bargaining with a rug dealer and visiting the Blue Mosque.

Undaunted by new challenges, Rhoads and Hetzel decided it would be exciting to swim from Asia to Europe. The Hellespont (Dardanelles) was initially considered, but finding that it would take a whole day to get there, they decided that they could still say that they swam from Asia to Europe if they swam the Bosporus. Rhoads describes the adventure:

We got a boat and picked a place where the current runs from the Black Sea about 5 miles an hour . . . so we sighted a cup shaped place and started swimming. I swam across. Ted stayed in the boat with the boatman. I went back and he swam across. . . . It took me 27 minutes, it took Ted 25. I suppose it was the better part of a mile.[40]

They would recount their shared experience of swimming the Bosporus for the rest of their lives.

Rhoads and Hetzel decided to split up at this point, Rhoads going to Salamanca to visit a Friends Work Camp and Hetzel flying to Athens.

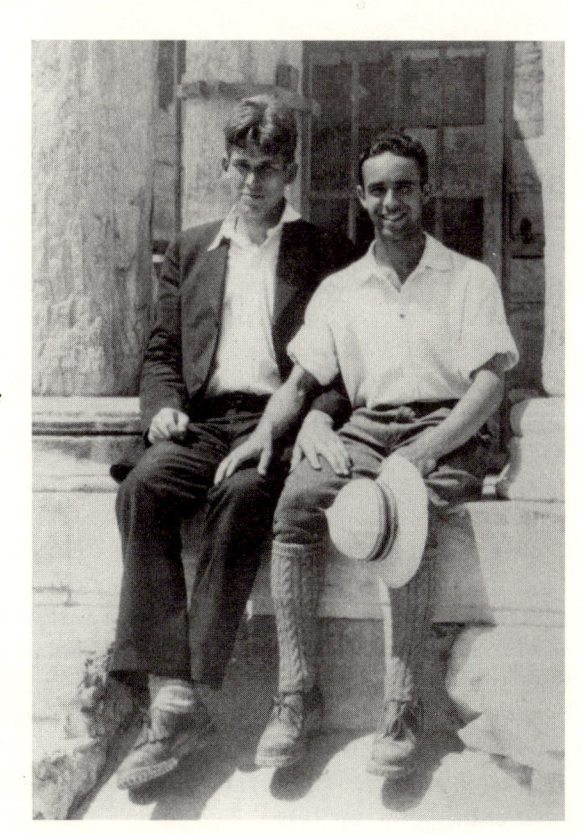

On the Acropolis—Temple of Athena Niki—with Ted Hetzel (right) in 1927.

They met up again in Athens and booked passage on a boat, sailed through the Corinthian Canal, then past Corfu to Brindisi. It was there that they took a train to Rome, up to Switzerland, and back to Wurzburg, where they sold the boat and picked up their outboard motor. Taking another train, they landed in Paris where they split up again. Ted, wanting more exercise, rented a bike and peddled from Paris to the French coast. Jonathan, wishing to attend a session of the League of Nations, telephoned a cousin who was associated with the Friends Service Committee in Geneva. His cousin was successful, and they managed to sit in on a session of the League and saw Neville Chamberlain.

Rhoads then took a train to Cherbourg where he joined up with Hetzel for the final leg of the trip home. The entire trip took 14 weeks and cost $1100, minus the $200 for the outboard motor.[41] Upon their return to campus they were the envy of their classmates, although, as Ing Richardson recalls, the rumor went around that because of the low elevation of the outboard motor, Rhoads and Hetzel only viewed the mud banks of the canals. The outboard motor followed them to campus, where it was occasionally tuned up in a bathtub in Lloyd Hall.[42]

Lloyd Hall was Jonathan's home for his senior year, where he roomed with John Woll. There was a common room with a fireplace, steam heat, and electricity; and each student had an adjoining bedroom of his own. Known for his fastidiousness, Woll was not, in some respects, the most "suitable" roommate for Jonathan, as Woll's entry in the yearbook reveals:

John's [Woll] life has been a drama in 2 acts, the second of which may be called a tragedy, unless a better name can be found for a methodical man's having to room with Rhoads. . . . Books, clothes, and vic records are strewn indiscriminately around the room. Woll's ears have been considerably enlarged by having his fingers stuck in them while he tried to concentrate during roughhouses. Even his hitherto sacred desk has been known to be messed up.[43]

The only required course in the senior year was ethics, taught by the famous Quaker historian and philosopher, Rufus Jones. As early as September Jonathan's course curriculum reflected some thought of going into medicine. The University of Pennsylvania Medical School required two undergraduate courses in English, and Johns Hopkins Medical School required German and French for entrance. Rhoads took contemporary drama and German. In addition to his honors courses in the theory of numbers and organic chemistry, he elected to take a course in elementary biology.

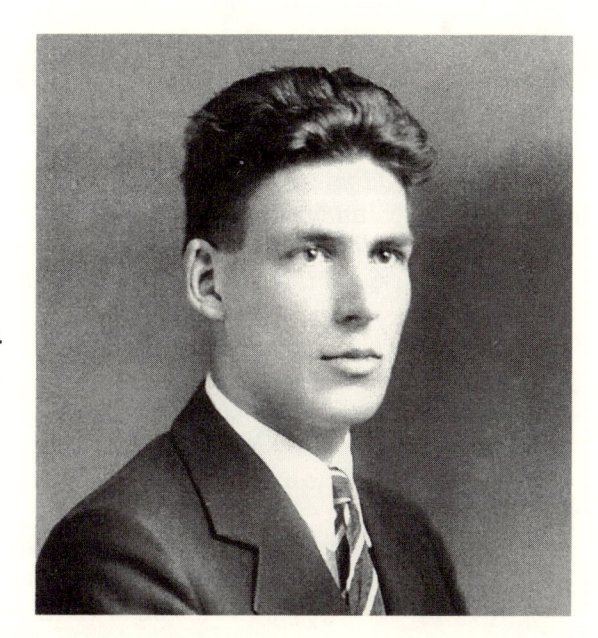

Rhoads' senior picture, Haverford College, 1928.

The instructors Rhoads most admired were Legh Reid and William Meldrum. Cited by Robert Stevens as one of Haverford's greats, Dr. Reid was affectionately called "f(x)" by his students. Educated at the University of Gottingen, then considered the "mathematical center of the world," he wrote his thesis under the direction of David Hilbert, thought by many to be the greatest mathematician of his time. Later, Reid published a book based on Hilbert's lectures on the theory of numbers with a preface by Hilbert.[44] A Southern gentleman with traditional manners, Reid also had a fine sense of humor. Rhoads recalls one incident in his classroom:

One student, unable to solve a problem, was asked by Reid, "Mr. Nichols, how many hours did you study last night?" The student replied, "Three hours, sir!" "Well," said Reid, "Three hours are not enough for you!"[45]

William Meldrum was Rhoads' professor in chemistry. Chairman of Chemistry from 1917 to 1956, Meldrum had graduated from Harvard and studied under the only Nobel laureate who graduated from Haverford, Theodore Richards. Meldrum coauthored four widely used textbooks on physical and analytical chemistry.[46] Meldrum was highly regarded by his students and colleagues and was a tough taskmaster. Rhoads recalled that

Meldrum let it be known that if you wanted to get into medical school you had to have a "B" in Chemistry or he wasn't going to recommend you.[47]

Meldrum also displayed a fine sense of humor and gamesmanship when he invited his students to his home and in the way of entertainment conducted the Chemistry Club Question Contest, which Rhoads won:

He placed 8–10 little white square boxes with a round hole cut in top and then cotton under that so all you could see [was] cotton. You were supposed to smell them to say what was underneath—what chemical. I was quite successful in that I had a pretty good nose for chemicals.[48]

Because he was in two honors courses his senior year—preliminary honors in chemistry, which required an additional 150 hours of work, and final honors in mathematics, which required 250 additional hours of work—his extracurricular activities were limited to the Scientific Society and pole vaulting. As president of the Scientific Society, Jonathan secured lecturers on such diverse subjects as airplanes and aviation, the development of dams in the Susquehanna River, the production of biological products and their uses in the prevention and cure of disease, x-ray spectroscopy, and birds of the island of Haiti. In sports he earned another letter in pole vaulting and was unbeaten in the dual meets.

Of significance in 1928 was the exam administered by the Carnegie Foundation to test how much knowledge was retained by college students. Most colleges in Pennsylvania participated. The overall exam consisted of 4 separate exams of 3½ hours each. Haverford College came in first, and Jonathan Rhoads had the second highest score in the state. On the basis of this showing he appealed to President Comfort to submit his name for a Rhodes scholarship, but this ambition was never realized.[49]

The yearbook entry for Jonathan Rhoads is revealing, for it describes some of the habits and interests he continued to have throughout his life:

Jonathan's accomplishments are many and varied. He is always first in the dining room, has never been known to complete a chemistry experiment, knows more math than $f(x)$, . . . never studies until the day before the examination, has never been known to pass up an opportunity to eat, and smoked his only cigarette to win a bet for an opera ticket. . . . He has had the added distinction of having aptly defined Philosophy 1 as "saying things everybody knows in words nobody understands" and of lifting his huge bulk eleven feet in the air with the aid of a bamboo pole, thereby winning a track letter. Where he will end up we hesitate to say, but he will probably succeed in inventing a radio-controlled auto if premature death is not incurred through his indulgence in amateur experimental aeronautics.[50]

A questionnaire conducted by the yearbook staff asked, "Who is the most sophisticated?" The answer was satirical:

Stokes and Rhoads led the rest by actual count, and we don't understand it because when we framed this question we thought the latter would poll a unanimous vote or else it wouldn't have been asked.[51]

In spring of 1928 Rhoads decided to forego a career in aeronautical engineering and apply to Johns Hopkins Medical School. In his application he cited his accomplishments as reporter for the school paper, his activities with the Chemistry Club and Scientific Society, and his managerial work for the track team; other interests listed were the Liberal Club, the chess team, the Radio Club, and a class debating team. He asked Professors Meldrum and Pratt (Reid was on sabbatical) for their recommendations.

Dear Dr. Baker:
In reply to your inquiry concerning the fitness of Jonathan E. Rhoads to represent Haverford College in the Johns Hopkins Medical School I regret to say that I cannot give him an unqualified recommendation. He has an excellent mind, in fact, a brilliant mind, but he has several times indulged in procrastination to a very serious extent. If he was certain to work steadily I could recommend him very highly but that is so uncertain that I hesitate to do so. In all other respects I consider him excellently qualified.

Yours very truly,
W.B. Meldrum[52]

And Pratt, his biology professor, wrote:

Jonathan Rhoads is a young man of the finest character and very good ability. He is not a star student so far as marks go, although he is in the top third of his class. In Biology however he is an "A" man and is one of the outstanding members of my classes. His work with me has been marked by persistent industry guided by intelligence. I recommend him highly for admission to your Medical School and am perfectly sure he will make good. I am also sure he will be a credit to Haverford College. He is a young man of powerful frame, being six feet or more in height and an athlete.

Yours truly,
Henry S. Pratt[53]

Graduation for the class of 1928 came on June 9th. Jonathan Rhoads graduated with honors and was inducted into Phi Beta Kappa on the strength of his character and grades. He was called to Baltimore for an interview 10 days later—an interview which, it would appear, gained him acceptance to Johns Hopkins. An admissions officer writes:

Mr. Rhoads lacks some four semester hours in Biology, which he is willing to make up by summer school work. When questioned about his deficiency in French, he said that he had studied this language some six years in preparatory schools before entering college and could read it on sight. He is a tall, strongly built boy, with an interesting and pleasing personality. . . . I should be inclined to reverse my previous decision and to admit him.[54]

I came to medicine as a last resort. I decided I couldn't do anything else.
                                                      Jonathan Rhoads, Jr.[1]

THREE ~

CAN WE GIVE HIM BACK HIS $18? ~
HOPKINS AND INTERNSHIP

It was not until the spring of his senior year at Haverford that Jonathan Rhoads decided to pursue a career in medicine. He had seriously contemplated going into aeronautical engineering, a new exciting field buttressed by the success of Lindbergh's flight over the Atlantic. Some thought was given to a career in mathematics when a visiting professor from Penn offered to help him secure a fellowship.

Rhoads said that medicine was a profession he thought he did not want to go into; however, there is evidence that this was on his mind as far back as Westtown School. He told Ing Richardson at Backlog Camp, "I'm heading for medical school and I have to make this job last for a lot of summers."[2]

His course work at Haverford also reflected some thought of medicine as a possible vocation, and while his roster did not strictly follow the prescribed pre-med curriculum, there was little deviation from it. In the end he chose medicine because he thought he could be more independent as a doctor and, as the son of a physician, was fully aware of its drawbacks. Reflecting on this further, he noted that medicine was a profession that "would be an enjoyable career at almost all levels of success."[3]

In May of his senior year at Haverford, he applied to 4 eastern medical schools: the University of Pennsylvania, Johns Hopkins, Columbia, and Harvard. In his application to Hopkins, he explains his choice of medicine as a life's pursuit:

I want to study medicine, because I have seen somewhat more of a physician's life than of the life of men in other professions as my father was a doctor. Biology, physiological chemistry, and physics have interested me a great deal and the medical sciences present a very wide field of interest. Social usefulness and ethical practice seem to be more in line with professional standing in medicine than in other professions or in business.[4]

He was accepted at two of the four schools: Pennsylvania and Hopkins. Harvard had filled its class, and Columbia put him on their waiting list. He chose Hopkins, which was one of the premier medical schools in the nation. Indeed, Hopkins was the leading contributor of faculty to other medical schools in the 1920s and 30s.[5] Rhoads' goal was to carve out a career in academic medicine, but if he failed, he thought he might practice general medicine in Germantown, as his father had before him. Hopkins offered a path leading to a career in general practice as well as academic medicine. Having spent the first 21 years of his life in Philadelphia and its environs, a change of scenery was in order but not so far from Philadelphia that he couldn't frequently visit his recently widowed mother and his sisters. Acceptance to Hopkins was contingent upon completing a course in biology and passing a French proficiency test. The summer following graduation from Haverford, Jonathan enrolled at the University of Pennsylvania in a course in comparative anatomy, where he met and became friends with D. Sergeant Pepper, the son of William Pepper, dean of the medical school.

While Jonathan sought a change of scenery, there remained one constant in his education—Quaker influence. Johns Hopkins (Johns was his great grandmother's maiden name) was an influential Quaker merchant in Baltimore. A bachelor all of his life, Hopkins left the bulk of his estate to found a university and medical school along the lines of the great European models, which were superior to American institutions of the time. Hopkins' vision embraced the enduring Quaker values of education and care of the sick. Upon his death in 1873, he bequeathed $3.5 million to the university and $3.5 million to the hospital: "A University for there will always be learning and a hospital for there will always be suffering."[6]

In addition, there were stipulations attached to his bequest, including a board of trustees composed largely of Quakers and a provision revealing his religious roots:

The hospital is to care for "the indigent sick of this city and environs, without regard to sex, age, or color. . . . The poor of the city and State, of all races, who are stricken down by any casualty, shall be received into the hospital without charge. . . . Their care is to be by surgeons and physicians of the highest character and the greatest skill."[7]

The great William Welch is credited for revolutionizing the medical curriculum at Hopkins and influencing, by example, the curricula of medical schools throughout the United States. Turner writes in his history of Johns Hopkins:

From the start, Hopkins was a university in the 19th century German pattern—an institution which fostered and emphasized creation of new knowledge [research] rather than the process of imparting the knowledge and skills already known [teaching].[8]

By the time Jonathan arrived in Baltimore in the fall of 1928, the curriculum revision of 1927 was in force. One of its main features was that the number of students in each class was reduced from 90 to 75. This was a radical departure from every other medical school in the country.[9] The only examinations given were at the end of the second and fourth years, and the most striking feature of the curriculum was the increased amount of elective time. The number of elective courses increased with each year so that by the end of the second and third years, the fourth quarter (a quarter equalled 8 weeks and there were no summer courses) was entirely elective; and in the fourth year, the third and fourth quarters were entirely elective. Another unique feature of the new curriculum was the opportunity to spend time in the senior year at another institution (Jonathan Rhoads took 2 months at Harvard).

Turner speculates that the expansion of elective time was in response to the "new trend toward specialization." This trend blossomed in the 1920s with the addition of research laboratories in clinical departments,[10] but it really wasn't until after World War II that specialization took hold. Kauffman, in *The Healer's Tale*, points out that in the 1930s, 75% of physicians were general practitioners and only 17% were specialists.[11] The new curriculum had its drawbacks, but it proved successful enough that a number of its graduates went on to have distinguished careers, many of them becoming specialists and leaders in their respective fields.

Prior to the Depression, Baltimore was the seventh largest city in the United States, a booming manufacturing town and the nation's third most active port. Its population was nonunion, predominantly white and 18% black. It was a segregated city, and there were no black librarians, streetcar drivers, firefighters, or police officers.[12] It was a city of home owners, characterized by monotonous rows of red brick housing with white marble steps and arched entrances. In 1930 Baltimore accounted for one-half of Maryland's inhabitants, including more than half of the state's black population.[13] Tuberculosis and syphilis were rampant in certain parts of the city.

Located at 600 North Broadway in East Baltimore, Johns Hopkins Medical School and Hospital were several miles away from the main campus of the university. East Baltimore was largely poor and black, but there was a sizable white middle-European group that was predominantly Polish.[14] Because marriage was frowned upon at Hopkins, and indeed at most medical schools of the time, Broadway, with its many boarding houses, was home to generations of single Hopkins medical students. Speakeasies also characterized life along Broadway. Indeed, Baltimore was a center of resistance to prohibition, with its internationally famous citizen, H.L. Mencken leading the fray. Baltimoreans, unlike their northern neighbors in Philadelphia, flagrantly defied the Volstead Act (prohibition against alcohol), and patrons could partake of spirits, mostly beer, without fear of reprisal by the police.

East Baltimore was not without its dangers: Turner describes it as a community "in which the straight razor and the jackknife were prime instruments of social policy."[15] Coming from provincial Quaker Philadelphia, the 21-year-old Rhoads was exposed to more than just a change in scenery.

In October 1928 Jonathan Rhoads moved to 1254 Broadway, 6 blocks north of the school. Tuition was $400 a year, and the required microscope cost $200. No scholarships or loans were available to students. Jonathan's father had left him an eighth of his estate, which enabled him to pay for medical school and to travel around the world at the end of the second year despite the Depression. It was common to belong to one of the four fraternities that were near the hospital so that members could eat lunch or dinner, learn of the experiences of older students, and shoot pool. Jonathan joined Nu Sigma Nu, located at 518 North Broadway, which, along with the historic Pithotomy Club, is the only other fraternity of the original four remaining today. As the few female medical students ("hens") had no sorority, 800 North Broadway served both as a residence ("chicken coop") and a social focal point for them.

There were 72 students in the Class of 1932, three less than the maximum of 75. Of the 72 only seven were women. The class was distinguished by graduates from highly regarded undergraduate schools such as Hopkins, Yale, and Princeton. There were three Haverford graduates enrolled in the medical school. Forty states and five foreign countries were represented; however, most students were from the eastern United States: 44 from New York, 37 from Maryland, and 25 from Pennsylvania. In a letter to a friend Jonathan noted that "there are many Phi Beta Kappa keys in evidence here."[16] Comparing the admission practices of the day with those of the present, Dr. Rhoads writes:

In those days, you got into medical school and the crunch was to see whether you could stay in. Now if you get into medical school, about all you have to do is show up everyday and you'll get a degree because the sifting out beforehand is so intense.[17]

While the new curriculum had many attractive features, the policy of not administering exams until the end of the second and fourth years left students uncertain about their academic status. In a letter written to Royal Davis, a fellow classmate at Haverford and a medical student at Columbia, Jonathan describes the practice as "nerve racking and rough." In the same letter, however, he remarks on the more positive aspects of life at Hopkins:

Hopkins is analogous to Haverford. While you are there it is hard to see why it has its reputation. It is very different, however, in that they experiment freely with teaching methods and they maintain an atmosphere of entire freedom and at the same time of responsible work.[18]

In an interview years later in his life, Rhoads compares his experiences at the two schools once again:

Medical school at Hopkins was rigorous but the work was no more demanding than the college courses at Haverford. The difference was not that the bright students were brighter, but that the lower one-half or two-thirds of the student body I had known in college were in absentia.[19]

The preclinical faculty was considered the best in the country, if not the world. Of the four heads of the basic science departments (anatomy, physiological chemistry, physiology, and pharmacology) three were members of the National Academy of Sciences.[20] The first of the two preclinical years was committed to lectures, laboratories, conferences, and demonstrations. Required courses dealt with structure and function. Like many medical students, Rhoads became quickly bored with the drudgery of dissection. He writes to Davis:

I expect by now you are dissecting gallstones out of the kidney or kidney beans out of gallnuts but we are merely pegging away at the back musculature which I have got into one great blur of ends of muscle fibres torn, cut and jagged. None the less I've located the more essential muscles. . . . About the most interesting job we've tackled so far is the cervical and brachial plexuses which we got out fairly well. As usual I disdain technique for its own sake and I hate to twiddle around cleaning muscle off carefully and separating skin from meaningless connective tissue and pottering with cutaneous nerves, etc.[21]

To break up these days he made frequent visits to the dog surgery unit and autopsy room, where he was "rewarded with the sight of a 2½ inch kidney stone."[22]

While medical school was demanding and intense, it was also boring at times. To relieve the boredom Rhoads spent a fair amount of time reading nonmedical literature and attending movies. He read the Bible from beginning to end and went to the movies two or three times a week, seeing Ginger Rodgers and Fred Astaire and Tom Mix ("terrible"). Additionally, he drove his $40 Ford and planned trips over the spring and summer vacation.

His fascination with cars and his legendary driving habits were evident to his friends even then. He was a peripatetic explorer of the area and an indefatigable motorist. His good friends Ted and Becky Hetzel visited Rhoads in Baltimore and joined him on one of the many trips around Baltimore and the Chesapeake Bay. Comparing the driving habits of Hetzel and Rhoads, Becky observes:

Ted was always a careful driver. He knew about a motor and what he could do, and what he couldn't do. Jonathan didn't care.... He used to drive like a fiend![23]

In addition to cars, boats played a prominent role in Rhoads' life. Exploring the Chesapeake and its estuaries proved to be another diversion from the very taxing work at school. Jonathan and a friend and fellow medical student, Solon Daveron, decided to purchase a boat for further adventures. Daveron, nearly 9 years his senior, was from California and had previously been in business in Costa Rica. Driving down to the Magothy River, which flows into the Chesapeake, they came across a private club where they found a boat with an inboard motor for sale. It ran and didn't leak too much, so they bought it and stored it at a nearby slip. When they took their physiology instructor, Gemmill, out on the Chesapeake, the boat's motor died and they were all stranded. Rhoads speculated that his instructor's dim view of this experience may have played a part in his poor evaluation in physiology. By March he writes to Royal Davis that because of a "dissatisfied state of mind, I'm going on the bum this summer."[24]

In addition to the boredom, the first year of medical school was, in at least two instances, not smooth sailing. Rhoads received a letter from the Dean that his performance in physiology was deemed "poor" and better work was expected of him. His intellectual ambition not totally satisfied at medical school, Jonathan sought to compensate for his poor showing in quantitative analysis at Haverford by electing to take analytic chemistry at Hopkins. He hoped to spend summers at the University of Chicago obtaining a Ph.D. in biochemistry. Instruction at the main Hopkins campus in Homewood was sporadic, and the lab was across town from the medical school. Under these unfavorable circumstances progress in the laboratory was less than successful. A letter from the Dean to Professor of Anatomy Weed recounts:

One of the first year students in the School of Medicine, Mr. J.E. Rhoads, obtained permission to take a special course with us in Analytical Chemistry, but his work is so unsatisfactory in every respect that the instructor wishes to throw him out. Would your feelings be hurt if this action were taken? He has already paid his laboratory fees of $18 and this, of course, would be returned to him.[25]

While this particular instructor was not impressed with "Mr. J.E. Rhoads" (or Dusty as he was known to his friends), many of his classmates were. They describe him as "a good student"[26]; "the most inquisitive member of the class"[27]; "the most intelligent and nicest . . ."[28]; "courteous and helpful"[29]; and "quiet, reserved, very serious and conscientious with a wry humor, impressive with dignity."[30] Harris Schumacker, a long-time friend and colleague, recalls the Rhoads of that time and captures his demeanor and intelligence:

The amazing thing is that I recall him as exactly the same sort of person he is today and has been for decades: quiet, deliberate, dignified, courteous, and wise. He had the same tendency to hesitate a moment before responding—a moment during which one could almost see something going on in his mind, quickly analyzing, judging, reaching a decision and organizing thoughts so that the words which followed were well chosen, brief, and to the point, with a penetrating logic that commanded attention and brought respect.[31]

His political views during this period appear to be what they are today—Republican. Writing to Davis about his friend Daveron, Rhoads says:

He knows some of the Hoover crowd in California and was quite ardent for Smith, but I think that H. Hoover will probably do fairly creditably as Pres. certainly far better than anything recent. I think Al should be given the credit of forcing the Republicans to put up a good candidate.[32]

Christmas vacation in 1928 consisted of visiting friends Becky and Ted Hetzel and his former roommate at Haverford, John Woll. He tells of meeting his chemistry professor at Haverford, Meldrum, who "slyly sought to encourage me to greater industry by mentioning the fact that I was the sole representative of the alma mater in the class of 1932 at Hopkins."[33]

He visited Penn to see Murphey (a Haverford classmate and medical student) and Dean Pepper, observed a brain operation, watched Deaver remove an appendix, and visited Lankenau Hospital.

While the academic year ended uneventfully, it was during the summer of 1929 that he would meet his wife to be, Teresa (Terry) Folin, and Dr. Isidor Ravdin, his future mentor and the man most responsible for his career. Jonathan returned that summer to Philadelphia to work with Dr. Joseph Stokes at the University of Pennsylvania. It was Stokes, a Quaker and friend of the family, who took over the practice of Jonathan's father following his death. He then moved on to university work, where he eventually became chairman of pediatrics. Stokes put Jonathan to work in his laboratory that summer for $50, where one of his duties included testing the pH of gastric juice in infants. He recalls one aspect of this experience:

So when there was a newborn child, Miss Keasey would give us a call and we'd go over to the nursery and put a fine tube down the poor little thing's mouth and suck the juice out. . . . Nobody said, "boo!" to the child or the mother or anyone else![34]

In addition to this assignment, he was sent to Ravdin's lab to assist him with an ongoing study of pernicious anemia, this being the year that it was identified and reported by Minot, Murphy, and Castle. Ravdin, who was 13 years his senior and 35 at the time, immediately impressed Rhoads and many others with his charisma and energy.

Rhoads' cousin Mary Evans, a classmate and friend of Teresa (Terry) Folin at Vassar, introduced them at a party that summer. Terry was the daughter of Laura Folin, a graduate of Vassar, and Otto Folin, professor of

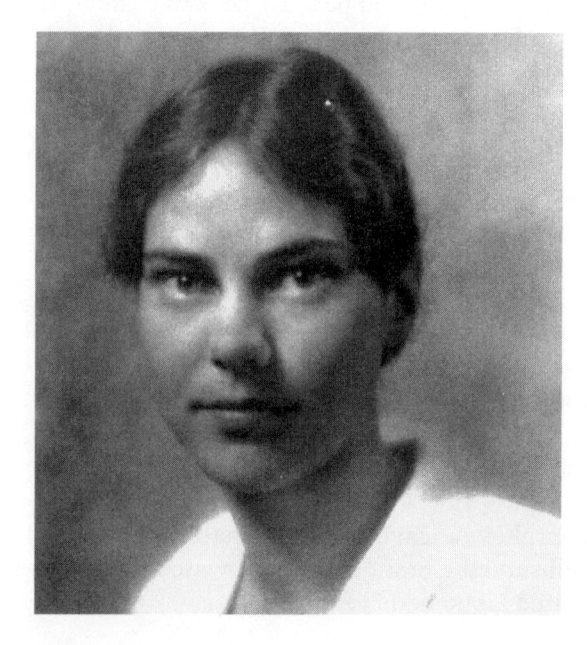

Terry Folin, 1930.

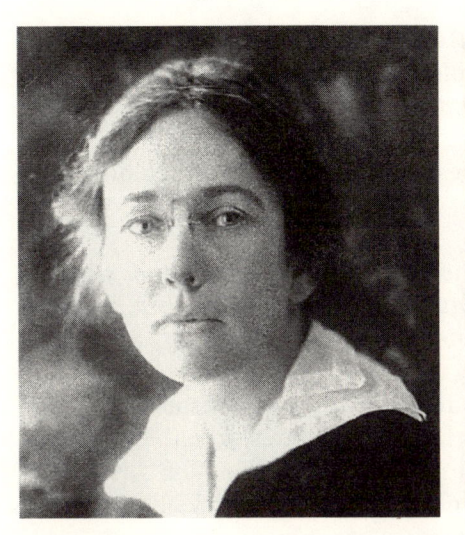

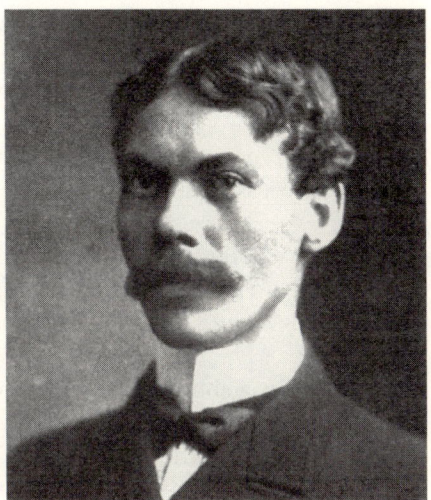

Laura Folin. *Otto Folin.*

biochemistry at Harvard Medical School and world renowned for the discovery of the Folin-Wu method of measuring blood sugar. Terry was attending Boston University School of Medicine. Graduating from high school at the age of 16, she went on to major in French at Vassar, where she graduated with honors in 1928. It was not surprising that she was attracted to Jonathan, who shared many of the same personality traits and interests as her father. Meites, in his biography of Folin, describes the professor:

Otto may have had simple tastes, but he was a highly complex man. . . . He was a man of few words because he liked to think things through before he spoke or wrote. . . . His was a slow, deliberate approach to solving a dilemma.[35]

Schaffer, in his monograph about Folin, mentions some of these qualities as well: "modesty and quiet humor, tranquility and kindliness, candor combined with a distaste for controversy."[36]

Jonathan and Teresa also had other traits in common. They came from highly educated, intelligent families, and both had lost a sibling to childhood illness. Teresa's paternal grandfather was a tanner, as was Jonathan's grandfather. Their families had very active households and frequently entertained relatives, friends, and colleagues. Sunday dinner was a ritual both families observed faithfully. They shared a special affection for their respective summer homes: the Folin's in Kearsarge, New Hampshire, and the Rhoads' at Maple Grove in New Hope, Pennsylvania. However, while religion played a central role in the Rhoads' household, this was not true for the Folins. Meites observes:

For the Folins, who were unenthusiastic Unitarians, the church ceased to be a focal point of intellectual stimulation. Laura (Teresa's mother) . . . now avoided church affairs entirely.[37]

Jonathan's attraction to Terry is best expressed by him when he recalls his first impressions of her:

She was an intriguing person with her father's eyes, her mother's height and academic aptitude, and a great sense of gamesmanship, which I think she inherited from both parents.[38]

Thinking it a shame that such an intelligent person was not attending one of the best medical schools in the United States, Jonathan, for reasons not clear to him, looked up Otto Folin's entry in *Who's Who* and dispatched a Hopkins catalogue, anonymously, to Terry. They would renew their acquaintance later.

Jonathan returned to Baltimore in October 1929, changed boarding houses, and moved to 1538 Broadway, the home of the Paulus family. The move to 1538 from 1234 Broadway proved to be a good one. His previous student home was rather impersonal and unhealthy, as some of its residents fell victim to tuberculosis. The warm and protective atmosphere of the Paulus' home made the students feel as if they were part of the family.

Boarding with Rhoads at the Paulus' home were fellow medical students Wilbur and David Sprong and Howell Wright, a fellow Haverfordian. David, the younger Sprong, had been Rhoads' "cadaver partner" in first-year anatomy. Rhoads and the fourth-year student Wilbur Sprong, spent many evenings studying and comparing notes on preclinical subjects. Wilbur's evening garb in the boarding house consisted only of underclothes, and when he was cold, a bathrobe so that Jonathan soon took to calling him "Mahatma." The Sprongs were strong and robust. Wilbur was a wrestler and participated in intercollegiate matches. He was also a talented hypnotist, although as Jonathan wrote to Esther, "he was so chary of practicing the art that I never witnessed a seance."[39]

In October 1929 the stock market crashed. The course of the world changed for most of the next decade and up to 1942, when the United States entered World War II. Much has been written about the crash of 1929 and the resultant Great Depression. Hoover, considered an able administrator but a poor politician, presided over the early years of the crash at its nadir—1929 to 1932. One in four people were without work. Between 1929 and 1932, 11,000 banks failed and $2 billion in deposits were wiped out. However, the initial reverberations of the October 1929 crash were not immediately felt in Baltimore, as noted by Mencken in his memoirs:

The great stock market crash of 1929 had only slight repercussions in the Sun *[newspaper] office, largely, I suppose because it had only slight repercussions in Baltimore. The town was in a favorable position to withstand the shock and in truth it actually withstood it better than any other large American city. This was mainly because its activities were widely diversified and few of them depended on Wall Street financing.*[40]

Indeed, Hopkins, Turner notes, was in good economic shape at the beginning of the Depression,[41] but as it wore on, signs of "depression mentality" pervaded the halls of the hospital. The existing physical plant was maintained, but

. . . notices went up to turn out unused lights, surgical dressings were used less lavishly, the annual report was reduced in size and patients were pressed more vigorously for higher payments.[42]

Most medical students were largely unaffected by these conditions, although Wilbur and David Sprong were not so fortunate. Unlike many of their fellow classmates, they worked their way through college and medical school in a variety of ways, such as transporting the mentally ill from institution to institution and working day labor jobs. With the crash of 1929 funds targeted for the University of Chicago dwindled, and Jonathan dropped his pursuit of a Ph.D. in biochemistry.

It was during the second year that Rhoads was taught by William MacCallum, the great pathologist and successor to William Welch. MacCallum, a Canadian, graduated from Toronto University at the age of 16 and went on to Hopkins, where he graduated from the institution's inaugural class. His *Textbook of Pathology*, last published in 1944, went through seven editions.[43] Rhoads writes to Davis that "MacCallum is an admirable fellow" and recalls that he was a good lecturer. He required his students to write an 11,000-word essay on a particular subject of their choice, encouraging them to search out other libraries for early references. Rhoads chose jaundice as his subject and diligently searched libraries in Philadelphia, New York, and what was then the Surgeon General's library in Washington, D.C. He recalls finding a puzzling case in which the patient was jaundiced on one side of the body but not the other. MacCallum was impressed with Rhoads' essay and sent him a note that his paper was "more carefully studied than the others."[44]

While anxiety regarding the second-year exams pervades his correspondence with Royal Davis, it did not preclude occasional trips outside Baltimore and ventures into "unrelated" reading. Weekend trips to the Smokies, the Shenandoah Valley, Luray Caverns, and Monticello marked travel during the school year. *Dracula*, Mencken's *In Defense of Women*, Turgenev's *Fathers & Sons*, a 2-volume work of *The Life and Letters of Woodrow Wilson* and Theodore Dreiser's work *Dreiser Looks at Russia* were among the books read, along with some antivivisection literature.[45] He went to many symphonies in Baltimore and Washington and attended a lecture given by Clarence Darrow, the lawyer famous for his ingenious defense of Leopold and Loeb and William Jennings Bryant's foe in the Scopes trial.

Toward the end of the second year, students were required to take a course in normal physical diagnosis, presumably as a transition to the upcoming clinical years. "Patient" experience was confined to examining fellow students. One in the group, Henry Schwartz, was designated the "ideal body form." The problem, as Rhoads remembers, was that you couldn't tell what was normal if you didn't know what was abnormal. The course was not one of the more fruitful in this year at Hopkins.[46]

As the year wore on and the exams loomed large on the horizon, Rhoads expressed his apprehension to Davis:

I'm so scared about these damned Hopkins' exams that when, as, and if I pass them, I don't give a damn if I get a zero in every National Board I ever take but that is chiefly because "Sufficient unto the day is the evil thereof." . . . Good day Mr. Davis and pray for me to Aesculapius, Panacea and Hygeia.[47]

Indeed, 1930 was a physically and psychologically demanding year. In addition to preparing for the second-year exams, Royal Davis and Jonathan Rhoads were studying for the upcoming national boards. National boards were administered at the end of the second and fourth medical school years and then again at the completion of internship, with the purpose of qualifying young physicians for licensure in all of the states except two. Typically, planning for another extensive trip underscored all of this activity. The decision to go to Russia and Japan came about during the year, when he opined that once hospital work commenced there wouldn't be time to take extended trips. Thus, the summer following his sophomore year seemed as good a time as any. He had two objectives. First, he wanted to see his sister Esther, who was working as a Quaker missionary at the Tokyo Friends School in Japan. Second, he wanted to visit Russia. This was sparked by the thawing of relations with the United States and his intense curiosity after reading Dreiser's book. He writes to Davis:

I want to sail from Vancouver on 6/26. The exams come 6/24-5-6 so I hope to take those on the 24th & 25th at least in the West. To get West, however, it will be necessary to leave about the 19th. Exams here should be over by the 4th. . . . The idea is that I want to go to Japan and see my sister and anything else possible.[48]

And again,

I posted a letter to Moscow to find out if I could go across the USSR to Vladivosktok. After all, a trip to Japan isn't to be turned down without due consideration.[49]

All that we know about his experience with the second-year exams is that he passed them. Regarding his exam in clinical microscopy, he tells Davis:

At any rate we had an exam in Clinical Microscopy which consisted in looking thru 20 microscopes (without moving the fields) and writing down what we saw. I believe I crashed thru w a 65 and those in authority have been spending weeks deciding if 65 or 70 is passing. My position has not been an enviable one.[50]

He recalls that the physiology professor, Kenneth Gemmill, after noting that he passed the written physiology exam, insisted on an oral exam to ensure he knew his subject matter. There was one "fatality"—his boating friend, Daveron, flunked out at the end of the second year.

Having passed his exams and having taken the national boards, Jonathan set out on the long-awaited trip to Russia, China, and Japan. His mother arranged for him to join up with a "medically" oriented tour group. They left on the *Europa* and crossed the Atlantic to Bremerhaven, Germany, and went on to Lubeck. Subsequently, they took a steamer to Helsinki, and after spending a day there, the group boarded a train first stopping at Leningrad (St. Petersburg) and then proceeded on to Moscow, where they stayed for 5 days.

At that point the group and Jonathan parted; the group went out through Poland, and Jonathan took the Trans-Siberian Railroad across Russia and into China. On the train he befriended an art student who was the only other English-speaking passenger. The student, Isamu Noguchi, was on his way to Peking to study calligraphy and then visit his father in Tokyo. The conversation turned at one point, as Rhoads recalls, to anatomy, a subject of mutual interest:

The thing that I remember that he told me was that he could diagnose pregnancy from the hypertrophy of the trapezius muscles. As the baby got larger, the woman held her head back further in order to balance herself.[51]

The train trip took seven days, and they went into Manzhouli in Northwest Manchuria and then on to Harbin. Noguchi and Rhoads parted company in Harbin, which was populated with many "White Russians" who had been driven out of their country by the Bolsheviks. Noguchi went on to study under Brancusi and became a famous sculptor. Their paths crossed many years later when, in 1983 after reading a magazine's list of the "Top 25 Older Americans Still Working in 1982" and seeing Noguchi's name (Rhoads was also listed), Rhoads wrote to him and asked if indeed he was that same student. They reunited at a dinner in New York in 1983, 53 years after their shared railway adventure.

The train took Rhoads on through Changchun, Shenyang (Mukden), and Tianjin (Tientsin) before finally arriving in Beijing (Peking). With only 49 hours in Peking, not knowing the language, and with a good exchange rate in force, he decided to hire a guide. He recalls:

The guide arrived with a car, a chauffeur and a footman and those people escorted me around.

I didn't ask for a footman, he sort of came with it. I stayed in a hotel that was popular with Germans. . . . I saw a great deal at the time because of all of the equipment I had.[52]

Leaving Peking, he travelled back toward Shenyang with the notion of taking the train from there to Seoul, Korea, and down to the straits. Halfway back to Shenyang the rail line was washed out and the trip came to a halt. There were many missionaries aboard the train, including a woman physician. Because conditions were quickly becoming unsanitary, the physician insisted that the station master move the train a quarter of a mile so that the threat of cholera and dysentery could be reduced, but her efforts were to no avail. The prospect of how soon the situation would be remedied grew dim, and a group, including Jonathan, on the advice of an Englishman who seemed to know his way around, opted to take a branch train down to the sea.

After arriving at the port, which was controlled by local Chinese warlords, they found a Dutch company willing to transport them to another rail line. Thinking they were in good hands, given the lore of Dutch navigational expertise, they boarded the boat in rough seas and proceeded with their trip. It soon became evident to the passengers that something had gone awry. After consulting with some Chinese men on nearby junks, they discovered that the captain couldn't read a chart and they were 60 miles off course.

In time, Jonathan along with the rest landed back in Shenyang, cleaned up, and took the train down through Korea to the coast and across the strait to Shimonoseki, Japan. Esther, who had been waiting there for three days, returned to Tokyo but left a note with the station master for Jonathan. Upon his arrival he was able to telephone her, and they agreed to meet in Nara. He spent a full month in Japan, visiting Kyoto, Tokyo, and Sapporo. At the end of the summer he returned on one of the Canadian Pacific ships, landed in Vancouver, and proceeded home, interrupting his journey with a brief visit to the Henry Ford Hospital in Detroit, where he met with two members of the original tour group. The world trip at an end, Jonathan returned to Baltimore to find that Terry Folin was now a member of the third-year class at Hopkins.

The third year of medical school was the first of the two designated "clinical years," characterized by a decrease in the number of formal lectures and an increase in small group conferences, discussions, and patient contact. Student exposure to patients in the third year was largely confined to the outpatient clinics, and inpatient contact was generally reserved for the final year. In 1930 there were 229,839 outpatient visits to the Johns Hopkins Hospital—34% were without charge and the average receipt for patients who could pay was $0.47.[53] Mencken, in his series about Johns Hopkins Hospital, describes the patient population:

The intentions of the founder have never been forgotten, and the Johns Hopkins is still preeminently a refuge for people who can't pay the whole cost, or even any of the cost of their care and treatment. It has, to be sure, some rich patients, and they naturally tend to get into the newspapers, but taking one day with another, it deals mainly with the poor.[54]

Through the efforts of Lewellys Barker, Professor of Medicine, an affiliation with the Bay View Hospital was established to introduce third-year medical students to physical diagnosis. The Bay View Hospital, situated to the southeast of the Hopkins' complex, was part of the Baltimore City Hospital System, and Bay View was originally established as an asylum for the city's mentally ill and chronically ill patients. Eventually, the hospital complex was expanded to accommodate "broad medical care for the indigent sick of Baltimore City."[55] Rhoads tells of his experience there:

You saw rather advanced disease out there. For instance, an aortic aneurysm had beaten its way through the sternum and was about to burst. They had the experience out there of having them burst and the blood would fly way up (the walls, ceiling) and the patient expired. These were due to syphilis. They had a great deal of tuberculosis.[56]

The students were exposed to many types of contagious diseases, and Rhoads recalls that the school authorities really did very little to protect them. However, Turner points out that because of the high incidence of pulmonary tuberculosis among students in 1911, steps were taken, although not immediately, to require entering students to undergo a special examination for pulmonary T.B., with regular inspection of the boarding homes along Broadway and its environs.[57]

Of the Class of 1932, 11% ultimately contracted tuberculosis. More than 50% of the students were exposed to tuberculosis, either from airborne or bovine sources. One of the Sprong brothers eventually died from tuberculous meningitis. Rhoads comments on the plight of medical students:

It was not a very healthy environment but it was an interesting one. I think we all had gone into medicine for better or worse. Medicine was not a money making game in those days. . . . If we survived, well and good, and if we didn't survive, that was part of our lot.[58]

While Jonathan did not fall victim to tuberculosis until many years later, illness did take its toll when, in late December 1930, he awoke with a fever of 103 degrees. After reporting to student health he was admitted to the hospital. Diagnosed with mastoiditis on Christmas Eve, he was operated upon emergently. The anesthetic was Avertin, which was new and administered rectally (later deemed too dangerous to use). The medical student again became the patient when it was decided that he subsequently needed a tonsillectomy. Less serious but no less bothersome was the reappearance of severe bouts of acne during these years.

Other acutely infectious diseases were ever present in addition to tuberculosis. Students saw and diagnosed many of the prevalent diseases of the time: diphtheria, rheumatic fever, all stages of syphilis, and pellagra. There were almost no effective treatments available at the time. Diagnosis, symptomatic care, and bedside comfort were the trademarks of the profession. A short list of chemotherapeutic agents included arsenicals, bismuth, and gold.[59]

The academic year 1930–31 was generally uneventful. His correspondence to Davis was brief and reflects his growing ruminations regarding marriage and matters of everyday life: the purchase of a new radio installed in Germantown, a spring trip down to the Carolinas with a cousin, and a discussion about his long-time friend and fellow Westtonian, Helen Bell.[60] Although he was seeing Terry Folin more often, it was not until the fourth year of medical school that their friendship blossomed, when Jonathan went to Harvard Medical School for two months for an elective course. This experience also led to increasing contact with the Folin family.

In the fall of 1931 and the beginning of his senior year at Hopkins, Rhoads was 24 years old, 6 feet 3 inches tall, and weighed 180 pounds. The summer was spent once again at the University of Pennsylvania in the laboratory of A.N. Richards. The group included Dr. Joseph Stokes and Dr. Carl Schmidt, a pharmacologist who, along with Seymour Kety, was later responsible for landmark studies on the measurement of blood flow of the brain. By 1931 Schmidt was already known for his work on ephedrine with Dr. K.K. Chen.[61] Some of this research had been conducted in China at the Peking Union Medical College, which Rhoads had visited the previous summer. Rhoads was welcomed into the research group. Dr. Joseph Stokes was interested in the relatively new anesthetic Avertin. One of its interesting properties was that it was slow acting and provided a period of analgesia often lasting for some time after the operation. Rhoads explains:

Dr. Stokes thought that this might be a useful drug in managing convulsions, such as those seen with tetanus or strychnine poisoning in children, and that the dose perhaps could be increased beyond the point at which respiratory failure would occur if the patient were supported with a mechanical respirator.[62]

The results of his work that summer were disappointing. The drug adversely affected blood pressure as much as respiration so that the animals could not survive a large dose of strychnine with Avertin, regardless of whether they were on or off the respirator. The one rewarding experience that summer, which called on his considerable mechanical ability and talent, was the construction of a respirator based upon the principle that Drinker outlined in Boston.[63]

The fourth year of medical school was stimulating. Students at Hopkins spent the majority of their time on the inpatient wards. Besides their everyday duties, considerable thought was given to where they would apply for internship. Rhoads had decided as early as his freshman year to return to Pennsylvania to practice medicine. Pennsylvania licensure required a rotating internship which was not offered at Hopkins. Three hospitals in Philadelphia interested him: Pennsylvania Hospital, the oldest hospital in the United States; Philadelphia General Hospital, a huge public hospital; and the Hospital of the University of Pennsylvania, just next door in West Philadelphia. In recalling his visits to these hospitals, he slyly notes that he stopped by their cafeterias to see which had the best food.

Internships then, unlike today, were sought after individually, and there was no matching system. This exchange of letters reflects the almost informal arrangement for choosing interns:

I am writing at the request of Mr. Jonathan E. Rhoads who is applying for an interneship [sic] at the University Hospital next year. . . . He is industrious and intelligent and I am sure he would make a satisfactory house officer.[64]

In response:

The Interne Committee has not yet decided how many men they will take from medical schools other than our own. . . . If I remember correctly, he is a resident of Philadelphia and a graduate of Haverford College. Naturally, I might be apt to be a little prejudiced in his favor with that background.[65]

The Hospital of the University of Pennsylvania filled most of its intern positions with graduates of its own medical school who were chosen by staff members. Three or four positions were reserved for graduates from other schools and were chosen by the dean. Perhaps because of his summer experiences at the hospital, his close relationship with Stokes, his friendship with Sergeant Pepper (son of the dean), and his Philadelphia and Haverford background, he won one of the few prized positions there. He writes to Davis:

I got the Dean's office here to write to Pepper stating my qualifications for a job at the University Hospital. Pepper did not deign to communicate with me but in the course of time his assistant whom you recollect is Thorpe caused it to come to my ears via the Dean's office here that I had an appointment. I was surprised and pleased both to a rather extraordinary degree.[66]

That part of his future settled, he planned a Christmas trip to Florida with his mother and sisters. Writing to Davis, Rhoads relates:

I have since been enabled to devise at least tentatively certain plans for the immediate future. Last summer I sowed the seed of driving to Florida during the xmas vacation in the maternal and sororal minds. This I have recently watered and it has sprouted nicely.[67]

In December 1931 we begin to learn about Terry Folin and Jonathan's growing relationship with her. This was clearly a very happy time, which is reflected in a letter regarding a Christmas party they attended:

I may as well append here an account or anamnesis of the party. As Terry and I drove back afterwards arriving in Balt. at 3:20 a.m. I'm somewhat in a fog. Biddle and Ruth, Miss Pegasus, my cousin Betty and Elizabeth Marsh were there together with Phil Rhoads, Dan Test, Mr. Trueblood and another from Temple Medical School, an agent from New York and John Forsythe. We cooked steak and ate it cum baked spuds and then we blew feathers into each others faces, played porch hockey, struggled with puzzles which were vaguely reminiscent of crosswords but different. Then we swapped travel yarns and the abler voices sang carols. Sounds rather simple but an extraordinarily good time was had by all or at least by me. . . . Monday I face my nemesis in the person of Dean Lewis, Surgeon in Chief at J.H.H. at ward rounds.[68]

Lewis succeeded the great William S. Halsted in January 1925 after serving as chairman at University of Illinois for a mere 6 months. "In the five years following 1920, Lewis was offered every major vacant surgical chair in the country."[69] He was 6 feet tall and had an imposing presence. He was in wide demand as a speaker and belonged to all of the major medical societies in the United States. He was said to have a remarkable memory. Turner points out, however, that Halsted and Lewis could not have been more different in personality and interests:

The one [Halsted], spare, ascetic, withdrawn, known well to few except his small circle of intimates, uninterested in the general run of students, a surgical investigator of note, and a cautious and often slow operator; the other [Lewis] a strong, vigorous, outgoing man, skillful and quick in both surgical diagnosis and operation, and a somewhat terrifying but dedicated teacher. . . . He had done little investigative work before coming to Hopkins and did not pretend to do any after his arrival.[70]

It is strange that a medical school that was deemed to be in the vanguard of surgical research would recruit Lewis as chairman. But as Lewis said of himself, "I would rather teach than anything else." Turner describes him as "a great teacher, though a formidable one for those ill-prepared."[71] Rhoads remembers his experience in Lewis' famous Friday surgical clinics:

He would bring in a patient or two and he would get some poor student in the front row and show everybody how little they knew. Never got me—I was always in the back row. He was sort of a gruff guy. . . . I left there thinking surgery was one of the last things I would go in to.[72]

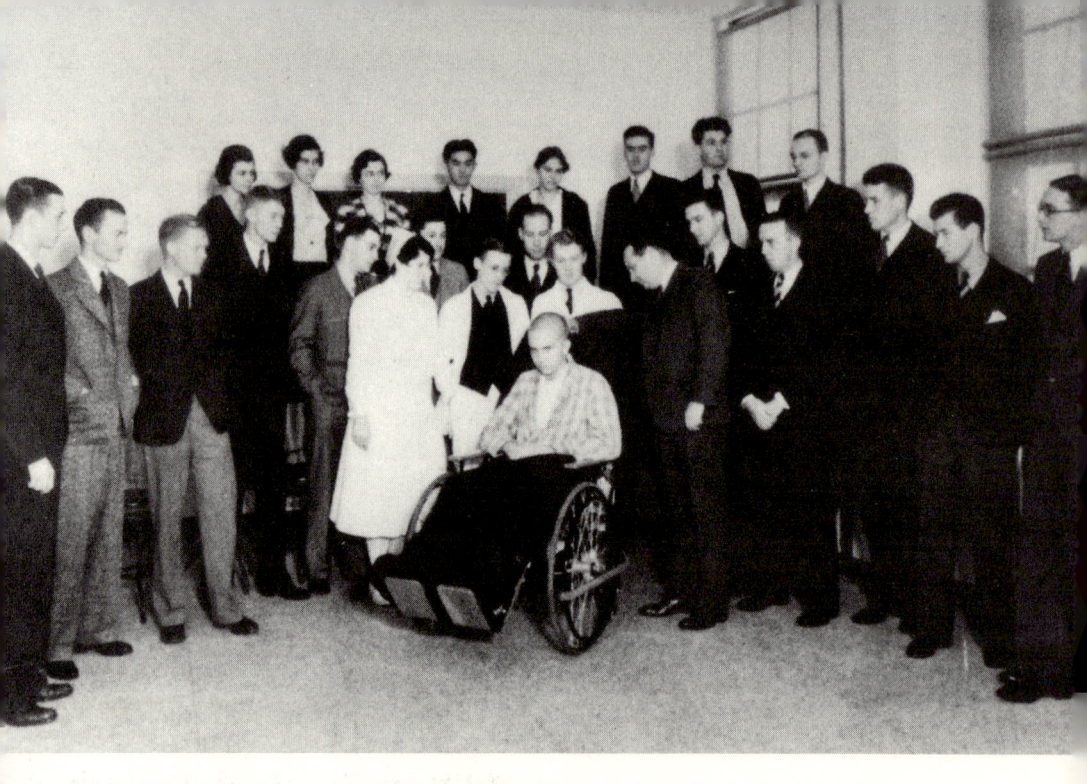

Jonathan Rhoads as a medical student at Hopkins. The famous neurosurgeon J. Walter Dandy is on the right of the patient. Rhoads is in the back row (third from the right). His future wife Terry Folin is in the center, back row.

Another Rhoads' experience with surgeons at Hopkins was albeit a brief encounter with the famous neurosurgeon J. Walter Dandy. He remembers Dandy as a "mean chief" who also humiliated his students:

He would say to the resident, "Isn't anybody trying to help me? You just killed this patient!" And so forth. . . . He was merciless.[73]

Rhoads did not like his experience in surgery. He found it largely mechanical, with limited patient contact, and very impersonal. And perhaps the confrontational atmosphere of surgery at Hopkins offended his Quaker sensibility. Instead, he directed his interests toward psychiatry, to which he devoted some of his elective time.

Interest in Freud's theories had been growing since the early 1900s, and it was firmly rooted in the curricula of universities and medical schools in the United States by the time Rhoads entered Hopkins in 1928. The Curriculum Revision of 1927 required a course in psychiatry each year. The two dominant figures at Hopkins in psychiatry were Adolf Meyer and Esther Richards. Born in Switzerland, trained at the University of Zurich and later at the University of Chicago, Meyer was appointed head of the Phipps Clinic in 1909 and remained there until his retirement in 1941. During the height of his career he was considered the

North American equivalent to Freud.[74] Rhoads recalls his impressions of Meyer:

Adolf Meyer was rather a fascinating person. He believed that you could not do everything by analyzing dreams. You needed to have the whole life history of the person including their physical health history before you were to evaluate them. He spoke with a foreign accent. He was a bit weird. I think he saw the limitations of the Freudian approach.[75]

Turner echoes this sentiment when he describes Meyer as "enigmatic, shadowy and strange."[76] His major contributions were not in investigation, but the training of men who would become heads of the leading departments of psychiatry throughout the United States.

Esther Richards, like Meyer, was not known for her contributions to original research but for her clinical observations of the mental and behavioral problems of children and adolescents. Trained and educated at Hopkins, she was "short, stocky, energetic, amusing," and a popular lecturer. She remained at Hopkins until her retirement in 1951.[77]

Why Rhoads' interest in pursuing a career in psychiatry waned is not clear. He writes to the renowned psychiatrist in Kansas, Walter Menninger, many years later:

Without analyzing it, I suspect that one of the reasons I veered off from psychiatry was that I really didn't want to be like Adolf Meyer, famous as he was.[78]

In any event, psychiatry continued to occupy an important role in his thinking and activities. Many years later, as chairman of surgery at Penn, he emphasized the psychologic aspects of patient care and invited a member of the psychiatry department to join them on surgical rounds once or twice a month.

Rhoads' interest in psychiatry may also have stemmed from his Quaker background. Quakers have had a long association with the mental health movement in the United States, having founded the nation's first psychiatric institution, The Friends Hospital, located in Philadelphia. Rhoads has served on the Board of Managers of the Friends Hospital since 1952.

Taking advantage of Hopkins' elective program, Rhoads spent February and March of 1932 at Boston City Hospital and Boston Children's Hospital. This was one of the most rewarding experiences of his medical school years. At Boston City Hospital he came into contact with the brilliant and charismatic Soma Weiss, who later became chief of medicine at The Peter Bent Brigham Hospital, and Chester Keefer, who later became chief of medicine at Boston University. This sojourn in Boston also brought him into closer contact with the Folin family, cementing in many ways the developing relationship with Terry. It was Terry who introduced him to Ben Carey, a medical student at Harvard who worked in her father's lab. Carey showed him around and made him comfortable for his short stay in Boston. Rhoads lived in Vanderbilt Hall and took his meals there.

Rhoads' principal reason for coming to Harvard was to meet and be trained by Castle, who did landmark work on pernicious anemia. However, when Rhoads arrived, Castle was on sabbatical, and Weiss and Keefer proved to be more than able substitutes. Despite this disappointment Rhoads took electives in both medicine and pediatrics and appears to have done well. Recalling his experience, particularly at Boston Children's Hospital, he has said, "It was possibly the best month I had in my four years of medical school":

There were as many students as interns so that you were part of the service rather than an "on-looker." We went around with the house officer and the Chief and it was a very fine experience for that month. In most places where you were a clinical student clerk, the nurses looked upon you as a sort of necessary evil, but at Children's you were accepted by the nursing staff because you were an essential part of the team.[79]

Dr. Weiss writes of Rhoads in a letter to Assistant Dean Andrus:

He is very sincere, thinks carefully.... [He is] slow, steady, [and has] good fundamental knowledge.[80]

News of his election to Alpha Omega Alpha (medical school honor society) arrived via a collect telegram from Edith Robinson, his lab partner and good friend at Hopkins:

Dear Dusty,
You've just been elected to AOA along with the other apple polishers!
Edith[81]

Election to AOA at Hopkins was different from that at other institutions at the time. Grades were not given to students, but at the end of the second and fourth years, class standing was revealed to students as to whether they were in the upper, middle, or lower thirds. The decision to elect students to AOA was made by the Hopkins graduates who had gone on to residency appointments at the hospital.

The stay in New England afforded Rhoads two other opportunities: to get to know Otto and Laura Folin and to explore New England and its coastline. Jonathan was familiar with the work of Otto Folin, having been introduced to it in his course in biochemistry at Haverford.

Compared to the Rhoadses, the Folins were recent immigrants to the United States. Otto Folin came to the United States from Sweden when he was 15 to stay with his brother Axel, who lived near St. Paul, Minnesota. Laura's family, originally from northeastern Canada, moved to Winnepeg when she was 4 and eventually settled in St. Paul. Through great industry, persistence and intelligence, Otto Folin worked his way through the University of Minnesota and, after a series of appointments at various institutions, secured a key position in the Physiological Chemistry Department at Harvard Medical School, where he remained until his death. Laura was very interested in politics and attended political rallies and read *The New Republic* when she was not tutoring her children and attending to matters at home.[82]

Terry was the last of the three Folin children, which included a brother, George, and a sister, Johanna, who died of diphtheria when she was 12. In addition to introducing Jonathan to various friends at the medical school, Terry asked her parents to invite him home to meet the family. Jonathan heard a lot about Terry's father from the medical students who expressed admiration for Professor Folin. He liked him and especially admired his approach to biochemistry. He remembers Folin's keen sense of humor and kindness toward him during his stay in Boston.

The signs of his growing and more serious relationship with Terry were becoming evident. On one occasion Folin sought out Jonathan in the dining room at Vanderbilt Hall to let him know his daughter would be home the next morning. Rhoads joined the Folins for dinner that evening and drove Terry as far as Philadelphia, where she met his mother. He recalls:

I went down to Baltimore. I think she came down by train the next day. I gathered she wanted to interview my mother.[83]

Rhoads also relates his mother's impressions of Terry:

One was that she was seriously interested in me and the other was that she usually succeeded in getting what she wanted.[84]

Having secured a passing grade in pediatrics and honors in medicine at Harvard, Rhoads returned to Hopkins to complete the final quarter of his medical education.

The 1932 school year ended with medical school graduation and with Jonathan and Terry, David Sprong, and Katherine Schultz (two fellow graduates) taking a trip to the Great Smoky Mountains—the trip being, of course, the brainchild of the newly titled Dr. Rhoads. Having accepted an 18-month straight medical internship at Yale, Terry Folin returned to

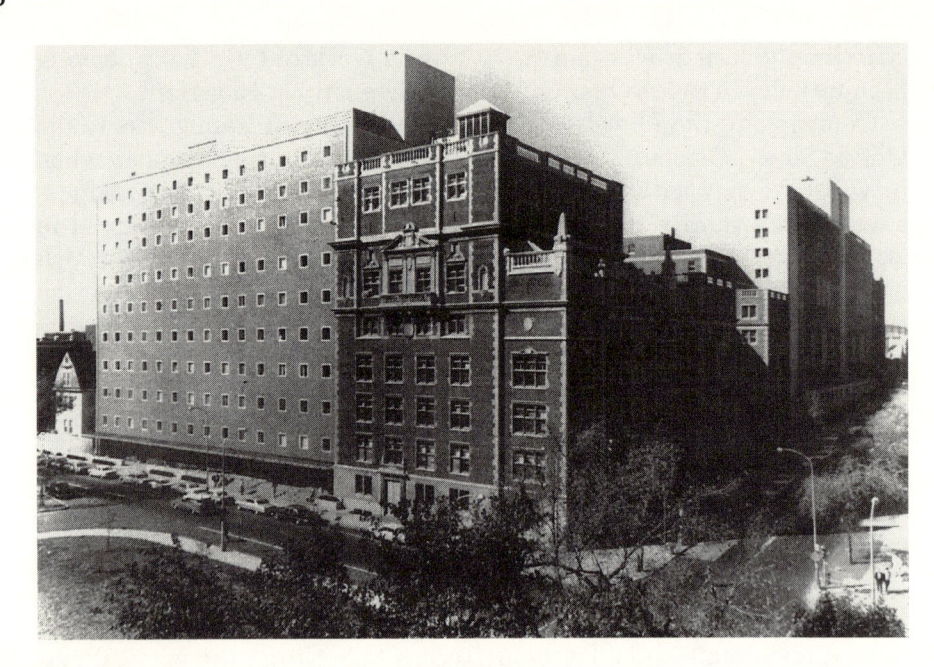

Hospital of the University of Pennsylvania (HUP) circa 1962.

her native New England. Jonathan Rhoads came back to Philadelphia to pursue his medical career at the Hospital of the University of Pennsylvania (HUP), where he would remain for the rest of his professional life.

Shortly after starting his internship, Rhoads recalls:

At times I feel as though life had become merely a succession of facts with very little personal interest attached. I am however cheered by a statement in a paper by Joe Stokes on general practice in which he says one is never so dehumanized as at the completion of his internship.[85]

Internship commenced on July 1, 1932. Of the 28 "internes" listed in the Board of Managers' report there were 27 men and one woman.[86] HUP took 14 internes each year for a 2-year period. Interns were required to buy their own uniforms (white coat, slacks, and shoes), but the hospital provided room, board, and laundry services at no cost.

Because there were few positions for advanced training in the specialties at that time, hospitals were "intern oriented." The intern was the first assistant at operations, and the "fellow" served as the second assistant unless he got to do the operation. Interactions between the interns and chiefs of service were direct and first hand. Interns performed their patients' blood chemistries and routine laboratory work at night. Work at HUP was hard and very confining. Rhoads recalls working 3 weeks straight without leaving the hospital and going 36 hours without sleep.

The HUP Board of Managers Report for 1932–33 reflects a profile of a hospital struggling, along with the rest of America, in the depth of the Depression. The only new work during the year was the construction of a G.I. clinic for fluoroscopic examinations. The salaried staff took a 10% pay cut. The daily charge to the ward (uninsured) patients was reduced to $3.50. The cost of an operation was cut almost in half—from $13.35 to $7.25. The average patient stay was 13 days. Ward patients accounted for 78% of the patient population. The average cost of an outpatient visit was $0.67.[87] While the interns felt overworked and at times underappreciated, Rhoads recalls:

We did not beef. . . . We knew we were more fortunate than our former classmates who were leading a precarious existence outside.[88]

Rhoads' close friend John Webster remembers how sad an existence John Furnas, one of their best friends and a fellow Westtonian, led during this time. Furnas was a seller of cash registers, which of course no one wanted to buy.[89] Generalized consumer demand became so low that retail prices got progressively cheaper. Dr. Rhoads remembers having a five-course meal in a nice restaurant for $0.50; gas was $0.11 a gallon; a semiprivate room at HUP cost $4.00 a day; and a private room $15.00.

During the first year interns were exposed to 2 months each of obstetrics; a composite rotation consisting of orthopedics, anesthesia, duty in the receiving ward and dermatology; urology; laboratory medicine; pediatrics; and nose and throat. One month into the internship he writes to Davis:

Being an obstetrician I deliver babies and as they are like tide and time I sometimes merely pick them out of bed. . . . Being human I make frequent errors, but being a Westtonian I quickly recover from such blows of fate and recoup my forces for bigger and better errors in the future. . . . Being unfortunate I have heard from scarcely anyone. I know only that the Folins got off for Sweden.[90]

By September duty on the obstetrics service was over. Rhoads summarizes his experience:

My obstetrics service is over—only about 50 deliveries some of which I was helped with, but we saw a fair sampling of pathology and operative deliveries and also a trifle of gynecological work. We had several nephritic toxemias, 3 hyperemesis gravidarum, 1 postpartum eclampsia, 1 placenta previa, 1 premature separation, about 5 or 6 breeches, 1 anencephalic monster, 1 transverse lie, 1 face presentation. I got fairly handy with outlet forceps, episiotomies and repairs of 2nd degree tears and applied axis traction forceps and aftercoming head forceps a couple of times under supervision. I also decomposed a breech. It was rather startling to reach up into the womb and hunt for feet.[91]

Rhoads' letters to Davis continue to reveal a man of wide and varied interests. Reporting his readings to Davis, he lists them along with a prècis for each:

Dostoyevsky's The Possessed *(not his best book but interesting contemporary comment on terrorists), highly spiced that I only read a little at a time;* Infant Nutrition *by Marriott (the title speaks for itself);* Osler's Aequanimitas *(a little goes a long way);* Droll Tales *by Honore de Balzac (I got left behind while passing from the particular to the universal);* The Autocrat *by O.W. Holmes (of this I hope to read more);* The Savoy Operas *by Gilbert (it is so sticky that the sheets no longer have a chance to be demure—but the operas are an ever present help in time of trouble); finally I started a novel of Mrs. Humphrey that is nearly too feeble to pursue.*[92]

While internship was very demanding and time off limited, Jonathan and his friend Helen Bell managed to set aside a weekend in June for a houseparty at the Bell's Pocono Lake cottage. Terry Folin came down from New Haven, and Royal Davis and his girlfriend and a friend named Uffie came from New York. He tells his sister Esther:

I succeeded in forgetting my bathing suit and so enjoyed myself without having to swim. Terry and I went up the lake (with motor) past the road bridge under the railroad bridge thru a strand of dead tree trunks that stuck up thru the water—to where the Tobyhanna again flowed. It was a heavenly morning. Presently the motor commenced grazing the bottom so we stopped—put into a place where the bank was grassy and basked in the sun. When the party broke up we were amazed to find that Helen and Min had held expenses for food, laundry down to 85 cents a piece—quite an achievement for 3 meals I thought.[93]

Quakers are known for their frugality and interest in finance, and Jonathan Rhoads was no exception. Frequently he broaches the subject of finance and economic theory in his letters to Davis. Rhoads and his close friend, John Webster, shared a joint interest in financial matters and stocks. Webster recalls one related amusing incident:

We shared an early subscription to Fortune Magazine *when it first came out and complained how much it cost—$10. I think his share was contributed by operating on our dog, so I had to pay for the magazine and then the dog ran away.*[94]

He writes to his sister Esther about the changing economic conditions of the time:

We are having inflation in quite a big way & it has many aspects $1 = 70 cents gold—the stock market crashing upwards. Gen'l Motors that I happened to buy at 12¼ in March is now 32½ and many other things proportionally which I did not buy. The 1929 feeling is getting in the air. So far retail prices have been affected only moderately so that inflation has not reduced our buying power much—but I suppose it will. Just as the Hoover administration with its deflation was one where one subsisted on his high grade bonds, so the Roosevelt inflation seems to be one where poor bonds and stocks will help us. In view of the violently changing conditions it is remarkable how Uncle Richard's doctrine of diversification that he taught Mother and she passed on to us seems to be justified. As I recall he recommended investment of substantial portions of one's estate in bonds, stocks and mortgages and there was in the background always some land.[95]

The "bank holiday" had been declared in March 1933. Rhoads recalls anticipating this and going down to the bank to withdraw some of his money, even though it was considered unpatriotic:

There was quite a line of people at each teller's window and they all looked a little ashamed of themselves but very determined, so I think I looked the way they did and drew out $100, $20 in gold and the rest in paper. I was not without money when the banks closed.[96]

It was about this time that Jonathan Rhoads wrote to President Roosevelt suggesting an ingenious solution to the country's economic problems. He opined that one of the biggest problems was that people with money wouldn't spend it, goods weren't purchased, and therefore no jobs were created. The solution, he wrote, was to date money. A person would have 90 days or 180 days to spend it and could save a portion of money which would not be dated; the amount would be regulated by the treasury. There would be free trade between the currencies so that if someone really wanted to save, he could buy the money at a premium for whatever it took. There was a very polite response from the White House, the national currency policy did not change, and Jonathan Rhoads' thoughts returned to medicine.

Having finished the first year of his 2-year internship, Rhoads was rewarded with a month's vacation. Writing to his sister Esther in July 1933, he expresses with growing confidence, great satisfaction and enthusiasm for his chosen profession:

I finished Nose and Throat July 1st, having been very busy the last 2 weeks or so. As my commission so to speak I got to do 44 tonsil cases. It was great fun. There was an assortment of cases that bled more or less and which were very good experience stopping. Since then I have been on the thyroid service, which is relatively light though one has to get up early on account of the bad habits of the surgeons who run it. The cases are quite similar yet each has its features and one gets more experience clamping blood vessels and tying knots than on most of the general surgical patients.[97]

In the same letter he tells Esther of his tentative vacation plans:

Plans are slowly taking shape. Finances are much in the air. The idea is to go with John Webster to Chicago to see the Fair, then up into Ottertail Co. Minnesota where there are many lakes & we hope a few boats and which is near So. Dakota, the 48th state. We may return thru Michigan, crossing the neck of Lake Michigan on the Ferry. John wants to be back in 2 weeks and save two weeks for a trip with Doris [his wife]. Soon after returning I am to change cars and start off with C & R and M [his sisters and mother] to do the Maritime provinces of Canada—East Port, Me—St. John N.B. up the river and across Riviere du Loup. There if facilities are cheap enough we may cross the river and drive up the Saguenay and around Lac St. Jean and back by another road to Quebec. We are uncertain about Montreal.[98]

While the Webster-Rhoads trip out West did not go strictly according to plan, they did manage to reach the Grand Canyon and visit various Westtown friends along the way. Using Webster's old Ford and Rhoads' canvas tent, they gradually made their way across country. The 17-day trip cost $110 between them. As Webster tells it:

In crossing Iowa it got so rainy and slippery—the roads weren't paved all the way out West—but the car kept slipping off the road and Jonathan would jump off and push the nose of the car to the center of the road. And then there was another time we came around a bend and there had been an accident. The car was turned over the wheels were still spinning.... People were thrown all over the place. Jonathan jumped out and looked the situation over ... found an old board and made a splint for an elderly lady and asked some young people who had come by there if they had any whiskey ... gave it to the lady ... jumped back in the car and away we went.[99]

They never did make it to the Chicago World's Fair, but Rhoads remedied this by tacking it on to the end of the trip with his sisters and mother, a trip distinguished by circuitous routes and visits to a dizzying number of sites in a short period of time. He writes to Esther:

Again back from a trip—this time only 4500 miles.... In addition to the indifferent condition of the roads the trip was distinguished by the fact that we made numerous stops and saw 21 people we knew.... The World's Fair at Chicago was really extraordinary—everything you could imagine. The transportation and electrical exhibits were especially fine.... We came home in 2½ days-about 20 hours driving. We seem to be getting poorer and poorer but are happy as usual.[100]

The second year of internship was divided equally between 6 months on the surgical service and 6 months on the medical service. It was during this period that Dr. Rhoads came into closer contact with the "greats" of surgery at HUP: Charles Harrison Frazier, Eldridge Eliason,

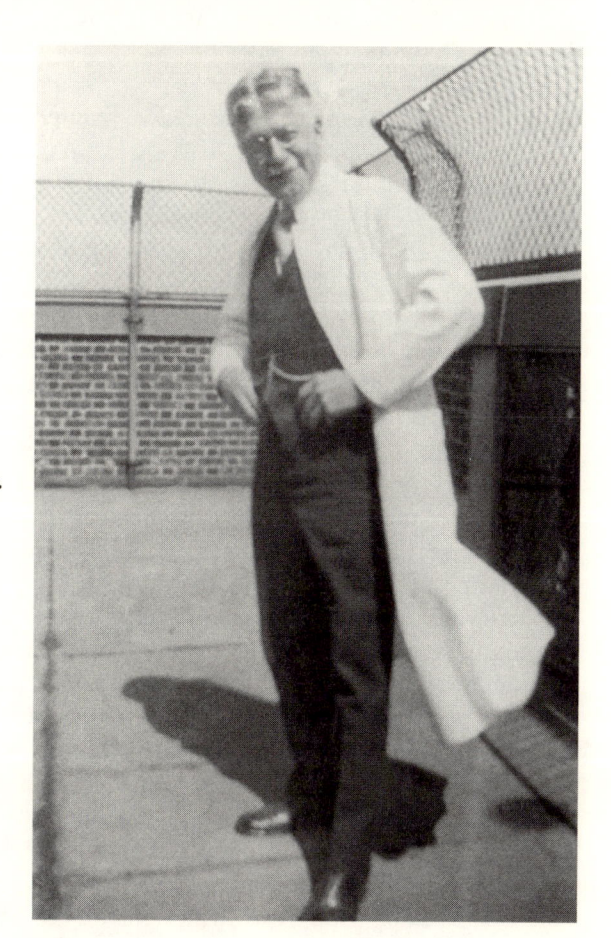

Charles Frazier.

and Isidor S. Ravdin. A fourth, George Mueller, left not long after Rhoads arrived.

The Surgical Clinic consisted of five divisions. Division A was headed by the chair of the department and the John Rhea Barton Professor of Surgery, Charles Harrison Frazier. This division was devoted to the young specialties of neurosurgery and thyroid surgery. Within the Department of General Surgery, Division B was headed by George P. Mueller; Division C by Eldridge Eliason; Division D (urologic surgery) by Alexander Randall; and Division E (research surgery) by Isidor Ravdin.

The Hospital of the University of Pennsylvania, until the arrival of Ravdin, was populated with physicians drawn from the blueblood families of Philadelphia and its wealthy Main Line. Frazier and Randall were from prominent society families, and Eliason came from an entrenched upper crust family in Maryland. Breaking with tradition, Frazier recruited Ravdin, a Jew of Russian and German extraction, who was brought over from Graduate Hospital to head the research division of the Department of Surgery. Pendleton Tompkins, a fellow intern with Rhoads in 1933, describes Frazier:

Although he was a medical giant, Dr. Frazier (we interns referred to him affectionately as Pop Frazier) was a smallish man with sparkling white hair and eyes as bright as a summer sky. He wore a cutaway with a white carnation, a gray vest, a pearl stickpin, striped pants, gray spats, glistening black shoes. . . . He was the epitome of elegance.[101]

Frazier's most famous contributions to neurosurgery were the development of a procedure for tic douloureux (inflammation of the facial nerve) and the cordotomy for the relief of intractable pain. He became the chief of surgery and John Rhea Barton Professor in 1922, succeeding John Deaver, perhaps the greatest abdominal surgeon of his time. Frazier was a tough and fiery chairman who pushed ahead to establish a surgical training program and a department of surgical research. He was also famous for throwing out interns and residents from the operating room (although only temporarily) when not satisfied with their performance. Interns and residents who were unfortunate enough to experience this humiliation formed what they called the Frazier Club. Rhoads, never having rotated through neurosurgery, was not a member. His limited contact with Frazier left him with the impression of a person who was austere but warmer than any of the surgeons at Hopkins. Ravdin was deeply fond of Frazier and admired him not only for his innovations in the practice of surgery and surgical education, but also for his many contributions to civic life.

Eldridge Eliason, the second in this surgical triumvirate, was a very imposing figure. Rhoads remembers him as handsome and very athletic: "He was kind of what you think of when you think of somebody being

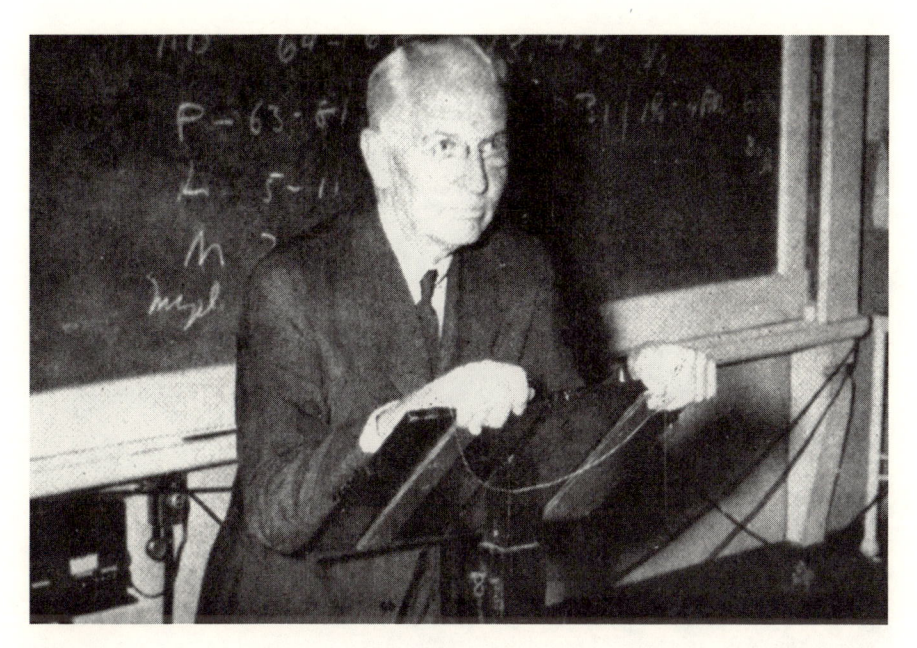

Eldridge Eliason.

aristocratic."[102] Brooke Roberts, now an emeritus professor of surgery at HUP and former resident, describes Eliason:

He looked as if he had almost been cast in Hollywood. He was an extraordinarily handsome man, elderly . . . snow white hair, ruddy face . . . wonderful athlete, gymnast and so forth . . . straight as a ramrod . . . although a bit of a martinet.[103]

Rhoads remembers him as a surgeon who, while more interested in technique and less enamored with the pre- and postoperative aspects of surgical care, nevertheless showed compassion for the plight of his patients, as is revealed in this anecdote:

Eliason was interested in patients, rather sensitive to their reactions. I remember one time we had a patient with a big area of gangrene or something and he wanted all the class of students, a dozen or twenty people to see it. And so they sort of filed in one at a time and Dr. Eliason was sitting off to the edge watching the expression of the viewers, and he pointed out to me that this was a very bad experience for the patient because each student or houseofficer that came up had a change of expression when they saw this awful mess. The patient of course was watching their faces. He was thoughtful about things and he was a great gentleman. Patients liked him.[104]

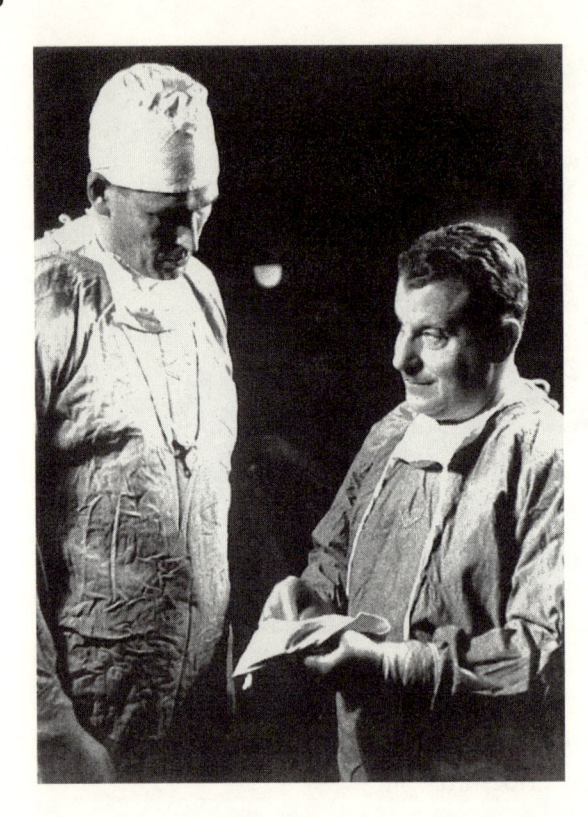

Rhoads (left) and Ravdin (right).

While Rhoads greatly admired Eliason, he became aware, in time, of the extraordinary capabilities of Ravdin, his warmth, enthusiasm, and personal charisma, and his tremendous energy. Ravdin was short and stout, and described by some who knew him as a stormy petrel, volatile, fiery, and sparkling. He was a man who had an uncanny ability to size up people accurately. Residents used to joke that "Rav" was a "one-man employment agency." Rhoads remembers Ravdin as a "complicated, tremendously intelligent man who was perceptive, persuasive, forceful and a remarkable leader."[105] Brooke Roberts recalls his experience on grand rounds with Rav (as he was affectionately called by all who knew him):

When Rav would run grand rounds, things would sparkle. He would get somebody up, he wouldn't make a fool of you, but he would ask you questions he was damn sure you didn't know the answer to and watch you squirm a little bit. . . . He wouldn't tolerate guys who didn't measure up.[106]

He infected all who worked around him with his enthusiasm and tremendous energy. Ravdin maintained warm relationships with most of his patients, and Rhoads recalls a dramatic example of this during his internship:

There was a man whose leg fracture I had reduced and cast, and he seemed to be pining away on the ward and no one could get him to cheer up. Dr. Ravdin perceived that he was a carpenter and had concluded that he never would be well enough again to continue as a carpenter. He was around 65, and this was sort of the end for him. Dr. Ravdin penetrated this and told him that he would be able to work again. Point of fact that he wanted him to come down and build a porch for him at the shore in the summer. His attitude just turned around, he began to eat, cheered up, his leg healed and he went down and built the porch.[107]

Another anecdote told to Rhoads years later by his fellow intern, Pendleton Tompkins, reveals once again Ravdin's uncanny insight into the motivations of people:

Dr. Ravdin enjoyed bearing down on me from time to time. One day I was at the back of the crowd making rounds at the bed of young girl, about 19, who had an extreme case of hospitalitis, and although recovered from whatever it was, absolutely refused to go home. Although I was silent and inconspicuous, Dr. Ravdin snapped around and said, "All right, Tompkins, what shall we do?" I replied, "Get a leech." Dr. Ravdin said, "Call Morgan's Apothecary and tell them to send two leeches." We put one on each thigh, they were about 1½ inches long and ¼ of an inch thick. In two hours each was more than 3 inches long and 1¼ inch thick. The girl got right up and went home. Never have I repeated so fast and complete a cure.[108]

Observing these surgeons and comparing them to the Hopkins' surgical faculty, Rhoads began to slowly consider becoming a surgeon. Whereas the Hopkins group seemed distant from their patients, the Penn group was both interested in surgical problems and patients as individual personalities. He got the sense that you could still perform surgery and build a lot of human relationships. Despite these benefits, surgery had its grueling side, too.

He writes to Royal Davis in September of that year:

I am on Surgery too. I must say I took a beating today with a straight 8 hrs in the operating room. I have not proved very handy there as yet.[109]

During this time his mother and sisters moved to their new home at 43 West Walnut Lane in Germantown. Always close to his family, Rhoads made as many visits as time would permit. His mother writes to Esther about him in October 1933:

Just had a supper visit from Jonnie. He is a dear. He looked very thin this summer and I was alarmed, now he has gained 12 pounds and is quite handsome. He is working with Dr. Eliason, who seems high on principles. Told how he advised an assistant not to take a drop of liquor, that it was better to abstain entirely as it so often got the better of you.[110]

In addition to doing his surgical rotation, Rhoads was assigned to teach a course in bacteriology to 37 nurses. His mother, expressing her approval of this, writes to Esther:

In connection with his class in bacteriology I rejoiced in his having this opportunity. I have always thought him a teacher and that he could teach in the U of P some future date. As he tells us about the general run of men, he is fine in character and the world might as well have the advantage of it. Thee sees I admire our children very much.[111]

By December 1933 Rhoads had decided to seek a surgical fellowship. Exactly when he made this decision is not clear, but as of the preceding spring, he was still undecided. Charles McLaughlin, a surgical fellow two years ahead of Rhoads, vividly recalls a conversation he had with Rhoads during the spring of 1933:

As Jon's internship moved toward completion I felt very strongly that he should apply for a surgical fellowship and confided this to Dr. Eliason who encouraged me to pursue it with Jonathan. On a beautiful spring evening, we walked for an hour or so under the trees on Hamilton Walk, which some may recall used to be behind the University Hospital and in front of the library and the research building. Every argument I could think of was presented to convince Jonathan to apply for a fellowship, and with some hesitation, either because of this or for some other reason, he ultimately accepted this advice.[112]

Interns were generally discouraged from entering surgery on the basis of a dire prediction that surgery would ultimately be replaced by better drugs. In any event, Rhoads' decision to enter surgery was not based on an impassioned need to be a surgeon, but on a practical and accurate assessment of his own abilities and interests and the inspiration of I.S. Ravdin. Rhoads writes:

Selection of a field of specialization was as slow as the decision to study medicine. I left medical school thinking that psychiatry would be a field in which it would be too difficult to judge one's results; neurology and neurosurgery were too grim. . . . I found Ravdin one of the warmest and most enthusiastic people I had ever met. The work was fascinating, the problems immediate and challenging and the results often very decisive, and for the neophyte, most instructive.[113]

Surgical fellowships or residencies were relatively scarce in the late 1920s and early 30s. In 1934 there were just two training positions open in the Department of Surgery at HUP. One was with Eliason, who had already promised that slot to Julian Johnson. The other, with Ravdin, was open, and it was for this position that Rhoads, along with several others, applied for in December 1933. He also interviewed for surgical positions at the Lahey Clinic and the Columbia Service at New York City Hospital but let Ravdin know that it was the opening at HUP that he desired over the others.

If accepted, a fellow was reviewed at the end of each year and was either renewed or fired. There were formal interviews and, as Rhoads recalls, the final decision took so long that the other applicants accepted positions at other hospitals and the opening with Ravdin fell to Rhoads. Looking back on his experience as an intern, Rhoads likes to quote what C. Everett "Chick" Koop said of his experience:

He wouldn't have missed his internship for anything, and he wouldn't do it again for anything.[114]

And so it was July 1934 that signaled the beginning of the remarkable association of I.S. Ravdin and Jonathan Rhoads.

"The surgeon should be an internist and something more, not something less." He was convinced that unless the surgeon had a broad interest in the medical problems of the patient he would always be looked upon by his medical colleagues as a craftsman, rather than a colleague—a circumstance which I am sure is true.

I.S. Ravdin on Harvey Cushing[1]

FOUR

MR. PIM PASSES BY
MENTOR, MARRIAGE, AND A MATTER OF CONSCIENCE

I.S. Ravdin was one of the most influential individuals in Jonathan Rhoads' life and his most important surgical mentor. By all accounts, Ravdin was a truly remarkable man. Isidor Schwaner Ravdin was born in Evansville, Indiana, an area largely settled by Germans, on October 10, 1894. Both parents were European and Jewish by birth. His father was a specialist in eye, ear, nose, and throat and was one of the earliest members of the American Academy. By the time his father had set up practice on his own, Ravdin was in high school and his older brother was attending Indiana University. As a schoolboy Ravdin excelled in the sciences but especially loved history. The family spoke German and had a good knowledge of German literature.

Ravdin started his young manhood as an itinerant salesman of Christian magazines. He traveled throughout the South, visiting the most prominent preachers in the area and persuading them to help raise advertising revenue for the magazine, and in exchange Ravdin published the preachers' sermons. He was amazed to see how anxious preachers were to have their sermons come out in print. As the year wore on, Ravdin became homesick and returned to his parents' home in Evansville.

Ravdin went up to Bloomington to see his brother, who was still in college. After he had visited a few days, some of the college men persuaded him to stay. With new determination he convinced the dean to let him take the courses if he promised to go into medicine after completing his undergraduate schooling. In support of his request, he reasoned that he had come from a long line of doctors: his grandfathers on both sides were doctors, and his brother was studying for medicine. Ravdin's application was accepted, and he plunged into his studies with enthusiasm. It was during this time that he befriended the famous preacher Billy Sunday, who managed to get Ravdin out of a few scraps at a local boarding house that was run by another evangelist. Through Sunday's efforts, Ravdin was permitted to continue to live there. Smoking and dancing were forbidden and Ravdin was guilty of both.[2]

Following graduation, he entered the University of Indiana Medical School. Disappointed with the courses and laboratories at Indiana, Ravdin considered transferring to another medical college at the end of his second year. His father had spent many months in graduate work in Boston and thought that Harvard was the best medical school around. Ravdin wrote to the dean and asked whether he might spend his third and fourth years there. He finally received word of his acceptance to Harvard, and he eagerly looked forward to finishing his training there. However, a Mexican named Pancho Villa changed Ravdin's immediate plans.

Ravdin had barely completed his second year at Indiana when he was notified to report to Fort Benjamin Harrison for induction into the Army. After notifying Harvard that he would be unable to attend medical school in the fall, he was sent to Mexico and served under General Pershing, whose troops entered Mexico in an unsuccessful pursuit of Pancho Villa. In time the recruited medical students were sent back to their respective schools to complete their training. At this point, the fates of Ravdin and the University of Pennsylvania became entwined. Dr. Herrick, a professor of medicine at the University of Chicago and a friend of Ravdin's father, came to Texas to inspect the medical students serving in the Army. Herrick was surprised to see Ravdin there and, after some conversation, suggested that Ravdin go to the University of Pennsylvania rather than Harvard. Ravdin had never heard of Pennsylvania, but Herrick convinced him that the tradition at Pennsylvania was a fine one. The more Ravdin thought about it, the more he was convinced that Herrick, for whom he had a deep affection, was right. He sent a telegram to the dean at Penn and told him that he had been accepted at Harvard but if he could get out of the Army, he would come to the University of Pennsylvania. Several days later he received a telegram that simply read: "Come ahead"—William Pepper.[3]

While Ravdin was warmly welcomed by his medical school classmates, he was required to repeat some of the courses he had taken at Indiana. As the country increasingly became involved in World War I, more interns left to join the Army Ambulance Corps. Charles Frazier, chief of surgery at Penn, faced with this shortage, recruited Ravdin and Emlen Stokes, still in medical school, to replace them. This was a remarkable opportunity for these young men. Subsequently, Ravdin was selected to act as chief resident when he was still only an intern. As with so many other things, he took on his responsibilities with great enthusiasm and soon won the respect of his fellow house officers. Ravdin and Stokes became immersed in Frazier's work and soon came to be known as "Frazier's men." Despite this, John B. Deaver, an attending surgeon at HUP, who was, according to Ravdin, "a great surgical individualist and perhaps the greatest abdominal surgeon this country has ever had," took to Ravdin even though he was tagged a "Frazier man." It was Deaver who gave Ravdin more surgical responsibility. With the advent of World War I, only 3 surgeons were left to cover the service, and within 6 months Ravdin was doing very complex abdominal surgery.[4]

The war came and went. Ravdin completed his residency and remained at HUP. Besides teaching him abdominal surgery, Deaver helped Ravdin in two additional ways. First, he arranged for Ravdin to become the assistant to George Mueller, then an up-and-coming surgeon in Philadelphia and, next to Deaver, the best abdominal surgeon in the area. Second, in 1927 Deaver arranged for Ravdin to spend the year studying physiology and biochemistry with some of Britain's most famous surgeons.

Armed with this knowledge, Ravdin returned to Philadelphia and was appointed to the new chair in surgical research that was established by Frazier. He quickly ascended the academic ladder and was appointed Harrison Professor of Surgery in 1935 and then, in 1945, Surgeon in Chief and John Rhea Barton Professor of Surgery after he returned from India. Ravdin was awarded the title of Brigadier General, and by 1956 he retired with the designation Major General, the only person in nonactive military service to do so. In 1956 Ravdin was called to the White House to consult and operate on President Eisenhower. After his retirement as Chairman of the Department of Surgery in 1959, he was appointed Vice President for Medical Affairs at the University of Pennsylvania.

Much has been said about Ravdin's extraordinary personality and intellect. Owen Wangensteen, the renowned surgeon at the University of Minnesota writes of him:

Bustling activity has characterized Rav's life in every sphere of his many absorbing attachments and functions from which he could not escape completely, even in the relaxed and serene atmosphere of his home. To spend a day with Rav was an engrossing experience. It was a revelation to see how one man deals effectively not only with the tangled skeins of day to day complexities devolving about running a large and active surgical clinic, but providing as well prompt and pithy solutions to scores of questions relating to his numerous obligations to important organizations.[5]

His research and national administrative activities were acknowledged in a festschrift published in the journal *Surgery* in honor of his 70th birthday in 1964. It was noted that he and his charming wife, Elizabeth, translated three volumes of Martin Kirschner's *Operative Surgery* into English. This was a monumental contribution to surgical literature.[6]

Ravdin's research accomplishments were indeed eclectic. In 1921 he published one of the largest clinical experiences with blood transfusions. Investigations with Tucker, Pendergrass, Lee, and others identified the most common cause of postoperative atelectasis (collapse of air sacks in the lungs), which was due to the abnormal accumulation of mucous plugs in the bronchi.[7] Working with Riegel, Morrison, Johnston, and others, he identified many of the important functions of the gallbladder, including absorption of water, and concentration of bile salts and pigments. Subsequently, they noted the important changes in bile composition with inflammation of the gallbladder.[8] In the 1930s, working with Goldschmidt, Vars, and others, Ravdin showed the damaging effects of hypoxia and certain anesthetic agents, such as chloroform on liver structure and function (*see* Chapter 7). Finally, and perhaps most importantly, Ravdin demonstrated for the first time that protein malnutrition was a significant determinant of adverse clinical outcome, particularly in patients undergoing gastrointestinal operations. These investigations provided the early impetus and foundation of the discovery of intravenous hyperalimentation.[9] James Hardy, a former resident of Ravdin and Rhoads, writes of what he deemed to be Ravdin's most important contribution to research:

One feature of Ravdin's research deserves special comment. . . . As an investigator himself he fully realized the value of able basic scientists in a clinical department — scientists deeply versed in biochemical and physiologic investigative techniques and analyses who knew how to do things. He respected and nurtured these scientists and in turn they accepted him as one of their own. He went to them, was at home in their laboratories.[10]

Indeed, many years later it was acknowledged that it was Ravdin, Wangensteen, Graham, Phemister, and Coller who took surgery away from its anatomical base to a physiological one.

Following World War II, Ravdin was one of the most influential physicians in the country in establishing the Cancer Chemotherapy National Program. He became president of the American Cancer Society in 1962, and he was directly responsible for the appropriation of major funding for chemotherapy from the National Institutes of Health. Most importantly, Ravdin was an untiring advocate of the importance of multicentered, controlled clinical trials to determine the effectiveness of cancer chemotherapy.[11]

He was tremendously successful in increasing the growth of the Hospital of the University of Pennsylvania. He was a major recruiter for faculty chairs and helped secure funding for the addition of two floors to the Dulles wing of the Hospital in 1940 and two and one-half floors to the Gates Pavilion in 1950. A decade later, the I.S. Ravdin Institute, consisting of 374 inpatient beds, operating rooms, and space for surgical and anesthesia research, in addition to the Hospital's central services, was established at HUP.[12]

Perhaps Ravdin's *modus operandi* is best expressed by Wangensteen:

Rav came to be known as a man who saw what was best to do, who knew how to do it and who knew how to get it done. Whether pleading the case for research before a Congressional Committee on Appropriations or participating in a meeting of his surgical peers, his presentation always reflected broad orientation, wise discrimination, courageous and steadfast fidelity to the cause he was espousing, expressed with a warmth of sincerity which engendered confidence and elicited sympathetic response from his listeners.[13]

In the summer of 1934 Rhoads started his work on Ravdin's service. The residency program at HUP in 1934 was a 3-year training course. By 1936, however, the American Board of Surgery came into being, and surgical training was expanded to 5 years. Jonathan Rhoads decided to go on with his "investment" mostly because Ravdin had a real gift for inspiring people:

He'd come in from a visit somewhere else, or from the laboratory or wherever he'd been and he would sort of light you up. The other thing I learned from him was that you shouldn't worry too much about the limitations of your abilities and proceed on the assumption that you were as good as anybody else, and just see what happened.[14]

The team would operate 3 days a week. On the other days they made early morning rounds and then started in the laboratory by 9:00 a.m. They returned to the hospital for brief office hours. The program was still tinged with the apprenticeship concept. The Ravdin and Eliason services participated jointly in scientific conferences. Patients were intermingled on the wards, giving the medical staff the opportunity of seeing interesting cases on the other person's service, even though they were not involved directly in their care. The arrangement, as Rhoads recalls, was in some ways "ideal." There was no intermediary between the resident and the chief. The chief assisted the resident through the early stages of his training and knew precisely what he or she was able to do or not do. Moreover, the chief was in an ideal position to increase responsibility accurately by direct observation of a resident's progress. Advice came from a mature surgeon rather than a senior resident 2 or 3 years his senior.[15]

Ravdin ran a very tight ship. He made rounds daily. Grand rounds were conducted on Sunday and consumed most of the morning, precluding any interruption for church services. All wounds were dressed and inspected; orders were rewritten and generally reviewed by the chief. At first, the resident was assisted at the operating table, but shortly thereafter he was permitted to do simple operations unassisted, except by an intern. When emergencies came in, which happened frequently, the patient was examined, laboratory tests were obtained, and then the chief was called. If the resident was instructed to proceed with surgery, and the case proved to be more difficult than anticipated, he was always at liberty to call his chief to come in and take over. Indeed, Ravdin told his wife when they were married that she could live anywhere she wanted so long as it was within 5 minutes of the hospital.[16]

Considerable time was spent in the lab, and the residents (or fellows, as they were known then) felt that they were working on the borders of what was known and not known. The fellows lived outside the hospital and came back after supper to see the patients. They were always on call unless signed out to another resident. About the second year, a new innovation of allowing a weekend per month off, from Saturday night to Sunday night, was initiated.

In August 1934 Charles Johnston, Ravdin's senior resident, writes to Ravdin regarding the new fellow Rhoads:

Rhoads is doing well and he is rather pleasant to work with. As regards his Hospital work I think he is working in nicely. I feel that he has a slight tendency to be ambitious. There has been no suggestion of friction such as we were used to in the past. He handles himself well at the operating table and takes suggestions pleasantly. I am trying my best to give him all the work that I possibly can but I have not felt free as yet to leave him entirely alone.[17]

Rhoads reports of his operating room experience to Esther that same year:

Today the first case of appendicitis that I have done quite alone and in the dead of night went home in what apparently is good health. It is a great satisfaction because she proved technically difficult and worried me quite a bit. A fracture I have been looking after has not done so well. After getting a nice reduction and maintaining it for 20 days, I told the parents to start taking the splint off at night to get some motion started in the wrist. When I saw him 2 weeks later, quite a bend had occurred which I am rather at a loss to explain.[18]

For the first year of his fellowship Rhoads lived with his mother and sisters at 43 West Walnut Lane in the Germantown section of Philadelphia.

As he ended up commuting three round trips daily, Rhoads moved in with a group of fellow physicians in West Philadelphia the next year, just a few blocks from the hospital. They leased a house at 251 South 44th Street from a Latin professor who was on sabbatical. Ironically, this was the same house that Ravdin and Pendergrass rented when they were starting out as fellows. His housemates were Bill Frazier (Charles Frazier's son), Bob Brown, Sarge Pepper (son of the dean), and George Gammon. The house came with a servant who did the marketing, cooking, and cleaning. The group kept a slot machine upstairs, hoping that they could lure people into dropping quarters into it—there were very few takers.

By March 1935 Rhoads' fellowship was up for renewal. He was required, along with Julian Johnson, to report on his laboratory and research activities to Charles Frazier. Frazier writes to Ravdin regarding Rhoads:

Dr. Rhoads informs me that his major work is the Study of Tensile Strength of Various Catguts in Contact with Body Fluids, and that this work will be finished this year. In addition to that he has given some time to the study of treatment of Fractures at the Massachusetts General Hospital in Boston; 2) he has constructed an original two-way traction apparatus and drawn the plans for a more finished product; 3) he has written for the Nurses' Quarterly *an article on Parenteral Intravenous Administration; 4) he has assisted Dr. Ravdin in keeping up his statistics of Acute Appendicitis; 5) he has assisted Dr. Ravdin in the preparation of an article for the* Surgical Clinics of North America—The Value of Biochemistry in Surgery. *This article appeared in February. 6) He is now preparing a technic book for the use of the residents. This will be kept in a small, special notebook that can be carried in their pockets and will contain material that is not in the technic book of the department. . . . On the basis of this record I beg leave to notify you that this man has been reappointed as a Surgical Fellow in this Department for the year beginning July 1, 1935.*[19]

In the year from June 1934 to May 1935, there were 8,750 surgical operations performed at HUP. The average stay of each patient was 13.7 days. The average cost per patient per day was $4.70. The average cost per outpatient visit was $0.94. The average cost of an operation in 1935 was $6.96. The surgical wards were extremely busy. Orville Bullit, the board chairman, reported to the Board of Managers:

With the exception of the Christmas season, scarcely a day has gone by when there has not been a waiting list for admission to the four surgical wards.[20]

In the fall of 1934 Professor Otto Folin suddenly succumbed to an infection resulting from prostatic enlargement. It was in the days following his death that Jonathan Rhoads and Terry Folin's relationship became closer:

I had then embarked on my surgical training and begged off a day to meet her in New York after the funeral. She and her father had been very close all of her life—reinforced I suppose by the untimely death of her older sister Johanna. . . . I remember we went out to Bledsoe's Island where the Statue of Liberty is, and in a cold breeze, and our love drew nourishment from her bereavement.[21]

Terry returned to her work at the University of Chicago, where she was a resident in Pediatrics, and Jonathan returned to Philadelphia. During the year, Rhoads used his free weekends to visit her in Chicago. In the summer of 1935 Terry and her mother invited him to their summer home in Kearsarge, New Hampshire. Situated on about 50 acres of property, the house was at the edge of a forest in an area dominated by mountains, trees, and wildlife. Across the Kearsarge Trail and up a general slope, a field topped by a huge boulder had been dubbed Mt. Teresa by the Folins.[22] That summer the couple decided to become engaged and marry the following year.

In July 1936 Terry cut short her training in Chicago, finishing two of the three years of residency, and returned to Cambridge, Massachusetts to marry Jonathan Rhoads. By marrying Terry, Jonathan was the first person in a long line of Quakers to marry out of Meeting. In the generation before, Quakers were disowned by the Meeting for marrying out of their close-knit community.

After the death of her husband, Mrs. Folin had sold their home, so Terry and Jonathan married in the home of Dean Chase of the School of Fine Arts at Harvard, who was a summer neighbor of the Folins in New Hampshire. Jonathan chose July 4th as their wedding day (this way he knew he would never forget their wedding anniversary).[23] About 40 people attended the service. John Webster came from Philadelphia to be Rhoads' best man. Rhoads purchased a "new" second-hand car, an 8-cylinder Ford coupe, for the couple's honeymoon. He christened it "Mr. Pim" after the popular play at the time by A.A. Milne entitled *Mr. Pim Passes By*. The choice of name was interesting. The major themes of the play—a plea for women's rights and an attack on aristocratic ways of life—are in tune with Quaker values.

Many years later, in addressing a group of young doctors at Roswell Park, New York, Rhoads described what he thought are important attributes in the wife of an academic physician:

If one can have as a marriage partner one who by her or his upbringing has been exposed to and understands the demands of an academic life, this may provide some assurance that the necessary support will be

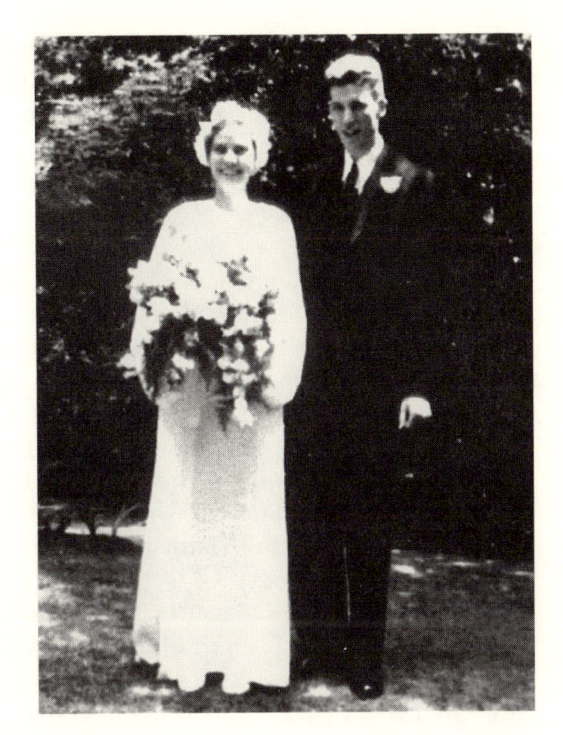

Marriage of Terry Folin and Jonathan Rhoads on July 4, 1936.

forthcoming. If one's partner shares in one's profession or in an allied profession, this may work out well. . . . It probably depends to a degree on what each partner really expects of marriage. . . . Also tied in with marriage and family life is the failure to be realistic in economic matters. The period of training and of gaining recognition is almost always a long one in academia and sometimes very protracted, so that most young couples live these years in straitened circumstances, years when their contemporaries from school and college are often making much more money. There are few assets a young scholar can have so valuable as a frugal spouse, and the reverse, an extravagant or spendthrift spouse is often an obstacle to the pursuit of academic goals, or indeed, to the pursuit of happiness in general.[24]

Where they would spend their honeymoon was known only to Jonathan Rhoads. He kept their destination secret, except to tell Terry that they would be driving north so that she would bring along an appropriate wardrobe. They jumped into Mr. Pim and sped off. Later his mother-in-law told him that everything was all right, except that their departure was a little abrupt. Rhoads was afraid that the car would get "unduly decorated" if someone followed them. However, Terry brought along a cache of firecrackers and fireworks, and lighting them with the cigarette lighter threw them out the window along the way. They traveled to Maine and to various places in New England and Canada, visiting relatives and friends. While the country was still deep in the Depression, Jonathan thought that Terry should have an overcoat, so they splurged and spent $40 on a fur coat made of rabbit. "It was nice and warm," Rhoads said later, "and I'm sure the rabbits were very comfortable when they had it."[25]

While on their honeymoon, Jonathan and Terry Rhoads learned of the death of Charles Frazier. They quickly returned to Philadelphia so Jonathan could help with the surgical responsibilities at HUP. The couple rented an apartment at 4045 Baltimore Avenue. Terry got a part-time job with Dr. Joseph Stokes at Children's Hospital, where she was assigned to investigate the comparative effects of irradiated evaporated milk and cod liver oil on the prevention of rickets in children. The Rhoads' first child, Margaret, was born on July 2, 1937. Shortly thereafter the family moved to the Victoria Apartments on 38th Street, which were owned by the University.

During the years 1936 to 1937 the hospital felt the impact of the death of Charles Harrison Frazier. Eliason succeeded Frazier as Chairman and John Rhea Barton Professor of Surgery, and Ravdin was appointed to a new chair in surgery created by the Harrison bequest. He was officially named The George Harrison Professor of Surgery and Director of the new Harrison Department of Surgical Research.

With the introduction of ether, surgery was changed from a cut and run procedure to a deliberate and careful procedure that could last many hours. Before the more sophisticated anesthetics, a good surgeon was a fast surgeon.[26] Scrubbing and rinsing in an antiseptic were common practices, and gloves were dusted with talc and used over and over again. Later it was discovered that talc contributed to the formation of adhesions (postoperative scar tissue). Instruments were boiled rather than autoclaved. Surprisingly, infections were not markedly prevalent, but when they occurred, they were more frequently fatal. Operations were hazardous—appendicitis carried a 5% mortality. Patients did not expect as much then as they do now, and dying was generally accepted. There were not as many restrictions on surgical practice then as now. Rhoads relates:

You had no committee on using patients for studies. You didn't get oral permission unless it was something they were going to notice. We didn't have any formal written consent forms, except the consent form from the hospital in which you gave your physicians permission to do what they thought was appropriate. . . . I think we would get a written consent for amputations.[27]

At HUP, Rhoads did the first three peritoneal dialyses for uremia in 1935. The Wangensteen suction was used, and William Abbott performed various clinical investigations with the nasoenteric Miller-Abbott tube. Surgeons at Penn performed one of the earliest operations for Crohn's disease in 1933. The first patient with islet cell adenoma of the pancreas was operated on in 1936. They encountered a case of Meigs' syndrome (fluid in the abdomen and chest associated with an ovarian tumor), which Rhoads reported on with Alex Terrell, giving the condition its name. Even with these advances, when Rhoads came into surgery in 1934, "there was a superstition that a person who said that he would not survive an operation would indeed die in the postoperative period."[28]

Rhoads became interested in blood clotting and its many ramifications. He recalls the fascinating aspects of his research:

We were confronted in the 1930's . . . with jaundiced patients who bled postoperatively. This difference in mortality between biliary tract operations in non-jaundiced patients and jaundiced patients was very great. Dr. Ravdin had a long series of cholecystectomies, around 10 or 12 years, without a death. A chap named Alex Ulin and I, and I think somebody else, went back over our records from 1922 up to about 1937 and we found the instance of the mortality in jaundiced patients in the first third from 1922–1929 was about 18%. We began to give a lot of glucose but not nearly enough to reach caloric balance, and [the mortality] dropped somewhat to I think around 11%, and then the final four years, 1933–1937, it dropped to 8%. In the third of these periods, when the mortality dropped we had gone to transfusing the patients pretty routinely.

I had a very dramatic instance of it. . . . Richard Cattel from the Lahey Clinic came to visit Ravdin, who took him on rounds. When we got outside one of the private rooms, there was a trickle of blood running out the floor boards under the door. We went in and [blood] was dripping off the side of the bed and . . . running out the drain coming out the patient's abdominal wall. The patient had been operated on . . . that morning or maybe the day before. So we transfused this lady and Cattel had had a similar experience. He said that he took the drains out. . . . I think there was a t-tube in because he had figured that the drains were irritating the place where it was bleeding. . . . She recovered but it was quite a moment when we took this famous visiting professor around and found the blood running out of the room.

So the next year in the Proceedings of the Society of Biology and Experimental Medicine *there was a report from Iowa from H.P. Smith and 3 collaborators saying that they had measured prothrombin (a blood protein important in the clotting process) with a Quick test and had given an extract of alfalfa and that they had been able to bring the prothrombin up. We went back into the literature. I can't remember* whether we waited until that moment to find the literature or whether we found some of it before. Armand J. Quick had been here at Penn in the 20's. Dr. Ravdin had known him.

Henrik Dam in Copenhagen explored the hemorrhagic disease in chicks which he had hit upon in 1929 when he was studying lipid metabolism, and he extracted the diet of chickens with fat solvents so as to get the fat away and fed them and some of them developed hemorrhagic phenomena. He persisted with his studies of fat metabolism and did not get back to investigate this hemorrhagic phenomenon for about 5 years, after which he said he had discovered a new vitamin. They spelled Koagulation with a K over there and that's how [vitamin K] got the K. He showed that it was present in fish meal and also in green vegetables and that these two forms had a different molecular weight. . . .

The man who showed that [vitamin K] required bile salts for its absorption was named Greaves, and he had worked with a biochemist named L.A. Schmidt in Los Angeles. They had already shown that bile salts were necessary for the absorption of vitamins A and D. They extended this to K.

This began to make sense, and so Quick wrote a letter to the editor of JAMA and postulated that the hemorrhagic tendency in jaundice was due to the fact that the bile, including the bile salts, did not get into the G.I. tract; therefore the vitamin K was not absorbed.

Now the reason that vitamin K deficiency had not been observed in normal chickens who were put on a vitamin K-free diet was due to coprophagia in chickens. Dam did this. You could take the stools from animals on a vitamin K-free diet and the animals would eat and it would cure the deficiency. So then he pursued that and showed that the colon bacilli and some of the other bacteria produced vitamin K in the G.I. tract. The reason that obstructive jaundice causes [vitamin K deficiency] is because the bile salts are not present to absorb the vitamin K which is formed by the intestinal bacteria. The reason that you sometimes got a prothrombin deficiency in people who were not jaundiced is that they had enough liver disease so that their bile salts had largely disappeared from the bile.

Well, in pursuit of these interesting phenomena, I borrowed a family car and set out on my vacation in the summer of '39. . . . I saw Quick in Milwaukee and then I saw Hugh Butt at Mayo, who had published a few months later than H.P. Smith, showing alfalfa extract was useful. And then I went and saw H.P. Smith and then Greaves and then across town to Doisy, who was working on the synthesis of vitamin K for which he finally got a Nobel Prize.

So I came home and we got rabbits that were being used for pregnancy tests, and they were being sacrificed anyhow. We'd get the brains and grind it up and smear it on a piece of cheese cloth stretched across a box *so it would dry out. Then, with a pair of scissors, you could cut a little square of this and put it in a test tube of saline, shake it up, and you'd have thromboplastin. So I ran the Quick test service in the hospital for nearly two years until the laboratory agreed to take it up. I wrote extensively on the subject. I suppose the reason I remember as much of it as I do is that I was asked to write a review for SG&O.[29]*

When Rhoads finished his residency in 1939, Ravdin gave him a part-time appointment in the Harrison Department with a stipend of $1500. He also suggested that he work with Dr. Walter Estell Lee at the Graduate Hospital. There were no office facilities in the hospital, so Rhoads sublet an office from Harrison Flippin, a physician who joined forces with a urologist in the Medical Tower Building at 255 South 17th Street. Flippin thought he could refer enough work to Rhoads so that he could pay his rent.

Rhoads had office hours 2 to 3 times a week. In addition to Rhoads' work at Graduate and HUP, Dr. Lee arranged staff appointments for Rhoads at Pennsylvania Hospital and later at Bryn Mawr, Germantown, and Children's Hospitals. He would on occasion send Rhoads to Memorial Hospital in New Jersey, which is where he first encountered air conditioning in an operating room. Rhoads later said that he thought air conditioning was one of the great advances in surgery. Rhoads likes to tell the story about George Mueller, one of the senior surgeons during the early 1930s:

In the summer, windows were left open to cool the operating room. This practice had some "dire consequences." . . . The story I heard when I came was that George Mueller, who was sometimes ill tempered, had been doing a breast amputation down there and he got very mad at his assistant. . . . He didn't catch the blood vessels fast enough. When the breast finally came off with a ring of hemostats on it, he threw it at his assistant and his assistant ducked and it went out the window onto Spruce Street. Some public person picked it up and brought it in. This got to the Board of Trustees and they wanted to fire George. They were talked out of it.[30]

Rhoads' assignment was to be Lee's principal assistant at Graduate, and every other month alternate with Dr. Harry Farrell, an associate of Lee's. A good deal of his work with Lee was to give spinal anesthesia. Ravdin's and Lee's operative techniques were very different. Ravdin standardized his operative methods so that the resident pretty much knew what to expect. Lee hated to do the same operation twice the same way, so no one could really help him except when he asked for things. At the time Lee probably had the largest surgical practice in Philadelphia. He was a strict Presbyterian, but Mrs. Lee was especially strict. Rhoads was called to meet him at his home one Sunday morning. He had brought the Sunday paper with him and offered it to Lee's wife, who responded: " Dr. Rhoads, we don't read the Sunday paper. We think there's enough evil in the other 6 days."[31] He served as sub chief at Pennsylvania Hospital, and every 5th and every 10th month he would have both services (Graduate and Pennsylvania) at once, which were very active.

In one month when Rhoads was on call at Pennsylvania Hospital, the team performed 85 to 90 operations. Pennsylvania Hospital at the time was largely charitable, whereas Graduate had a lot of private practices and drew patients from nearby wealthy Rittenhouse Square. Rhoads remembers his private practice wasn't "very brisk." A colleague and he compared their recent surgical experiences: his colleague had done two sebaceous cysts and Rhoads had done one. In addition, he had a few cases of appendicitis. Henry Royster, then new to the Ravdin service, relates his observation of Rhoads with a particularly difficult patient:

Dr. Ravdin was away and Jon was making rounds. We entered the room of a woman who was dying of cancer of the stomach. She talked very badly to Jon about her woes, pains, vomiting, etc. After we left her room I asked Jon why he did not stop the woman's diatribe, which was in some respects insulting. His reply, something I have used many times and which I shall never forget, is as follows, "If you let someone talk, don't cut it off, for you may learn something you didn't know."[32]

The year 1940 was a momentous one for the Rhoads family. With the arrival of Jonathan, Jr. (Jack) in 1938 and George in 1940, Jonathan and Terry had three children. It was also the year that Rhoads completed the requirements for his Doctor of Medical Science degree and wrote his thesis, "Plasma Proteins in Relation to Surgical Therapeusis." Two other events in this same year would prove to be major turning points in the life of Jonathan Rhoads.

On a May evening in 1940, I.S. Ravdin, who loved Chinese food, took his residents to Chinatown. Shortly after dinner, which included a considerable amount of egg foo yung, he had severe right upper abdominal, colicky pain, with fever, nausea, and vomiting. Ravdin had an attack of pancreatitis (possibly gallstone induced) the previous summer during a trip to Halifax. The symptoms appeared to be consistent with an acute attack of an inflamed gallbladder. Ironically, Ravdin was one of the world's major critics of gallbladder surgery. In fact, he was often fond of quoting an old medical saying: "You often die or get sick of the disease you study."

Nevertheless, he was in considerable pain and resigned to the inevitable conclusion that he would need an operation. The next issue was which of his colleagues, including Eliason, Lockwood, Erb, Kaplan, and a number of other very capable surgeons at HUP, should perform the operation.

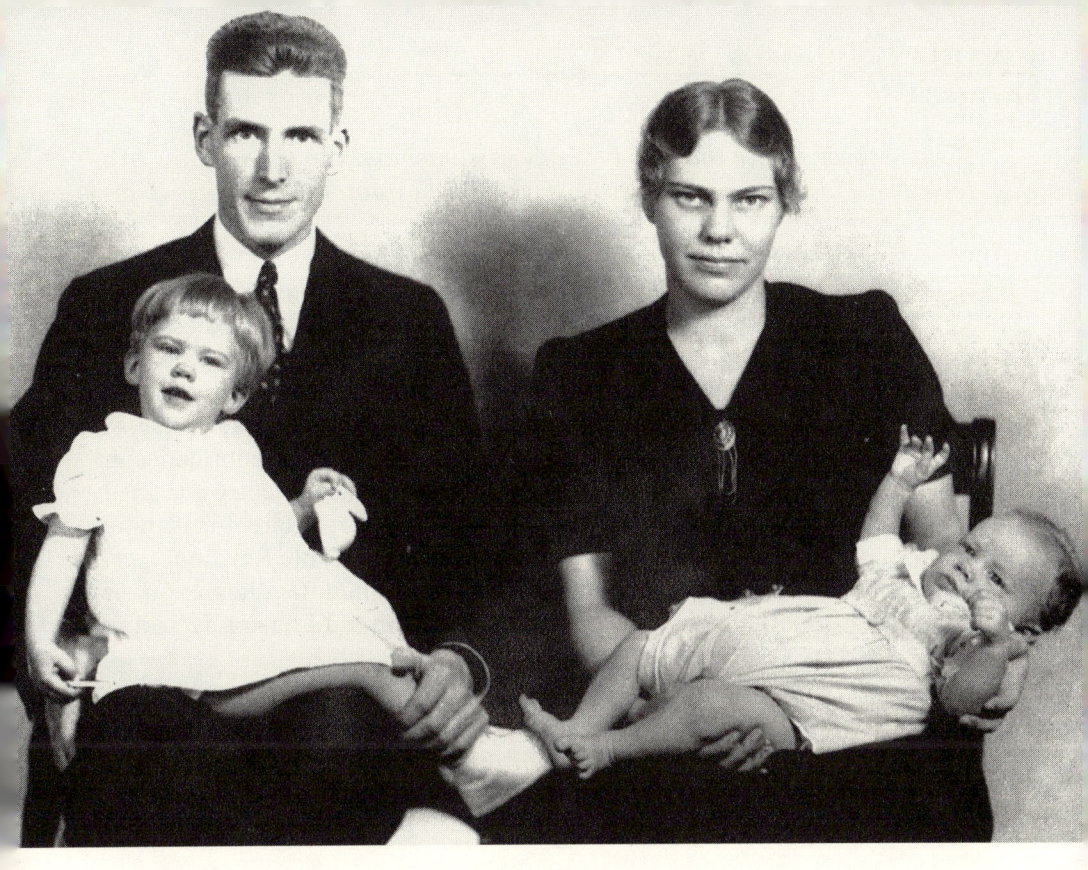

Jonathan Rhoads holding Margaret and Terry Rhoads holding Jack—1938.

After some discussion, Ravdin telephoned his long-time friend, the internationally renowned New York surgeon, Alan O. Whipple, and asked him to come immediately to Philadelphia. Whipple filled a suitcase with his preferred biliary instruments and rushed to Pennsylvania Station. When Whipple arrived at Ravdin's house at 2015 Delancey Place in Philadelphia, Rhoads was already there. Whipple examined Ravdin and said, " Rav, you're right. You've got an attack of acute cholecystitis and you should be operated on right away." Ravdin thanked him for coming to Philadelphia and confirming the diagnosis. He then spoke with his wife Betty and asked her to convey a message to Rhoads, who was downstairs in the living room. She said, "Jon, Rav wants you to operate on him." Upon learning of this decision, Whipple was visibly annoyed at having dropped everything to come to Philadelphia to confirm a diagnosis that he could have made over the phone. To add insult to injury, he was then passed over as Rav's surgeon of choice for a then-unknown, very junior surgeon, Jonathan Rhoads. Rhoads gulped and agreed to perform the operation; he could not very well have said he wouldn't. It was agreed that Eliason and Whipple would scrub in as well. Rhoads later opined that Ravdin wanted him to be the surgeon on the basis of the old story Roger Babson (a popular financial advisor at the time) told:

Roger Babson wrote that the best advertisement was in the window of a restaurant in Boston, which read "Fish's Restaurant. Mr. Fish eats in his own restaurant."[33]

Ravdin's unanticipated decision put Rhoads in a difficult position. If Ravdin suffered a major postoperative complication, Rhoads' professional reputation might be ruined. If Ravdin did well, the senior surgeons would probably conclude that the operation was less than challenging and that was why Rhoads was permitted to operate on the chairman. Despite Rhoads' concerns, Ravdin's decision was an example of his confidence in his young associate and the belief that his trainee was perfectly qualified to perform the operation. Rhoads later explained that the real reason he set up the surgical team this way was that it would enable Ravdin to persuade his patients to let Rhoads operate on them when Ravdin was out of town. Additionally, he probably didn't want to offend Eliason by asking someone from New York to do it.

As Ravdin was being prepared for surgery, the question arose as to which type of anesthesia should be used. At the time Ravdin was an outspoken advocate of spinal anesthesia. Rhoads worried that if Ravdin was operated on while under only spinal anesthesia, he would be sufficiently alert to oversee and direct every aspect of the operation.

Rav was pretty determined to take spinal anesthesia because of his advocacy of it. So he wasn't asleep, and he kept kibitzing me all through. . . . "Jon, what did you find? . . . Jon, are you through yet?" So far, I hadn't finished tying off the bleeders in the wound. There was a fair amount of edema down over the region of the pancreas. This was the kind of case in which we usually did a cholecystostomy [opening into but not removing the gallbladder]. We got the stones out and put a tube in and sutured it up and closed the wound. [34]

The operation went well. Rav was very pleased with the outcome, but with tongue in cheek he told Jonathan, "I'd rather have a lucky surgeon than a good one." Many years later after Ravdin's death, the question arose whether Dr. Ravdin had had recurrent gallstones (the reported incidence of recurrent gallstones following cholecystostomy is approximately 50% in 5 years). According to Rhoads, Ravdin had no long-term problems due to his retained gallbladder. Moreover, Rhoads attended Ravdin's postmortem examination and examined the residual gallbladder. It was quite shrunken, and there was no evidence of recurrent gallstones.[35]

As a postscript to this story, verified in Ravdin's papers, there is a letter to Whipple in which Ravdin told him that the tubercle bacillus was cultured from his gallbladder at the time of surgery. He asked Whipple to remove his gallbladder after he returned from Hawaii, where he had gone to convalesce after the operation. Ravdin asks him to maintain confidentiality and "not let the boys in Philadelphia know" about his request.[36] Ravdin, a consummate politician, probably asked Whipple to do this to smooth over the feathers he had ruffled in Philadelphia. The plans were dashed when Ravdin got a cold on the way back to Philadelphia and Whipple was out of the country. Ravdin never pursued the possibility of further gallbladder surgery to our knowledge.

By the summer of 1939 it was becoming more evident that the United States would be drawn into what would become World War II. Rhoads became increasingly concerned about Hitler's stepwise conquests in Europe. He listened to Hitler's charismatic and highly energized speeches over the radio. Interestingly, Rhoads read a considerable amount of Hitler's *Mein Kampf*, and he recalled a provocative theme—greater action accrued from the spoken word rather than the written word. Hitler cited Jesus Christ as an example of one who never wrote anything but who spoke extensively and whose words resulted in major action. Hitler concluded that if ideas and force were directly competing, force would inevitably emerge victorious.[37]

Though extremely concerned about Hitler's militant philosophy and cruel behavior in 1940, Rhoads recalls that, at the time, he did not fully appreciate the magnitude and severity of Hitler's atrocities, especially upon the Jews.[38] Moreover, the extent of these atrocities did not become fully known until the end of the war. Rhoads' disdain for Hitler's anti-Semitism intensified as he learned firsthand of the cruelties and injustices inflicted upon a number of Jewish academicians who were expelled from major German universities. Many of these individuals emigrated to the United States, and several German Jewish professors were subsequently hired by the University of Pennsylvania.[39]

There was considerable concern in the Quaker community about German aggression in Europe. They were alerted early on of Hitler's persecution of the Jews and sought a meeting with the Gestapo in 1938 to try to intercede on their behalf. Their efforts were unsuccessful, and they subsequently diverted their work to France and elsewhere in Europe, where they worked with many German refugees.[40]

In 1939, the peace churches—the Mennonites, the Quakers, and the Brethren—organized to present a proposal to President Roosevelt regarding conscientious objectors (COs). The proposal drafted by the three religious groups included two tenets: that a CO must register and declare that he was a CO at the time of registration, and that COs perform alternative service under civilian control which was "acceptable to a Christian conscience and conformable to the principle of the Gospel."[41] The American Friends Service Committee objected to this proposal in that it did not allow a provision for those who chose an "absolutist" position to the draft, which included a refusal to register or serve the military in any position whatsoever. This caused some dissension among the three groups. The Mennonites and Brethren took the position that this "absolutist" objection would jeopardize their efforts to gain legislation protecting the majority of COs. The position of the government was to favor a voluntary draft, as the country was still strongly isolationist and the state of the military was "a wreck." Friends decided to help defeat the Burke-Wadsworth Bill, or the Selective Service Act of 1940. In the original version of this bill, conscientious objection was accepted for only those who belonged to "well recognized religious sects whose creed of principles forbid its members to participate in war in any form." The snag for the Friends was that even if a person met this criterion, he was not exempt from service—it was up to the president to decide what he deemed to be the appropriate form of noncombatant service.[42]

Not long after Ravdin's return from Hawaii it became evident that the United States was preparing for war. At HUP, the Naval medical unit was formed under Dr. Richard Kern and the Army unit under Dr. Ravdin. Rhoads, like his father, was an absolutist conscientious objector to war. This expression of conscience came at a particularly difficult time. To publicly acknowledge that one was a CO was indeed a "lonely" position in the midst of growing patriotism. Rhoads writes:

The next three years were tense ones for everybody. World War II had started September 1, 1939 by Hitler's sudden invasion of Poland. The news reached Teresa and me over our car radio that morning as we had left early for our vacation. . . . I remembered enough of World War I to recognize the vortex-like effect of such a confrontation. I knew the medical profession and especially perhaps its surgical branches were highly motivated toward military service. I knew further that I would not join the armed forces, as it was a denial of my whole upbringing and belief.[43]

Rhoads felt that there was no moral alternative to this position of conscience, despite the possibility that his career as an academic surgeon might be finished. Ravdin's long association and strong identity with the military and his continued participation in the Army Reserve were additional factors that contributed to Rhoads' consternation. Rhoads was in a distinct minority even within the Quaker community. Some 75% of the eligible young men in Philadelphia Yearly Meeting served in the Second World War.[44] COs who refused to join the military, even as noncombatants, differed from 1-AOs who reluctantly joined the military as noncombatants. In support of his position as a CO, Rhoads believed that the overriding objective of all military personnel, including those caring for patients, was to get the soldier back to combat as soon as possible. Additionally, he was deeply concerned about an implied tenet of military medicine, namely, to care first for the lightly wounded, who could be returned more quickly to combat, and then to treat the seriously injured who required extensive care and were less likely to return to active combat. These priorities of war perceived by Rhoads were contrary to standard medical teaching that the highest medical priority should be given to the sickest patients despite the unlikelihood that they would return to combat.[45] In an essay many years later, Rhoads addressed the problem the Quaker physician (who adheres rigidly to the peace testimony) faced when confronted with military service during wartime:

According to official Army statements, the medical officer is first a soldier and only secondarily a physician. I am told that, unfortunately, this has at certain times in the past been almost too true. . . . In the United States, however, those who adhered to Friends' basic testimony on peace found no direct way in which to take care of military casualties without joining the Armed Forces and promising to carry out orders as received.[46]

Jonathan and Terry Rhoads visited the Ravdins one evening late in 1940 to advise Ravdin where he stood on the war:

I was apologetic that I had accepted so much from him toward a successful career, and that I was about to blow it. I believe I offered to resign. He listened carefully.

After a brief silence Ravdin said to Rhoads: "Well, someone has to stay behind and I will therefore declare you essential to the surgical service at HUP."[47] This declaration essentially made Rhoads' affirmation moot. Rhoads stayed with Lee 6 weeks short of 3 years, when he was called back to HUP to take over the Ravdin's service after Ravdin and his colleagues left for World War II. Rhoads, writing to the Procurement and Assignment Service in Washington, states:

I have agreed to carry on the clinical work and teaching of Dr. I.S. Ravdin, Harrison Professor of Surgery at the University of Pennsylvania Medical School and University Hospital, during his absence. This is a full time assignment and one which utilizes the training I have had to the fullest extent.[48]

Little did Rhoads or anyone else left behind realize how full-time an assignment it would be.

C. Everett "Chick" Koop, upon reflecting on the war years at the Hospital of the University of Pennsylvania, said to Dr. Rhoads, "Well, Jon, while they were fighting World War II, we survived the battle of Spruce Street!" Responding with characteristic Quaker understatement, Rhoads said, "Well, Chick, I don't look at it as a battle. I remember it as sort of a series of small skirmishes."[1]

FIVE —

THE BATTLE OF SPRUCE STREET —

THE WAR YEARS

World War II changed the lives of Jonathan Rhoads, I.S. Ravdin, and the Department of Surgery at Penn in dramatically different ways. America's involvement in the war officially began with the Japanese attack on Pearl Harbor, on Sunday, December 7, 1941. In his book *Surgeon to Soldier*, Edward Churchill describes the preparedness of the medical community in Honolulu:

Fortunately, in the spring and summer surgical teams had been organized by the Honolulu County Medical Society and were prepared to provide emergency care to the injured. On December 7, 1941 the station hospital at Hickham Field was immediately overwhelmed with casualties and many improvisations were made. The station hospital functioned as a divisional clearing station and evacuated by ambulances and trucks to the Tripler General Hospital. Wounds had been caused by high explosive fragments, machine gun bullets and secondary missiles.

Many patients (especially in those instances when an operation had to be postponed) had ample amounts of crystalline sulfanilamide packed in their wounds as a prophylaxis against infection at the time their injuries were inspected in the receiving wards.

Through the joint action of the Committee on Medical Research and the National Research Council and Surgeon General James C. Magee,

Professors I.S. Ravdin of the University of Pennsylvania and Perrin Long of Johns Hopkins were flown to Hawaii for the period of December 17–22, 1941. The primary purpose of the trip was to obtain information concerning the treatment of Pearl Harbor casualties.[2]

In a follow-up report, the importance of antibiotics was emphasized:

Finally, there can be little doubt that the local and oral use of the sulfonamide drugs contributed markedly to the splendid condition of the wounds and the absence of infection in these patients, which has been noted and remarked upon by all who have seen them. . . . In every instance when wounds are dressed they should be sprinkled with crystalline sulfanilamide until final healing has taken place.[3]

In a letter written on December 10, 1941, Ravdin designated Rhoads as his temporary successor just before he departed for Pearl Harbor with Dr. Long to assess the treatment of American casualties. The letter, addressed "To Whom It May Concern," was portentous in tone and content. Ravdin's will and bank accounts, along with a directive regarding the medical education of his son, make up the bulk of the missive. It ends with a recommendation of Rhoads:

No one is better fitted to continue my service in the Hospital of the University of Pennsylvania than is Dr. Jonathan E. Rhoads. He is an able surgeon, an excellent investigator, and a splendid teacher. He has every one of the qualities necessary for an academic career in surgery, and I hope the Faculty of the School of Medicine will consider this in their selection of a successor, should that event become necessary.[4]

Rhoads recalls Ravdin's trip to Pearl Harbor:

Right after Pearl Harbor he was sought out by the Roosevelt administration to go with Perrin Long of Johns Hopkins to Hawaii to help administer treatment of casualties. Dr. Long taught me in medical school and he was well versed on penicillin and sulfanilamides, and Ravdin was consulted for his expertise in transfusions and the treatment of shock. They were not allowed to take any baggage except a small carry-on bag. So the two of them got on a plane to cross from California to Hawaii and asked each other what they had in their bags. Each one had taken a bottle of scotch![5]

Many advances in surgery have resulted from the treatment of victims of wars. Thus, the advent of World War II provided many young surgeons with the paradox of considering their own mortality and the subliminal excitement of challenging operative cases. There was ample precedent for the American stigma against those men who remained on the homefront. Dr. Edward Churchill speaks of the intense pressure on those who stayed behind in WW I:

I explained what it meant to be in medical school, out of uniform, in time of war. I told them that in the First World War, I was a student at the Harvard Medical School. We students were given a bronze button— a caduceus—to wear on our lapel. I recalled going to the theater one evening with one or two classmates, sitting in the gallery and having people in the audience hiss as we clambered up the aisle during intermission. Young men who are not on active service, I emphasized, are exposed to intense emotional pressures.[6]

While their experiences were different, unique circumstances and unusual opportunities fell to those left behind. Robert Mayock, a medical intern at the time and later chief of pulmonary medicine at Penn, recalls the atmosphere at HUP during World War II:

Well, there weren't that many people who stayed. Most of the people who stayed accepted Jonathan's noncombatant religious preference. To my knowledge, nobody ever remarked about the fact that he didn't go. Don Pillsbury, a HUP physician stationed with the 20th General Hospital, briefly came back to HUP and then returned to India. In a newsletter he was noted to have said, "I just came back from my stay at the hospital [HUP] and things are in terrible shape. The records are poorly kept and the consults are not that good."

Mayock continues,

He was saying how bad things were. Well, of course that infuriated the people staying behind. He was in India and he came back for a short visit, and returned to India telling how bad things were at HUP. We kind of bridled at this, so somebody went to the hospital record room and got out all of Pillsbury's charts. The notes were short, there was no adequate workup and that sort of thing. I don't know if they published it or not, but they made it known that his charts were not much different when he was here. They [the 20th General Hospital] had a full complement and we were still working with half a complement.[7]

The physicians of the 20th General Hospital, led by Ravdin, left Philadelphia for Louisiana on May 15, 1942. There were only three remaining staff surgeons on the Ravdin service compared to its usual complement of seven.

The mood of the country and of the hospital had changed dramatically following Pearl Harbor. While the effects of the Depression were still being felt, people were doing much better and enjoying normal Sunday activities: going out to restaurants, movies, and museums. Suddenly, Americans were "running for cover," buying blackout paper, and looking for shelter in the event that the Japanese would attack the mainland. The hospital director, Dr. Robin Buerki, noted in his report that year:

During the past year every effort has been made to render the hospital as safe as possible from enemy air raids. A complete blackout system has been arranged which is ready for use at any time. A fire pump has been purchased . . . for use against incendiary bombs. . . . Costs continue to mount; an ever increasing number of necessary articles are becoming difficult to obtain or have disappeared from the market. . . . A ruling by the National Selective Service Act eliminated all two-year internships.[8]

The onset of rationing severely affected family and institutional life. Twenty essential items were rationed, including sugar, butter, meat, rubber, and gasoline. The rationing of aluminum affected the use of pots and pans essential to the hospital kitchen. The surgical staff reused rubber gloves and, when they were damaged, patched them up. Rationing of gasoline restricted the use of private cars, of which there were few. In one year, death by automobile accident dropped from 423 to 169 in the United States.[9] Physicians were allocated extra gas since they had to make house calls, which was frequently the case even for surgeons.

The onset of World War II also led to a marked exodus of U.S. physicians and surgeons from civilian practice into the military. Thus, there were fewer surgeons in the community to care for a continuously growing civilian population. At HUP, Eliason remained as the John Rhea Barton Chairman concurrent with Rhoads' appointment. William "Dutch" Dyson, a first-year intern at the time, recalls differences in the two services:

There were two services when Ravdin left and they did everything differently. Rav's service used cat gut and Eli's service used wire. Whatever one did, the other did the opposite. Rav's service used tubes and Eli's didn't believe in tubes.[10]

In May 1942, the Ravdin Service consisted of Rhoads, Harold Zintel, then a junior resident, and Dyson. In addition, there was John Lockwood, who was left in charge of the Harrison Department. Dyson was just finishing the first year of his internship and was scheduled to depart for military service at the end of June. He was a lanky individual with a keen mind and an indefatigable work ethic. In Dyson's view, these were busy, heady days:

I was in the first year of a two-year internship when in December of 1941, Ravdin got everybody together and made his big unit and they left on the 15th of May. The guys who were in their first year of internship were unable to go in that unit because they hadn't finished their one year and hadn't gotten their license yet. Christ, that left the ones who were left in a pickle.

There was Jonathan, Harold Zintel and myself, and surgery happened to be my last rotation in May and June. We never went home, we just slept in the nurses station, it was just awful. The new people hadn't come and the old people didn't finish their residency. Those were funny years, the wartime. We were just hanging on by the skin of our teeth. Really trying to do all the work in the hospital. All the second-year guys left and then I turned patients over to Chick Koop who had just finished his internship at Pennsylvania Hospital. So I went off and that left Chick, Jonathan and Harold.[11]

C. Everett Koop, who had been declared "essential" by Ravdin, was selected as the Harrison Fellow in general surgery before Ravdin left for India. He was therefore trained exclusively by Rhoads, who not only became his surgical mentor but also a life-long friend. He remembers Rhoads as being not only gentle and kind but generous in ways uncharacteristic of most surgeons. In his autobiography, Koop describes Rhoads:

A tall, Lincolnesque man with a low pitched voice and a laconic sense of humor, he was a master surgeon and a master teacher. His judgment and

Harrison Department—war years.
Top row—4th from left, Otto Rosenthal; 5th from left, Harold Zintel; 1st from right, Harry Vars.
Second row—3rd from left, Chick Koop; 2nd from right, Jonathan Rhoads.
Third row—2nd from left, Elizabeth Ravdin.

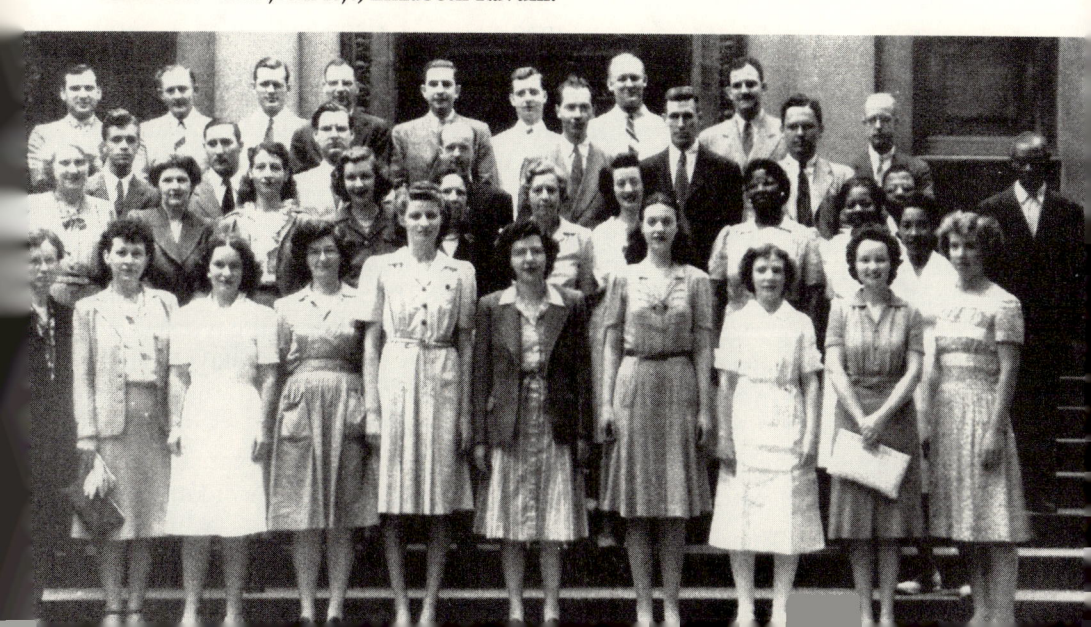

diagnostic skills were superb. His research background was well regarded and he was universally admired and respected in the field of surgery.[12]

One of Koop's first interactions with Rhoads was as an intern at Pennsylvania Hospital. Rhoads was called to operate upon a gunshot victim. Preoperatively, surgical teachers frequently query medical students as to which organs might be perforated when the bullet enters at a specific location and exits at a distant site. This is exactly what happened with the patient with the gunshot wound. Blood and air were coming from the lung at the entrance wound, and bile from the gall bladder and liver, combined with intestinal contents, spewed forth from the exit wound. The endotracheal tube was inserted for the anesthetic; every time the lungs were inflated there was a collective eruption of air, blood, bile, anesthetic gas, and intestinal contents from the gunshot wound.

Rhoads was positioned and poised at the operating table—gowned and gloved—and appeared to the intern Koop to be "about 9 feet tall." A severely injured patient such as this was not an unusual sight for Rhoads and not too unusual for the surgical resident. However, the medical student was startled by this "Vesuvius" erupting from the wound, and the student suddenly fainted and began to fall to the floor. In a seemingly effortless motion, Rhoads simply reached out, grabbed the falling student with one hand, and held his head while simultaneously moving his leg to catch the student's body, and he lowered him gently to the floor. After preventing the unconscious student from becoming seriously injured, Rhoads' sole comment was, "It looks like I've soiled my glove." Koop recounted that this was a perfect example of Rhoads' Lincolnesque, taciturn, totally laid-back attitude—always understated, yet always in control.[13]

The other member of the team, Harold Zintel, graduated from the University of Pennsylvania Medical School in 1938 and finished his internship 2 years later. He was appointed Harrison Fellow in general surgery at HUP in 1940. Zintel's talents as a surgeon were recognized early on by all of those who worked with him. In addition to the tremendous burdens of clinical practice and research, Zintel found time during the war years to rewrite the chapters in Mason's *Pre and Post Operative Treatment* because the original authors were overseas. This was a tremendous undertaking, as it consisted of rewriting 34 chapters.[14] Along with Koop, Rhoads, and Lockwood, Zintel was involved in the early studies of penicillin. He also investigated the effects of sulfanilamides on experimental peritonitis (inflammation of the abdominal cavity).[15] He was an expert swimmer and participated in the Penn Relays. When Ravdin left for India, Zintel was also declared "essential" to the service and remained behind.

John Lockwood came to HUP in 1936 and performed considerable teaching and research tasks for the department, although he did not have a very large surgical practice. He had a very imposing personality, and when he talked, everyone listened. He came from New York, where he worked with Alan Whipple and Frank Melanee. They sent him to England about the time that sulfanilamide was developed. Lockwood brought some back to the United States and treated President Roosevelt's son, who had a bloodstream infection. As a result, sulfanilamide became popular with the American public. By 1943, when penicillin became available, Lockwood performed studies with the newly developed drug.[16] There was very little available for use in experimental clinical research since most of it was going to the Armed Forces.

In his late 30s he suffered a heart attack and soon afterward, a saddle embolus (a blood clot completely obstructing flow to the lower extremities) developed. Ravdin was immediately summoned, and he performed a very dramatic life-saving operation. This innovative operation on Lockwood was the first of its kind and was reported in *Time* magazine.[17] By 1942 it was evident that Lockwood was physically unfit to join the military service, and he too remained at HUP.

It became increasingly evident to Rhoads that he would only be able to perform the many tasks required of him at HUP and Pennsylvania Hospital if he could enlist the help of his closest surgical colleagues Dyson, Zintel, and Lockwood, and then after Dyson's departure, Koop. Although few in number, these very competent and energetic young physicians were asked to provide the demanding operative and perioperative care for the complete surgical service. Robert Mayock describes the overwhelming circumstances they faced:

The atmosphere was different when compared to today. There were 26 rotating interns and a total of 24 residents/fellows for the whole hospital of 1000 beds. There were two interns on the Rhoads Service. When I was the intern on the Rhoads service, we had 104 patients.[18]

The small number of housestaff contributed to a good deal of stress among the young physicians. Mayock, Koop, and Zintel worked from 6 in the morning until 10 or 12 at night. Many times they worked 16- to 18-hour days. They had to start all of the intravenous infusions at night. One evening one of the interns had a patient who repeatedly pulled his I.V. out. The nurse called the intern, informing him that the patient had pulled out the I.V. once again. After restarting the I.V. for the fifth time that night, the completely exhausted intern finally got to sleep at 5 a.m. About 6 a.m., the nurse called the intern to attend to the same patient, who had pulled out his I.V. once more. The exhausted intern responded, "You know what you can do with the patient's I.V.—stick it up his ass!"

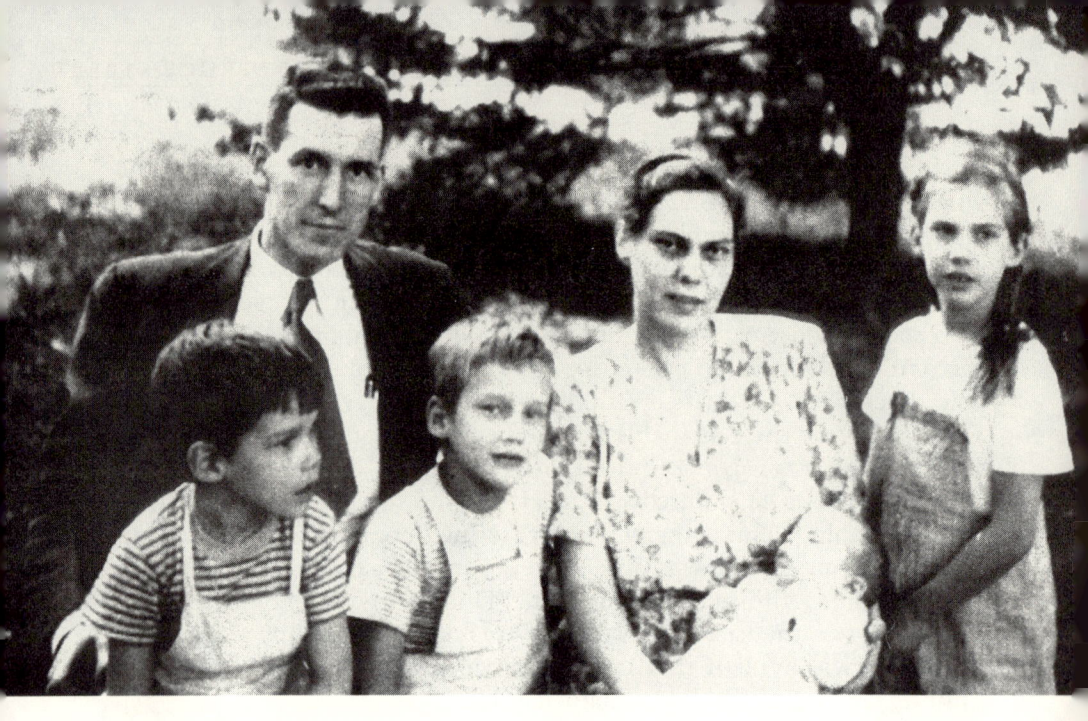

Jonathan, George, Jack, Terry, and Margaret Rhoads. Edward is on Terry's lap—1944.

The intern then rolled over and finally settled down for a short sleep. When Rhoads made morning rounds a few hours later, the patient was lying on his side. Rhoads inspected the I.V. and was somewhat taken aback when he noted the I.V. was infusing in the patient's rectum.[19]

Assuming the responsibility for Ravdin's large and complex surgical service was a major challenge for the 35-year-old Rhoads, who had only completed his formal surgical training 3 years previously. Typically, Rhoads' week consisted of three operating days and three days primarily devoted to research, teaching, and outpatients. The operating day began at 6 a.m. with inpatient rounds made by junior members of the housestaff.

Home to the Rhoads family was 4021 Pine Street, only a few blocks from the hospital. The proximity of his home to the hospital made it possible for Rhoads to walk to work. He would occasionally use his car to go to Pennsylvania Hospital to see burn patients and occasionally make house calls. By 1944 Jonathan and Terry Rhoads had four children: Margaret, Jack, George, and Edward. Along with their growing family, Terry continued her research at Children's Hospital, then located at 18th and Bainbridge Streets.

Rhoads supervised all of the nonprivate patients at HUP admitted to the Ravdin service in addition to operating upon Ravdin's patients and his own private patients under a partnership arrangement. Surgeons are happiest when they are busy operating; the large number of operations, the frequent referrals of complex cases, combined with the relatively few surgeons, contributed to an exhausting, yet exhilarating experience.

Rhoads reduced his clinical responsibilities at the Pennsylvania Hospital with the exception of continuing to work in the burn unit. According to Rhoads,

> We had this on-going burn project at Pennsylvania Hospital with Dr. Walter Estell Lee. Lee's interest in burns went back to World War I, when he was in the service and the Germans developed flame throwers. He took care of some of the men who were injured by flame throwers. I remember his coming out to the Westtown School and giving a talk on the treatment of burns when I was a student there. What he emphasized was the usefulness of paraffin mesh, which reduced the pain of changing the dressings. Ironically, I worked for him later on at Pennsylvania Hospital. As the war threatened and started, he arranged to have burn patients from all of his services sent into Pennsylvania Hospital. Referring hospitals included Graduate, Children's, Bryn Mawr, and Germantown. We performed many studies on these patients.[20]

Investigations were conducted on burn-induced changes in plasma volume using serial hematocrits. Topical treatments for burns such as tannic acid, silver nitrate, and triple dyes were examined as to their effects on plasma volume. The effects of steroids on plasma loss was also investigated. The rationale for the use of steroids in burned patients was partly based upon the Zeppelin (dirigible) disaster in 1936, when the hydrogen-filled airship blew up and burned most of the passengers. As Rhoads explains:

> We were hoping the steroids would decrease the leak of plasma under the burn. Some had been given to a few of the burned patients injured in the dirigible accident in New Jersey in 1936. One of those patients was doing badly and was given some cortical extract which Parke-Davis produced under the name Eschatin, I think. I think it was extracted from the beef adrenal glands.
>
> So we measured the effects of steroids on plasma volume as estimated by the determination of serial hematocrits. Using that rather elementary technique, we followed plasma loss in a series of burn patients. As I recall there were 11 controls and 11 patients treated with Eschatin. We put out a preliminary report in the **Annals** of Surgery, and Walter Lee was the Editor of the **Annals**, so there was no problem to get it published. Then we continued this study and by the time we doubled the number of patients it was no longer statistically significant. We published a second paper retracting our claim. It wasn't nice to have to take back what you hoped would be a breakthrough.[21]

Further studies in burn research were conducted with Miles McCarthy, Otto Rosenthal, and others in the Harrison Department of Surgical Research. Clinical studies were performed in collaboration with Jerry Walker, who subsequently identified the nonprotein nitrogen components in plasma and urine in burned patients.[22] These byproducts of protein breakdown increased significantly in patients with severe burns and were associated with a poor prognosis. Interestingly, some of the analytical methods used to perform these measurements were discovered by Rhoads' father-in-law, the renowned biochemist, Otto Folin. Additional burn research was performed in rats. Miles McCarthy was the principal investigator of these studies which examined the effects of various intravenous fluids on survival. The study concluded that plasma volume was maintained and survival was significantly increased with 1.3% saline solution when compared with 0.9%.[23]

In addition to his commitments at HUP and Pennsylvania Hospital, Rhoads shared emergency call at the Children's Hospital of Philadelphia. Because of the depleted surgical staff at HUP in 1942, it was necessary to delegate more advanced responsibilities to the younger trainees, such as Koop, who had only been a surgical resident for 5 weeks. As a rule, most first-year surgical residents do not actively participate in operations, especially if they are complex.

One morning Koop was assisting Rhoads with a stomach operation. Shortly after the skin incision was made, the anesthesiologist in the adjoining operating room stuck his head through the connecting door and said, "Jon, your gallbladder patient is intubated and ready for surgery in the next room." With distinct consternation Rhoads looked down at his gastrectomy patient on the operating table, glanced at the clock on the wall, and pondered the many unusual aspects of the patient with gallstones in the adjoining operating room. Somewhat reluctantly, he said, "Chick, why don't you go over and start that case and I'll come in and finish it up."

To understand why Rhoads permitted Koop, despite his very junior position, to begin the operation, it is helpful to recount the history of this interesting patient with gallstones. In addition to gallstones this elderly women had a devastating skin disease known as exfoliative dermatitis. She was a patient of O.H. Perry Pepper, professor of medicine, and it was his considered opinion (although everybody scoffed at him) that if her gallbladder was removed, she would also be cured of her exfoliative dermatitis. Rhoads and Koop saw the patient in preoperative consultation. She was very frail and quite ill, and there was considerable concern about whether she would survive the induction of anesthesia, let alone the operation. Her skin was repeatedly shedding; it continued to be infected and bled frequently. When he first saw the patient, Rhoads said, "Chick, find some way we can open that belly without carrying the infection into the peritoneal cavity." So Koop set out to help solve the problem. He saw the patient daily and scrubbed the skin overlying the abdominal wall with iodine, even though it bled. Surprisingly, the infection on the surface of the skin began to resolve.

Subsequently, Koop had an idea about how the skin infection might be contained at the time of surgery. He went to the Henrietta Cigar Factory on Walnut Street. The factory, owned by Mr. Eisenlohr, a wealthy patron of the University of Pennsylvania, was named for his wife, Henrietta. Koop purchased a large piece of cellophane, which was used to wrap cigars at the factory. He reasoned that the cellophane might be used as a protective cover for the abdominal wall to prevent the spread of infection into the peritoneal cavity at the time of the patient's gallbladder surgery. Two potential problems were evident: first, how to sterilize the cellophane, and second, how to make it adhere to the abdominal skin, which was very moist and slippery because of drainage from the skin infection. Numerous unsuccessful attempts were made to sterilize the cellophane. When it was put into alcohol, it became yellow and brittle; if placed into the autoclave, it melted; however, if the cellophane was soaked in the solution used to sterilize cystoscopes, it could then be dried between sterile towels, and it remained intact. The problem of the cellophane's slippery surface was solved with the use of rubber cement, which was cultured and found to be sterile.

At surgery, before the skin incision was made, the patient was "painted" with rubber cement, and then the cellophane was placed over the cement (this may have been one of the first examples of a sterile, transparent, occlusive drape, which is now commercially produced and used worldwide). Rhoads was pleased with the improvised dressing and inspected it the morning the patient was prepared for surgery.

Because the patient was already intubated in the adjoining operating room, Rhoads was faced with the dilemma of two operations at once. He was very aware of the tremendous amount of time and effort that Koop had exerted in preparing the patient for removal of her gallbladder. Patients with gallstones are usually overweight and are often technically difficult to operate on because of the obesity; however, this patient was unusually thin. After Koop opened the abdomen, he breathed a sigh of relief when he observed that the gallbladder was attached to a very long pedicle and thus easily accessible and removable. Koop glanced over his shoulder, and Rhoads was still in the other operating room. He then performed the cholecystectomy in the exact manner in which he had assisted Rhoads in approximately five similar operations.

Rhoads entered the operating room when Koop was placing the last skin suture, and he walked up to the operating table and put on a new gown and fresh gloves. Without saying a word, he removed the newly placed skin sutures and reopened the abdominal wall. Retractors were reinserted into the abdominal cavity, and the ligated remnants of the blood supply to and the drainage duct from the gallbladder (cystic artery and cystic duct, which had been tied off twice) were viewed. The liver bed, which had been sewn up tightly, and the two drains were carefully inspected. Rhoads then replaced all of the sutures exactly as they had been placed initially, closed the abdomen, and never said a word!

The following day Rhoads asked Koop to see a patient in the emergency room with a bleeding stomach ulcer. The patient needed an emergent operation, and Rhoads instructed Koop to proceed on his own with the partial removal of the stomach.[24]

Zintel and Koop were on alternate night call for surgical emergencies without any time off for almost 4 years. Sometimes they were both on call if there were very long and difficult operations or multiple surgical emergencies on the same night. During the war it was evident why surgical residents were called "residents"—they were literally residents of the hospital for as long as 72 hours consecutively. Many surgical residents did not have a day off for the first two years. An *esprit de corps* evolved on the service. Koop and Zintel were very proud that Rhoads permitted them to address him as Jon or Jonathan even though he was their senior in age, outranked them, and had more surgical experience.[25] It is possible that Rhoads' equal acceptance of his more junior colleagues resulted from his Quaker upbringing, which emphasized equality instead of elitism.

The attending surgeons did not receive salaries for their services to the hospital. Rhoads recalls:

We never charged patients on the Ward Service (nonprivate patients). This was taboo. The hospital never paid us anything for our services. It was sort of a privilege to work at the hospital. What we could collect from the private patients we could keep.[26]

Recognizing the importance of getting away from HUP for a short holiday, Rhoads asked the Koops if they would like to spend a few days at the family cabin in New Hampshire. The Koops readily accepted the invitation. Since gasoline was rationed, private transportation for long distances was very difficult and expensive. They took the train from Philadelphia to North Conway, New Hampshire, and hired a taxi to Kearsarge. Upon entering the cabin, it was apparent that it was infested with mice, as there were residual droppings in every room. Because mice were not Mrs. Koop's favorite animals, the Koops decided to sleep on the sun porch rather than inside the cabin. Before going to bed, they sat in front of the fireplace, and Mrs. Koop tucked her feet under covers to avoid an unwelcome nibble. Convinced that most of the mice were in the attic, Koop quietly positioned himself near the mouse hole in the stairs coming from the attic. When a mouse emerged from the hole, Koop, in an "act of chivalry," dropped a log on him, picked him up, and threw him out the door. When they returned to Philadelphia, the Koops thanked the Rhoadses and returned the keys to the cabin. Mrs. Koop asked Rhoads if he ever had any trouble with mice in their cabin. He replied characteristically, "Well, Betty, we have mice, but I don't recall ever having any trouble with them."[27]

One August day in 1942, Jonathan and Terry Rhoads left for Atlantic City for a much needed weekend vacation. After arriving there, Rhoads began having increasingly severe right lower abdominal pain coupled with a low-grade fever. As the pain intensified, he was certain that his symptoms were due to acute appendicitis. Harry Flippin was called, and he agreed with the diagnosis. Eliason, the most senior surgeon at HUP, and his senior resident, Lloyd Stevens, confirmed the diagnosis of acute appendicitis. Rhoads was prepared for surgery, and Eliason asked him which anesthetic he preferred. As Ravdin's protégé, Rhoads decided to go along with Ravdin's usual preference, namely, spinal anesthesia. This was, in part, an unfortunate decision. Bob Dripps, the anesthesiologist, underestimated Rhoads' large body size, and the amount of spinal anesthesia delivered was woefully inadequate. According to Rhoads:

Bob Dripps gave me a good big dose of spinal anesthesia and it worked all right for the skin and so forth. When they started to pull on my entrails it hurt, but I managed to survive that. Despite this problem, the appendectomy was performed uneventfully. The operation was in the evening and I stayed over in Maloney 407 for approximately a week. Terry came down and got me in the car, and I think I'm correct that I drove home. I stayed home about a week and analyzed the data of her research project at Children's. I performed the statistical analyses. She bought an old-fashioned adding machine that you could pull the crank on. I spent most of those days doing root mean squares on her data. Then I came back and I was all right. I got a burn from the adhesive tape, and it took longer for that to heal than it did for the incision.[28]

Somewhat later in the evening of Rhoads' appendectomy, Koop was operating on a patient with a large bowel obstruction. The operation was difficult, and he was trying to decide whether or not to perform a colostomy. As he pondered the decision, he looked into the amphitheater above the operating room, and Rhoads, in his hospital gown and bathrobe, was intently watching—it was only 5 hours after his surgery.[29] This was indeed a living confirmation of Rhoads' belief in early ambulation.

During the war years illness in the family was not limited to Dr. Rhoads. Mrs. Rhoads was admitted to HUP for pneumonia, and she was under the care of the noted internist, Bernard Comroe. Antibiotics were not readily available, and the conventional practice was not to use drugs such as the sulfanilamides until the susceptibility of the causative organism was established. Rhoads became highly concerned about his wife's condition because of increasing fever and worsening cough. Comroe prescribed sulfanilamide for Mrs. Rhoads because of her "rusty sputum." The antibiotics were effective, and the pneumonia began to resolve; however, shortly before discharge from the hospital, she came down with mumps. This additional problem extended her hospital stay, although there were no permanent adverse sequelae.[30]

Every Christmas the Rhoadses invited the faculty wives, known as "war widows," of the clinical surgeons and researchers to their home for a holiday dinner. Their husbands were overseas at the 20th General Hospital. Sometimes the only three men in attendance were Rhoads, Koop and Zintel. The Rhoadses traditionally served apple pie and ice cream for desert. On one occasion Rhoads said to Koop, "Chick, I think it's time for the ice cream. Would you help me with it?" Koop dutifully went into the kitchen and walked over to the refrigerator to find the ice cream. Rhoads said, "It's not in there, Chick. It's out in the yard." Despite the freezing temperature in December, Koop, dressed in his suit, and Rhoads, attired in a big hat with overhanging earmuffs, a large overcoat, and galoshes, marched into the backyard. Rhoads handed a snow shovel to Koop and informed him that the ice cream was buried in the snow. Rhoads started digging in a straight line, and Koop was instructed to dig in another parallel line. Koop's shovel finally hit something in the snow, and he said, " Jon, I think I've found it." Rhoads said, "No, that's Mother's turkey—put it back." After digging further they finally found the ice cream, which was enjoyed by all.[31]

The Rhoadses would on occasion invite friends and visitors to their home for dinner. While meat was rationed and difficult to obtain, dinner guests eagerly accepted these invitations. Occasionally, they would have a leg of lamb, and in one instance a grateful patient provided a unique gift as a token of appreciation for her medical care. Rhoads had operated upon this patient for large, painful congenital cysts of the liver. At surgery, he

Facing page: Terry (on stilts) and Jonathan Rhoads with son George romping outdoors in the late winter of 1942.

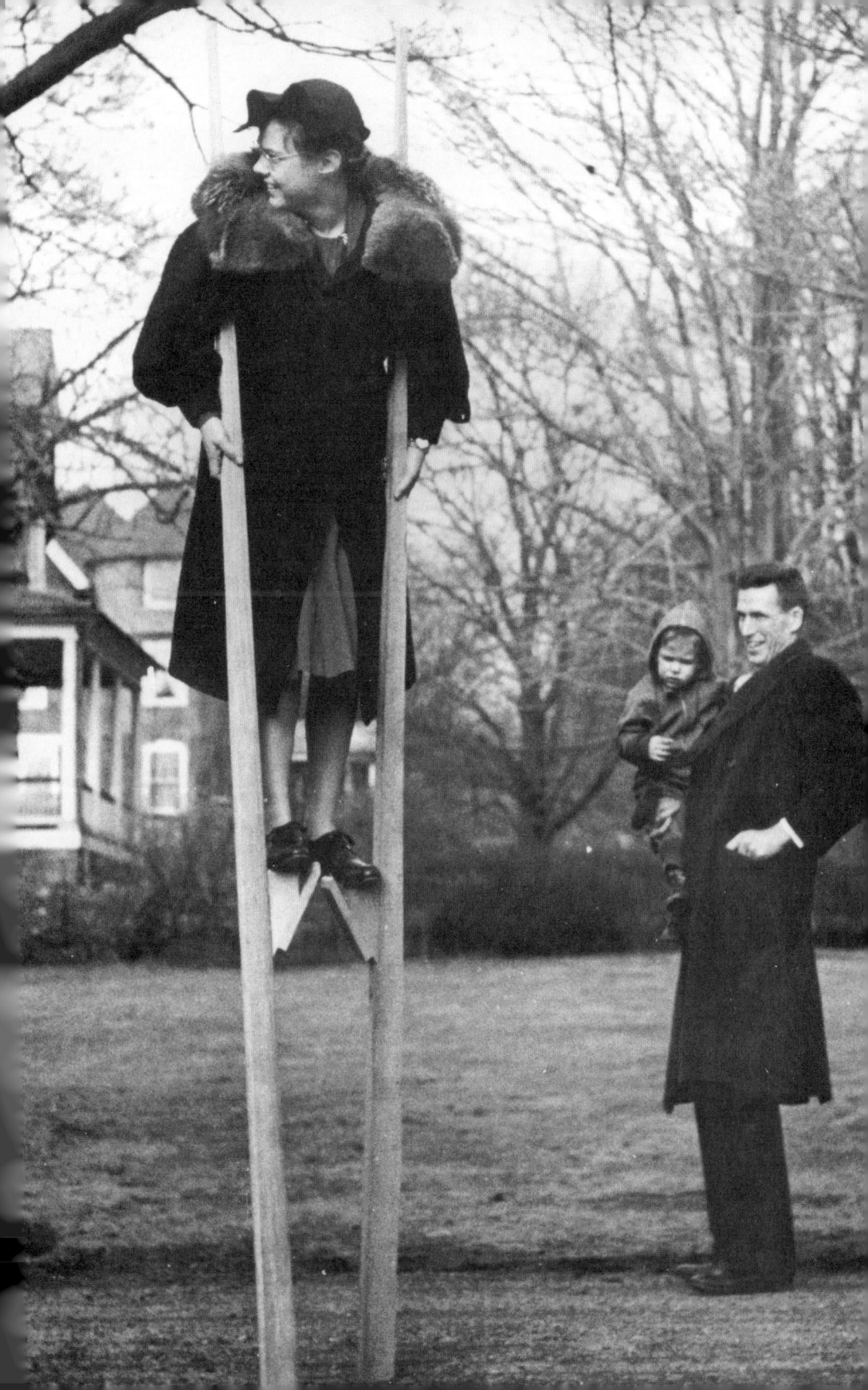

unroofed and packed the cysts. The cysts could not be excised because they were dangerously close to the highly vascular hepatic veins, and he was concerned that an attempt at excising the cysts might result in a fatal hemorrhage. During the operation he painted the inside of the cysts with a sterile formalin-based sclerosing solution from the pathology department and packed the wound in the liver with a roll of gauze, which exited through the skin incision. Ten days later it was time for the packing to be removed at the bedside. One of the residents attempted to remove it, and it was so painful for the patient that the resident had to stop. Rhoads was summoned, and the patient said, "If you get the packing out without hurting me, my husband [a farmer from New Jersey] will bring you a pig." Rhoads reasoned that the best thing to do would be to remove the packing under general anesthesia. The packing came out without too much bleeding, and the next day Mrs. Rhoads called her husband's office and said, "There's a pig tied up in our kitchen and I can't move it." In the true manner of a chairman, Rhoads dispatched his able assistants Koop and Zintel to solve the problem. The pig weighed more than 400 pounds. After a considerable struggle and realizing that the recalcitrant pig was so large that he could not be moved by two people, they prevailed upon a local butcher who had a shop on 40th Street to take the pig. The Rhoads', Zintel's, and Koop's homes were well stocked with pork chops, ham, and bacon for the next several weeks.[32]

With the exodus of many staff physicians during the war, the remaining surgeons at HUP were frequently called upon to perform operations for which they had little experience. One of these operations was for intractable temporomandibular joint disease. Another operation was to provide a surgical access for invasive diagnostic procedures. On one occasion, a neurologist at the Graduate Hospital asked Rhoads to perform a cut-down (opening into a blood vessel) in order to insert a small catheter into the common carotid artery to perform a cerebral angiogram (x-ray of the blood supply to the brain). Rhoads recounts:

There was a neurologist [who] . . . thought he could get a good picture of the vessels of the brain with the intra-arterial injection of contrast material that had recently become available. I think it was mainly developed to visualize kidneys. . . . He wanted somebody to put this contrast material into the carotid artery with the patient on the x-ray table so the pictures could be taken right away. The neurologist prescribed the dose of the contrast material, and I cut-down on the carotid artery and injected it. They got rather good pictures of the vessels of the brain, but the patient had a convulsion, so that scared us away from doing any more.

After telling this story, Rhoads said:

This was one of a number of things that I did when I was younger that I would never have done when I was older. It reminded me of Julian Johnson's old statement: "You can't both fly high and keep your feet on the ground."[33]

Years later, this technique was improved upon by others and became relatively routine, although attended by a small risk.

The surgical residents frequently asked Rhoads for help or advice concerning difficult problems in the operating room. Upon entering the operating room, he rarely said a word. He usually walked up to the table, put on a gown and gloves, stood directly behind the resident, and then gently moved him out of the way. Most surgeons operate with their first assistant across from them, but both Ravdin and Rhoads operated with their assistant on the right-hand side. This position was somewhat awkward for the assistants, who frequently ended up with a terrible kink in their backs after long cases.

Rhoads was a fast technical surgeon, which surprised many of his surgical colleagues. When witnessing his walk, listening to him talk, and observing his perpetual state of slow motion, the unsuspecting surgeon most likely would predict it might take Rhoads a considerable amount of time to repair even a hernia. However, he was a fast operator—neat, clean, and known to be a very motion-efficient surgical technician. Years later it was thought that the reason Rhoads became both a good and fast surgeon was that there were not enough surgeons for the large number of patients. One of his former surgical colleagues stated that the only thing he could be faulted for in the operating room was an excessive concern about bleeding. If a blood vessel was cut, the surgical assistant was asked to step aside immediately while Rhoads expeditiously stopped the bleeding.[34]

Rhoads was an advocate of early postoperative ambulation—considered to be somewhat heretical at that time. The standard of care in the 1940s was to keep patients in the hospital and often in bed for as long as 14 days, even after minor surgery. It was not unusual for patients to remain at absolute bed rest for 1 week after a hernia repair and for 2 weeks after removal of the gallbladder. Rhoads questioned this practice and believed that patients recovered more rapidly if they were active and ambulating soon after the operation. When asked about this issue, he responded modestly:

I don't think I can claim any leadership role in this. The first that I heard about early exercises I think was about the last year I was in medical school. I had a classmate named Leadbetter who came from Maine and eventually became Chief of Urology at MGH [Massachusetts General

Hospital]. He had an uncle who was an orthopedist in the Washington D.C. area and he was a proponent of early postoperative exercise and ambulation. In those days, patients with hip fractures were placed in traction for two or three months if they lived that long. A good many of them died of pulmonary emboli. Leadbetter's uncle conceived the idea that they needed exercise and arranged for the patients to receive regular range of motion exercises....

At HUP, Charles Kirby, a surgical colleague, was very interested in pulmonary emboli and I wrote two papers with him. He thought that early postoperative ambulation was not only important in reducing the incidence of pulmonary emboli after fractures but also following other types of surgery. He had a very active program which Dr. Ravdin backed. On Ravdin's service each patient was inspected twice daily for tenderness of the calf. Unfortunately, it was subsequently shown that a large percentage of pulmonary emboli occurred without any warning such as swelling of the calf.[35]

Another interesting report of early postoperative ambulation came from the Persian Gulf:

There was a missionary surgeon whose son, Timothy Harrison, married one of Oliver Cope's daughters. The son eventually joined the staff at Hershey but spent most of his time in the Middle East. I believe the father worked at a small missionary hospital on the Isle of Bahrain, which served nomads on the mainland. They performed a lot of hernia operations on the nomads, who would not remain at rest after surgery. They would have the operation and then get on their camels and just go. There was something in the surgeon's report about the patients seldom getting deep venous thromboses and pulmonary emboli.

I questioned the follow-up but I was told that there was no other hospital in the area for these people to come back to. Therefore, they presumed they should know about all of the bad results. It was remarkable; right after the operation, these patients would simply get on their camels and ride off![36]

It was not uncommon for Rhoads, a young, strong man over 6 feet tall, to lift patients out of bed, either placing them in a chair or helping them to walk on the first postoperative day. While making postoperative rounds, Rhoads would often chat with the patient a bit and inform the nurse that it was imperative to get the patient out of bed as soon as possible. Without much warning, he would proceed to the bedside, pull the covers out from under the foot of the bed, lift the patient with bed covers and whatever else was attached, and place him in the bedside chair. As a former colleague recalled, "This used to drive the nurses crazy because he often pulled the mattress, pad, and everything else off the bed at the same time as the patient was being lifted out of bed."[37] It was at least another 10 years before surgeons truly acknowledged the benefits of early postoperative ambulation to reduce deep venous thrombosis and improve respiratory function.

Rhoads was continually confronted with difficult surgical problems. On one occasion he had a patient with pancreatitis who suffered a long and complicated hospital course. Despite many disease-related problems, she recovered from a major operation, and she and her family were extremely grateful. One evening when Rhoads was making rounds with Koop and Zintel, they visited this patient. She and her husband, who had brought in a bottle of wine to celebrate his wife's discharge the next day, asked the surgeons to have a toast with them. The husband produced some old-fashioned paper cups that were cone shaped on the bottom and could not be set down. Approximately 3 teaspoons of wine were poured into each of the cups. Koop drank his down, and Zintel followed suit. Everyone toasted Rhoads, who sipped at his wine but did not finish it. Later that evening Koop returned home and finished supper when the telephone rang. It was a call from Rhoads. He said, "Chick, Jon here. I don't think I should make rounds tonight; I had a little bit too much to drink this afternoon."[38]

Rhoads was widely respected for his surgical judgment, which included not only making intraoperative decisions but also solving difficult perioperative problems. Good judgment is perhaps the most important quality of a surgeon. It is based upon not only knowledge, but also sensitivity, intuition, and experience. Surgeons are often faced with difficult decisions on a daily basis. Rhoads was extremely good at knowing when to be aggressive and when to back off and continue to observe the patient.

Dorothy Bender (later Maxwell) finished her internship at HUP in 1944 and became HUP's first female general surgical resident there, largely due to the efforts of Jonathan Rhoads and Eldridge Eliason. As an intern, she was so impressed with Rhoads' demeanor, his excellent surgical skills, and teaching ability that she decided to go into general surgery. This was a very unusual move for a female physician at the time. Female interns and residents lived on the top floor of the Piersol Building. Bender remembers Rhoads' unflappability under the most trying circumstances:

We had a thyroid patient, a young woman. We started the case on time and Dr. Rhoads was uncharacteristically a little late. When he arrived he stuck his head in the operating room at the same time the young woman went into cardiac arrest. At that time we didn't have closed resuscitation and so we opened the chest on the side of the heart. . . .

Rhoads said, "Oh my!" and promptly got scrubbed and dressed. The anesthesiologist was a very young man and very distressed. We finally got everything quieted down and everything was stabilized. The anesthesiologist turned to Dr. Rhoads and said, "Dr. Rhoads, what are we going to tell the patient?" Rhoads replied in his quiet, laconic way, 'Well, we'll tell her that her heart stopped and she can't but be grateful that it started again." Typical of Rhoads, he wasn't ruffled by the things that happened. . . . He was never out of control.[39]

In addition to his duties as acting chief of the service, Rhoads assumed a very heavy teaching schedule. The onset of the war required more information to be taught in a shorter time. The academic year of the medical school was reduced from 12 months to 9 months. There were two graduating classes in 1943. In addition to the need for instruction of medical students, the war led to a need for instruction of military physicians. Rhoads recalls teaching for 7 full hours one day:

I gave 7 one-hour lectures one day. Groups of people would come in who had joined the Army Medical Corps. We would brief them on what we did with sulfanilamide and later with penicillin. Additional topics included the treatment of shock and burns. They would be here for 3 to 6 weeks.[40]

Despite a heavy operating schedule and research commitments, the quality of Rhoads' teaching remained high, as is reflected in the comments of one of his students who wrote to him anonymously:

This type of communication may not be strictly up to par, but I'd like you to know how some of the boys, and especially myself, feel about your lectures to the third-year class on Friday mornings. I want you to know that your lectures are the finest, best organized, and best presented lectures that I've ever attended in this school. I can say, sir, that I've really learned in principle, at least, more from your talks to us than from any other instruction that we've had thus far. I only wish it were my privilege to learn my practical surgery from you as well—I would really know something of the art.[41]

Like many excellent surgical teachers, Rhoads used the operating room as a classroom. While performing an operation he frequently discussed the scientific rationale for the operation in addition to the technical nuances of the surgery. During the procedure, he simultaneously talked about similar cases and instructed those at the table about variances of the current operation when compared to his experience with similar surgeries. Rhoads was a strong advocate of using patients and clinical events to teach surgical principles. Many years later he expressed some of his thoughts about teaching:

There is, however, another medium of teaching that is increasingly important in the medical field. This is teaching by practice or example rather than by precept or lecture. Particularly in the years of hospital training, students and young doctors learn much more by what they see than by what they are told. Here those who make a habit of careful practice, especially if they can explain what they are doing with clarity and sincerity, can excel as teachers.[42]

In the late 1930s Rhoads became interested in various methods of dialysis for the treatment of renal failure. He later began these investigations with peritoneal dialysis. He recalls:

We did peritoneal dialysis here when I was a resident. Subsequently, I got permission to treat a patient who was going down with renal failure. I think the patient was on Dr. [Peter] Randall's father's service at Abington Hospital. He was Chief of Urology. I got a large amount of urea out of the blood. The patient subsequently died. There was some reason to believe that the patient had acute renal failure; however, at autopsy it was noted that he had chronic, terminal renal failure. I thought that I had better not get a reputation for laying too many patients away, so I quit.[43]

His previous experience with peritoneal dialysis provided the foundation for investigations of hemodialysis during the war. Early in 1945 Rhoads was emergently summoned to the Pennsylvania Hospital to see a woman with toxemia of pregnancy. She was a few days postpartum and had developed liver failure followed shortly by acute renal failure. For many years before caring for this patient, Rhoads had been interested in whether hemodialysis might correct abnormal amounts of blood urea and other toxic byproducts of acute renal failure.

Shortly before seeing this severely ill patient, Rhoads purchased some special Visking tubing, a product primarily used as a substitute for sausage casing and known to have excellent properties as a dialyzing membrane. Rhoads and Henry Saltonstall, a young surgical resident and member of a prominent New England family, boldly decided to dialyze the toxic nitrogenous waste products from the blood in this patient, who would certainly die of combined liver and renal failure. An arterial catheter was inserted, and the blood flowed through the special tubing that was rolled around a wire test tube rack, which was immersed in a basin of the dialyzing solution containing sodium, chloride, glucose, calcium phosphate, and potassium. Gelatin was substituted for plasma protein. The dialyzed blood was then collected and returned to the patient by way of gravity into an arm vein. This archetypical hemodialysis technique was highly successful in extracting urea from the patient's blood. Approximately 20 grams of urea were recovered, and the abnormally high level of blood urea nitrogen was significantly reduced.

The patient was heparinized before the procedure to prevent clotting within the tubing; however, the heparin was not neutralized at the end of the procedure. Unfortunately, the patient had a severe hemorrhage on the evening after the dialysis. Saltonstall transfused her; however, she died shortly thereafter. Although she did not die of the hemorrhage, there was concern that something in the dialysis procedure contributed to the bleeding. The death of this patient discouraged Rhoads from continuing with renal dialysis. Rhoads recalls:

Saltonstall had to transfuse her and she went downhill and died of toxemia. Somehow, I lost the pictures and we never wrote it up. That was before we had heard about the work from Holland around 1942 or 1943.[44]

Shortly thereafter, extensive research in renal dialysis began worldwide. The technique was made clinically relevant by W.J. Kolff, who developed the procedure in Holland under great difficulties during the war. Kolff's initial experience included 11 patients with only 1 survivor, but he did observe improvement of a temporary nature in some of the others. When Kolff visited the University of Pennsylvania shortly after the war, he asked Rhoads why he had not continued the investigations of renal dialysis. Rhoads replied that although the patients he had treated had been diagnosed initially as having acute renal failure, it was shown subsequently that they had chronic renal disease and therefore did not improve with dialysis, in part because of the chronicity of the disease.[45]

In addition to many administrative responsibilities, Rhoads maintained his involvement in research during the war. With the departure of John Lockwood in 1944, who had accepted a position at Yale, Rhoads was appointed acting director of the Harrison Department, and he continued in this position until Ravdin returned in late 1945. The appointment to yet another major administrative position was thought to be due in part to his special relationship with Ravdin. As Rhoads tells it:

I was asked to take over when he [Ravdin] left. I suppose this decision may have been influenced by Betty Ravdin [the wife of I.S. Ravdin] who served as an Assistant Dean. The Dean was aging and I believe Betty was calling many of the turns. She would never, of course, admit it. I remember A. Newton Richards, who was Vice-President, called me in and told me that when I took over the laboratory that I had better change my attitude and be very tight with money.[46]

As the result of limited funds and few personnel, the number of basic science investigations decreased. Emphasis was directed to the military effort because of several war contracts with the National Research Council. One of these contracts was designed to develop blood substitutes for the treatment of shock, and another investigated the nutrient requirements and optimal sources of protein repletion for wounded soldiers.

The Harrison Department was deeply engaged in a classified project on the pulmonary effect of poison gases. Rhoads was not involved in these studies because of his noncombatant status. The deleterious effects of phosgene on pulmonary function in dogs was investigated. Phosgene, a very poisonous gas, produces severe alveolar (air sac) destruction with ensuing pulmonary edema and death. Mary Gibbon, the wife of the famous cardiothoracic surgeon John Gibbon, was involved in the study in collaboration with Dr. Brunner, a physiologist, and Charlie Chapple, a pediatrician who subsequently invented the isolette (a special bed to treat critically ill neonates).[47]

A considerable amount of collaborative research was performed with William Abbott, who contracted leukemia while in the Army. He returned home to Penn and performed many important physiologic studies of the gut. Abbott was very innovative, although not necessarily prudent. His studies were performed with the use of his long tube that was passed into the small intestine. Abbott frequently experimented upon himself by swallowing self-made intestinal tubes and used contrast x-rays to confirm the location of the tube. One of the aims of these studies was to correlate the site of intestinal obstruction with the site of abdominal pain. He placed an external marker on his abdomen at a measured distance from the umbilicus and radiographically confirmed the position and migration of the tube. The tip of the tube was advanced into different segments of the small bowel, and then the balloon on the end of the tube was inflated to simulate intestinal obstruction, which in turn produced abdominal pain at fairly reproducible sites. These studies were carefully performed and recorded. They showed that peristalsis was not limited to forward movement, but consisted of to-and-fro mixing motions in the bowel. Additionally, Abbott demonstrated that vomiting due to intestinal obstruction was not really associated with reverse peristalsis but resulted from forward peristalsis against the obstruction.[48]

Rhoads also performed studies of penicillin with John Lockwood in 1944:

Lockwood got a lot going with penicillin. He essentially "controlled" penicillin in the Delaware Valley. Most of it was going to the Armed Forces. There was a limited amount for clinical research; therefore we gave it sparingly. We gave 12,500 units every three hours or 100,000 units every 24 hours. We got wonderful responses even with these small doses. Harrison Flippin, who had been through the medical residency here for one year and with whom I had shared an office, did a lot of work with penicillin at Philadelphia General Hospital. They had an enormous amount of lobar pneumonia coming into PGH and it worked like a charm. They wanted to publish a hundred cases and they were up in the 90's somewhere when they had this written up. The manuscript was sent to JAMA, and the editors held their press run until they got the 99th and 100th cases. The figures were amended accordingly. I think the last cases got a favorable response on about Saturday and the report appeared in the JAMA on the following Thursday. Additionally they found that despite unfavorable in vitro tests, it [penicillin] worked well against this bacillus (anthrax) that produced large skin lesions when leather workers scratched their necks while working with animal hides[49]

Rhoads was also involved in early studies on the use of antibiotics. These works were based upon some of the seminal studies of investigators at Rutgers. Dr. Katharine Evans, who later married Rhoads in 1990, participated in these studies while training at the Philadelphia Municipal Hospital. While an intern, Evans worked with Franklin Murphy to treat anthrax patients with penicillin. Interestingly, penicillin was not effective against anthrax *in vitro* yet it worked very well *in vivo*. One of Evans' tasks was to ensure that the penicillin infused without difficulty in a continuous delivery throughout the night. This responsibility was indeed a challenge and often resulted in sleepless nights. Some of the preliminary studies on penicillin were published from Penn in 1945. A more detailed report was published from the Mayo Clinic about the same time.[50] The superiority of the Mayo Clinic paper was brought to Rhoads' attention by Ravdin.

Because of the high quality and peer acceptance of these investigations, combined with acknowledged clinical, teaching and administrative skills, Rhoads was elected to the Society of University Surgeons, the Society of Clinical Surgery, and the American Surgical Association in 1942 and 1943, one of the youngest men to be so honored.

Many years later, Rhoads expresses his thoughts concerning research:

While the qualities that make for success in research are intellectual, they are generally bound up with qualities of character that often seem to play the definitive role. The successful scientific investigator is a person of great dedication to a given task. He must be willing to stick at *it through many difficulties and discouragements. He must often be willing to work very much alone and without the daily appreciation and thanks that do so much to sustain the practitioner through the long days and night hours that his work entails. Yet, at the same time, he must not be too dogged in his determination. He must be looking for the way around obstacles and he should be constantly on the alert for pearls scattered along the wayside. He needs to be possessed of unusual judgment about when to stop and pick up such pearls (serendipity) and when to press on toward more ultimate goals.[51]*

Though Rhoads had many research successes, he lamented some of the shortcomings and failures:

One's failures can sometimes be more illuminating than one's successes. Examples are my failure to follow-up on peritoneal dialysis in the treatment of uremia first reported in 1938, my failure to publish an early case of extracorporeal dialysis in another patient with renal shutdown, and my failure to affect the immune system by thymectomy in 3-week-old rabbits. Thymectomy after birth was later shown to have a profound effect on the immune response. Knowing when to stay with one problem and when to give in and turn to another area of investigation will always be a matter of judgment but also of luck. In general, I favor persisting with one set of problems if the long-term goal seems worth the effort and the possibilities for progress are still open. One can probably spend a lifetime searching for new knowledge and not find anything of importance, but one thing appears certain: if you do not do research, you will not find.[52]

With the end of World War II in 1945, Ravdin and the physicians of the 20th General Hospital returned to Philadelphia. Robert Mayock remembers what a relief it was:

After the War, when they returned, they said the 20th General was going to take over this hospital [HUP] . . . and they were right in a way. Actually nobody was even fighting with the returning physicians. . . . We were all exhausted. We needed all the people we could get.[53]

Of those soldier-physicians who returned, most wore a small button called the ruptured duck. It was frequently worn, especially during job interviews, and distinguished those who served in the war from those who did not. Francis Wood, one of the physicians with the 20th General who later became chief of medicine at HUP, addressed his medical residents at a dinner that year:

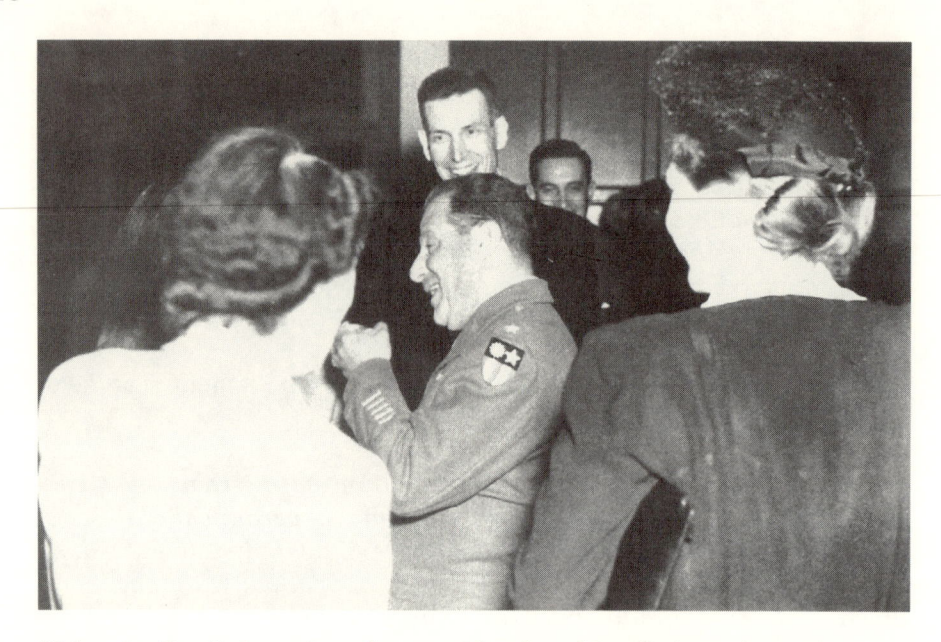

Welcoming Ravdin home from the war—Rhoads and Ravdin (center).

You know, since I've come back from the service I've been thinking. I realized that after seeing the number of patients [who] were here and the shortness of the staff and the fact that they did so well, I realized they were probably working hard or maybe harder than we were in Burma. I've decided to stop wearing my "duck."[54]

The war had also taken its toll on the physicians of the Ravdin surgical service who had remained behind. As Zintel said to Koop many years later:

Well, Koop, what the war years did for us was it gave you ulcers, I lost my hair, and Jonathan came down with tuberculosis.[55]

The compleat physician is one who has had a major operation and has successfully gone through a severe prolonged illness. May I wish you both of them.

Joseph Stokes—Addressing the graduating
U of P medical school class of 1941[1]

SIX

THE CHIEF, THE COW, AND THE CORTISONE

SICKNESS AND HEALTH

Dramatic changes occurred in the Department of Surgery at HUP following the return of Ravdin and his colleagues in 1945. Ravdin resumed his clinical practice almost immediately, and the amount of surgery that he performed during the summer of 1946 approached his pre-war levels. Rhoads had functioned well as a surrogate for Ravdin's patients, who, in turn, welcomed his charismatic personality and clinical acumen. Ravdin performed 133 operations in the month of July, and Rhoads' total was 123 in the month of August.

Shortly after his return, Ravdin invited three of his closest surgical colleagues at the 20th General Hospital to join the Department of Surgery at HUP. Ironically, each of these individuals—Cletus Schwegman, Julian Johnson, and William Fitts—would remain at HUP for their entire professional careers. Of the three, Schwegman, a Kentuckian, was the only one who had not attended medical school at Penn, instead having graduated from the University of Cincinnati.

Schwegman's initial contact with Ravdin was quite auspicious. He had recently attended the Army Chemical Warfare School in Aberdeen, Maryland. Schwegman was asked to give several talks on chemical warfare to the group while the 20th General Hospital was in transit by ship to India. Although he only knew a little more about chemical warfare than his surgical colleagues on board the ship, Schwegman prepared his presentations in an assiduous and scholarly manner. The clarity of presentation and the organized content of the talks immediately caught Ravdin's attention. By fiat, Schwegman was made a member of Ravdin's team. Upon arrival to the 20th General Hospital, not only were Schwegman's qualities as a teacher recognized by Ravdin, but his skills in the operating room were highly regarded. Following his return from India and not knowing quite what to expect when he joined the staff in January 1946, Schwegman recalls:

When I first came to the HUP I was provided with a bed on the upper floor of the administration building, which is no longer standing. We were never assigned a specific bed; you simply occupied any bed that was empty. Our meals were provided by the hospital. I lived like that for some months.[2]

William "Bill" Fitts was born in Jackson, Tennessee, where he spent most of his youth. He later attended Union College and the University of

Surgery department—late 1940s.
Top row—1st from left, Gerry Walker; 2nd from left, Nick Gimbel; 3rd from left, Chick Koop; 3rd from right, Brooke Roberts.
Second row—3rd from left, Dottie Maxell; 2nd from right, Martin Rhode; 4th from right, Jim Hardy.
Front row—1st from left, Charlie Kirby; 2nd from left, Henry Royster; 3rd from left, Julian Johnson; 4th from left, I.S. Ravdin; 1st from right, Clete Schwegman, 2nd from right, Bill Fitts; 3rd from right, Harold Zintel; 4th from right, Jonathan Rhoads.

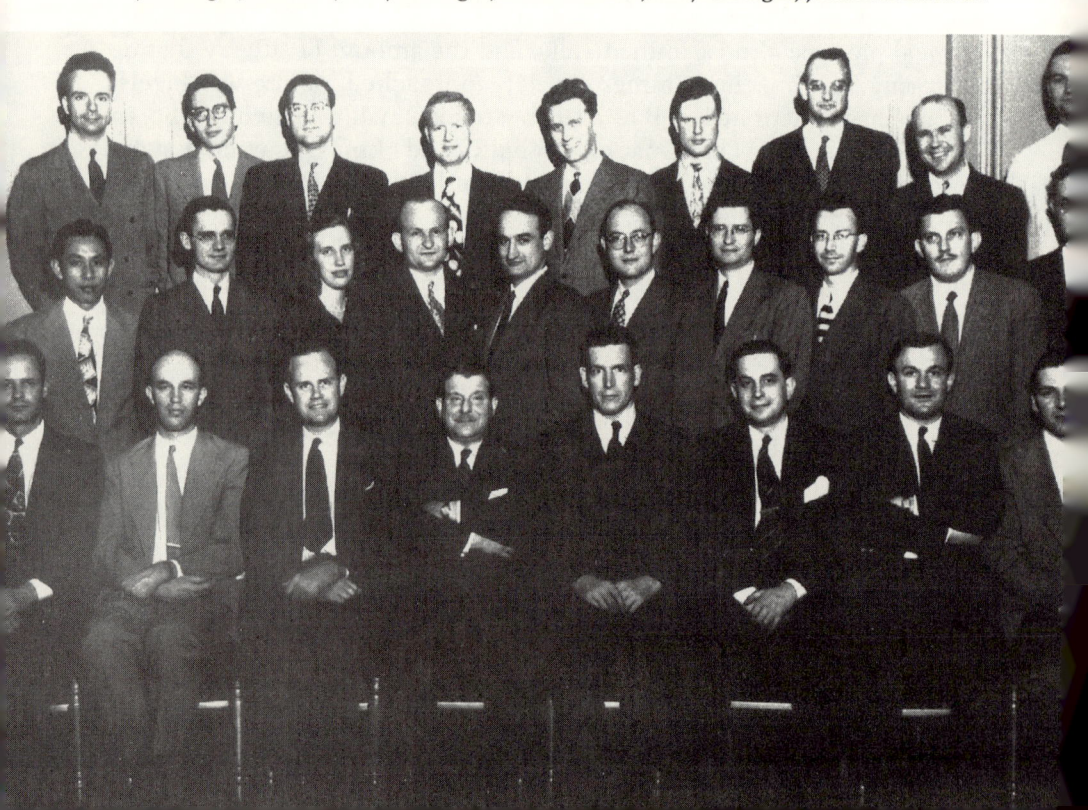

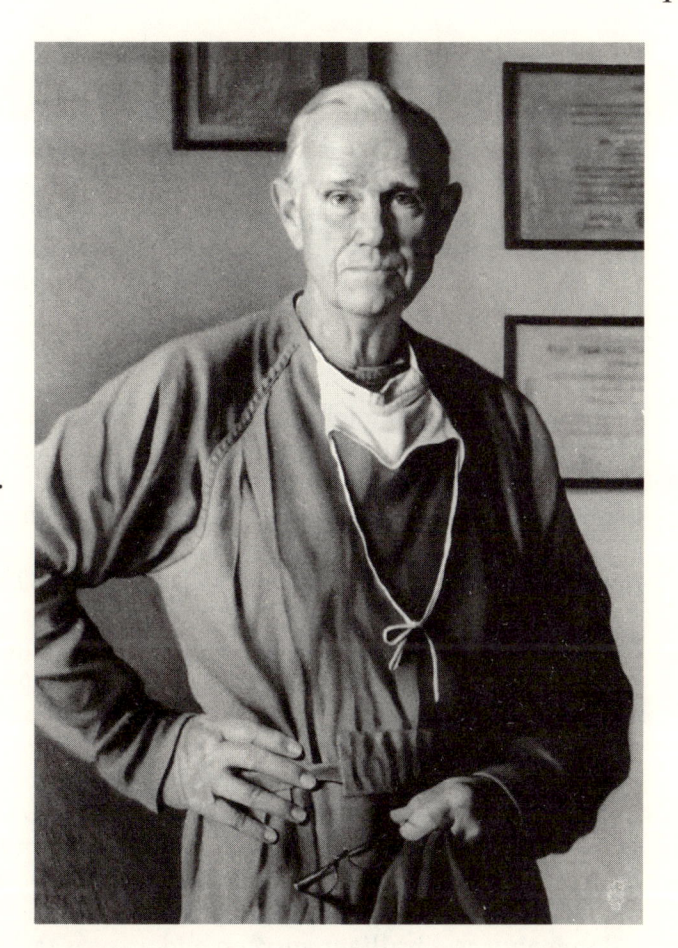

Julian Johnson.

Pennsylvania School of Medicine, where he was Alpha Omega Alpha. As a medical student he won the Spencer Morris Prize, given to the best student in his class. At the 20th General he was assigned to the fracture component of the surgical section. While in India, Ravdin commented that Fitts probably performed more onlay grafts for delayed union of the tibia than any surgeon in the United States.

In 1946 Fitts returned to HUP and finished his surgical training. He was then persuaded by Ravdin to pursue an academic career with a subspecialty interest in trauma. He became a nationally and internationally recognized expert in trauma. He was selected editor of the *Journal of Trauma* in 1968 and president of the American Association for the Surgery of Trauma in 1972. In 1972, Fitts was appointed the John Rhea Barton Professor. He died tragically in 1980 following an emergent operation for impaired blood flow to the intestine.[3] His legacy has been perpetuated with the recent establishment of the William T. Fitts Surgical Education Center in the Department of Surgery at Penn.

Julian Johnson was Ravdin's choice to play a major role in the reassembled surgical faculty. Johnson graduated from the University of Pennsylvania Medical School in 1931 and interned at HUP for two years. During one of these years, he was a co-intern with Rhoads. Never one to waste time, Johnson finished his internship on June 30th at 6 p.m. and was married at 8 p.m. by his father-in-law, a Presbyterian minister, in Bridgeton, New Jersey.[4]

Ravdin, Rhoads, and Johnson officially became major partners within the department. Ravdin decreed that Johnson would specialize in cardiac surgery, a suggestion Johnson welcomed with characteristic enthusiasm. Johnson's wife, Mary, recalls the group's interaction:

It was Rav's idea. We had the Jew, the Quaker and the Southern Baptist. Very interesting combination. When Rav operated on me for my ulcer, Julian insisted on being there. It may have been hard on Rav. I did have trouble afterwards. I think he cut the vagus nerve. [Note: This is a normal component of certain anti-ulcer operations.] But anyhow, he had to be there; I guess a lot of surgeons would say they wouldn't want to be there. Julian's explanation was that he would like to have operated on me because he knew he was the best surgeon. He had to bow to Rav, I guess. Jonathan did my gallbladder, and he operated on Julian too when he had cancer of the sigmoid colon. So we knew each other inside and out![5]

Johnson was a brilliant surgeon and a stern taskmaster, as Leonard Miller, a former resident notes:

In June of my internship, I was dead tired. There were no I.V. teams. You had to draw all the bloods and change all the dressings and put in all the tubes before you went to the operating room. Julian used to do the thoracic and abdominal aneurysms, the first to be done at that time. One day I overslept. So I didn't put the Foley catheter in the guy who was going to have his aneurysm resected. I got to the operating room all unshaven. There's Julian passing the Foley himself in the operating room. So I walked in and I said, "Dr. Johnson, I apologize. I guess I just overslept. Let me take over for you." I knew I was in trouble because Julian was humming the Red River Valley, *which was a sign of trouble. He didn't say anything to me. He just continued to hum. So I repeated, "Dr. Johnson, it's my job; here, let me take over." He continued to hum. I tried a third time and he turned to me. He had these crescent-shaped glasses and he looked at me over the glasses and said, "Len, I'm not going to say anything to you now. But I've got five more years to make it up to you."*[6]

Thus, the triumvirate of Ravdin, Rhoads, and Johnson began their long and successful collaboration.

Because of Rhoads' increasing recognition as a surgical educator and researcher, he was invited to Poland at the end of the war by the United Nations Relief and Rehabilitation Authority. This program included several highly regarded teachers from medical schools in the United States who were invited to go to post-war Eastern Europe to instruct and update their beleaguered medical colleagues about recent advances in medicine and surgery. Rhoads, who was about to become the father of 6 with the impending birth of twins, felt a sense of duty to complete this mission because he had stayed on the homefront during the war. Prior to leaving for Poland, he was surprised by the results of his requisite chest x-ray performed by the Public Health Service in Philadelphia:[7]

They said I had to go down to get a chest x-ray at the U.S.P.H.S. I didn't know they had a station in Philadelphia. So I went down there and came back, and the next day I was working in the dog lab and I got a phone call and the doctor said, "Did you know you have moderately advanced TB?" I said, I didn't know anything like that.

I had worked all weekend and put in a pretty good week, and I had prepared papers ready to take to Poland. I hurried over to see Dr. Philip Hodes, who was in x-ray then. I knew him well. He had been a year ahead of me in the internship. So he took another film and confirmed it. I was not ill and found this hard to believe. They couldn't find my initial chest film taken 10 years before.

So I got in touch with Ravdin and, of course, David A. Cooper Sr. . . . Cooper had been through a bout of tuberculosis and had been to Saranac [a tuberculosis sanitorium in New York] and had subsequently gone into pulmonary medicine. So he looked me over and said that I had better slow down and stop taking night calls. So then I slowed down and did that, and this was the beginning of May, and in June he said that I had better knock it off and I went up to the country [New Hope] and rested a good deal in bed. Bedrest on the farm in New Hope was accompanied by a cream-rich diet after which I was never able to feel my dorsalis pedis [an artery in the foot] pulses. My mother was living [at New Hope] then and she filled me up with food and I got fatter and fatter.[8]

Rhoads continued bedrest at the Folin's cottage in New Hampshire. Despite being confined to absolute bedrest, Rhoads recalls the unique setup of his room: "I had things set up so I could cook without getting out of bed."[9] Following a one-month stay, he returned to Philadelphia for further tests:

They had me come back to the HUP overnight about the first of August. Cooper had one of the interns put a tube down into my stomach; I guess the chest x-ray hadn't changed materially. So gastric washings were obtained inasmuch as I didn't have any sputum. I remember I was a very bad tube swallower . . . coughed, sputtered and spat all over the intern. I don't know whether he got TB or not. They didn't see any bugs in my gastric washings and they put it into a guinea pig, and around the beginning of September they called me to say that the pig was positive.[10]

Rhoads was formally hospitalized in the Eisenlohr Pavilion at HUP in September under the care of David Cooper. Cooper, a North Carolinian, was respected for both his clinical acumen and humanistic qualities. At the time of Rhoads' hospitalization, Cooper's wife of many years was acutely ill with paralytic poliomyelitis, of which she died several days thereafter. Despite this tragedy, Cooper was back with his patients almost immediately.

Streptomycin was newly identified as an active agent against the tubercle bacillis, and Cooper proposed that Rhoads receive it. The drug was procured through Merck and Company. The dosage for long-term administration was not known, and Rhoads was empirically given 1.8 grams per day intramuscularly. As he explains:

Over a few weeks I began to lose my sense of balance and had trouble keeping my gaze level when I was jiggled as when riding in a wheelchair. There I sat and he gave me 3/10 of a gram anyhow, 1.8 grams a day, and I lost my position sense rather completely. So when I trundled in a wheelchair, I couldn't keep objects in line. . . . They were all bobbing up and down all over the place. I had a Bárány test which made me violently ill, which it is supposed to do. It is a test where they squirt cold water into your ear and it does something to your 8th nerve. They also put you on one of these wheels that turn you around.[11]

Impairment of the equilibrium component of the eighth cranial nerve was confirmed by standard tests; however, the hearing component of the nerve was not significantly affected. In later life, Rhoads' equilibrium never fully returned to normal. Concerned that the medication had reached toxic levels, Cooper discontinued the drug. Rhoads remained hospitalized at HUP approximately 4 months before leaving for the Presbyterian Sanitorium in Albuquerque, New Mexico.[12] The possible financial and emotional consequences of Rhoads' illness and the likelihood of prolonged hospitalization were major concerns to his family. Caroline, writing to Esther, reports:

Went to see J this p.m. and I had quite a nice visit with most of the family out of the room, but only briefly. J and I discussed world affairs and then he read me letters from sanataria of people who had been away. . . . Dr. Cooper will see him soon and it will be settled. It will be hard for all of us when he goes away. Cousin Charles Rhoads had quite a talk with them. He had called M [mother] before and asked if J needed financial help, which I felt was kind.[13]

Ravdin continued Rhoads' salary during his illness, and Miss Berrang, director of the hospital, did not charge him for the long hospitalization. At the same time Rhoads was diagnosed with TB at the end of the summer of 1946, Terry was pregnant and quite rotund. Rhoads later learned that Ravdin had bet his wife, Betty, a dollar that Terry was carrying twins.

On October 7, while Rhoads was still hospitalized, he received a phone call from the obstetrician, Robert Kimbrough, informing him that Terry was in labor, although the estimated date of delivery was not expected for another 5 or 6 weeks. Rhoads asked how large he thought the baby was, and Kimbrough replied that he wasn't exactly certain but it was large enough to have a good chance for survival. About three hours later, Kimbrough called Rhoads again and told him, with some chagrin, that he was the new father of twins. Each baby was an ounce or two under four pounds, requiring additional hospitalization for a couple of weeks after Terry was discharged. Fortunately, both children survived and matured normally. Kimbrough, who had been the obstetrician for one of President Franklin Roosevelt's grandchildren, was one of the most distinguished men in his field, and he received a certain amount of "good natured comment" from his staff for letting the twins take him by surprise.[14]

Kimbrough wasn't the only one surprised by the birth of the twin boys—Caroline writes to Esther of the family's reaction:

I am almost overcome by twin nephews! Terry is pleased that they are identical. She thinks they can have fun. She seemed fine this afternoon. . . . I fear Grandma Folin will be done out by the children. . . . It's all most exciting. Mother was nearly as excited as Margaret over the twins![15]

Although thrilled by the birth and good health of the twins, Rhoads recalls:

At the age of 39 I was in bed at the University Hospital and had a family of six children. Assuming that I should be responsible for them until each reached the age of 21, I calculated that I had 101 years of minority to provide for.[16]

The twins were named Charles and Philip. Rhoads remembers his first glimpse of them:

I first saw the twins when they were brought from the Pennsylvania Hospital when Dr. Herbert Volk, then an intern, took me down in a wheelchair to see them in their baskets. They were still slightly icteric [jaundiced] and still I suppose only between four and five pounds of weight and about 4½ weeks old.[17]

Another unforeseen medical emergency occurred in the Rhoads family about a month after Jonathan's tuberculosis was discovered. Terry developed a breast lump that was sufficiently suspicious for carcinoma to warrant a biopsy. Adding to this concern was the knowledge that when carcinoma of the breast appeared during pregnancy, the prognosis was dismal. While waiting for the final pathology report of the breast lesion, Rhoads reflected that his own diagnosis of tuberculosis seemed comparatively minor. Fortunately, the lesion turned out to be benign, and she recovered uneventfully.[18]

Terry was actively engaged with family activities during the months Rhoads was hospitalized at Penn. Rhoads recalls:

We had a sort of word game we played. I can't remember whether it was a crossword puzzle or what, but anyhow, after she got the children to bed, she'd call up on the telephone and we kept the phone line open about 30 or 45 minutes and played this game.[19]

Cooper strongly recommended that Rhoads be transferred to a sanitorium specializing in the care of patients with tuberculosis. Rhoads was faced with the dilemma of selecting the sanitorium:

[Cooper] thought I should go away. He said I could go to Saranac or I could go to the southwest. So I got some statistics out and I didn't want to go to Saranac; it's cold up there in winter and I had a friend who was an intern a year ahead of me who landed at Saranac and he told me they put you out on a porch with an electric blanket, and you could stay warm except for your face but your visitors couldn't stand it for over 5 minutes. So it turned out that the choice seemed to be between Phoenix with 1100 feet altitude and Santa Fe at 7000 feet and Albuquerque at

5000 feet. I chose Albuquerque. The Presbyterians ran a TB sanatorium there, and Dr. Cooper arranged for me to go.[20]

Rhoads was admitted to this facility in Albuquerque on January 9, 1947. Writing to Esther shortly after his arrival, he comments:

I do enjoy flying, though 80 pounds of baggage goes such a short distance that I arrived with only 1 book, 2 pairs of pajamas and had to leave the rest of the supplies to come later. . . . The Professor [Ravdin] insists on carrying me along as though I were working so we have no financial problem this year except to save as much as we reasonably can in case things don't go well in the future. . . . Dr. Cooper seemed to think that the x-rays made 2 days before I left were definitely better. I don't know what the x-ray department thought.[21]

He later describes the treatment plan envisioned by Dr. Cooper:

Cooper's plan was for me to stay here 3 months—6 weeks in bed and 6 weeks of getting up and around—then return to Philadelphia. For part of April, May and June, working 2–4 hours a day and then go away and take gradually more exercise in the summer and return to doing a day's work again in the fall.[22]

Rhoads' health began to improve during his stay in Albuquerque. Ravdin and Rhoads frequently wrote to each other. Rhoads writes to Ravdin in January 1947:

All seems to be going well here. Dr. Werner [the physician in charge of Rhoads' care] was once a patient of your father. It seems that he lived in Evansville [Indiana] from 1898 to 1914 and had a submucous resection done about 1914. He recalls seeing you and your brother at the time of the operation. He understood you were at the University of Indiana at the time.[23]

During Rhoads' convalescence, he took correspondence courses in the history and philosophy of education and in educational psychology. While these courses "occupied time," he thought that they were of dubious practical value. He writes of his surroundings at the sanitorium:

We have a ground floor bedroom with 3 windows facing west over a garden toward a cottage. To the S.W. are purple hills and sunsets. There is also a glassed in porch on a N.W. corner from which you can see the mountain (N.E.). We are not far from the airport or from the University of New Mexico. I have a private bath, the meals are good, and I supplement a little as I have a huge appetite despite my 207 pounds.[24]

By January 1947 the twins had tripled their birth weights. Rhoads, describing pictures of them to Esther, remarks:

They look terribly solemn. I hope they are not without joy in their souls but perhaps they are.[25]

Later in the month he writes to Ravdin of his progress:

Yesterday I was surprised and pleased to see the familiar face [Ravdin] in the paper which is enclosed. There has been much more news of Pennsylvania and Philadelphia in the press and the radio here than I expected. . . . The time is passing satisfactorily here and I am continuing on bedrest as at the University Hospital. Sometime this month, Dr. Werner plans to get another x-ray and I will let you know what they have to say about it.[26]

Ravdin, writing to Rhoads, reports on the state of the department:

It seems to me that I am nothing but a traveling salesman these days, but thank God we have enough to do and there is enough coming in to live on. I am sure of one thing, that we will not go to a home for the indigent. Marjorie [Ravdin's secretary] is making a face but I am accustomed to this, for Betty [his wife] has done it for many years. I did have an automobile accident and I still can't get down on my knees, but since I have learned to say my prayers without getting on my knees, I suppose I am all right. . . .

In spite of all of my infirmities I am still going and you need not worry about me. Between Betty and Marje, I am leading a dog's life. They cook up all sorts of things; then each in her sly way begins to pester me. Maybe Marje won't sign this letter for me. . . . Ravdin, Rhoads, Johnson and Company have about seventy-five patients scattered around various parts of the hospital. I am sure that we have over one hundred waiting to come in.[27]

Schwegman describes his added clinical responsibilities during Rhoads' absence:

When Rhoads took ill, I had a double burden because I tried as best I could to maintain his practice for him until he fully recovered. I had, therefore, whatever patients were truly his plus those who were truly mine. That meant that it was sort of double duty.[28]

Ravdin, writing to Rhoads, sets the "rules" for Rhoads' work schedule upon his return to Philadelphia:

I shall ask Dave [Cooper] just how much work you can do when you get home. But I am going to lay the law down now. The night work is and will continue to be done in the main by our juniors. They are doing a good job of it, and you are going to get eight hours sleep a night if I have to lock you up myself. I have decided that for my remaining years I am going to keep the rest of you fellows well and for that reason I am going to dictate the policy of work.[29]

Commenting on Rhoads' latest x-ray results, Ravdin tells him:

You don't know how happy I am that your films are all right, but I really and truly believe that you should not do any work until the first of May. I can't see the slightest sense of your coming back here until the weather is stabilized, for a bad cold at this time is just the worst thing you could get and would set back all of us indefinitely. . . . Terry tells me everything is well at your house so that all you need worry about is getting well.[30]

Many years later Rhoads reflected on being a physician-patient:

A physician learns so much about the psychology of illness by being sick himself. Apart from a variety of minor afflictions, I have been through a mastoidectomy, a tonsillectomy, an appendectomy, pulmonary tuberculosis, removal of a parotid tumor and a supposed subendothelial myocardial infarction. [Later in life he had deep venous thromboses and pulmonary emboli.] While I had the good fortune never to be desperately ill, these meanderings through or near the valley of the shadow of death have done a lot to let me know the kinds of things which go through people's minds when illness is diagnosed.[31]

In May 1947, Rhoads returned to Philadelphia. He writes to Esther regarding his new routine and daily events:

Things here chug along in much the same groove. I work in the mornings mostly at the lab and spend most of the p.m. in bed. Then I am up from about 5–9, eat supper and occasionally take the kids for a short ride. Also I often help make bottles in the pressure cooker. . . .

The time at the lab has been largely engrossed with editorial work. We got one paper straightened out in the proof. . . . A long thesis was gotten into acceptable shape for Koop to get a graduate degree. Zintel and I have just finished a chapter of a book. . . .

Experimentally, I tried out a paper stapler as an instrument to sew intestine together. It works to an extent in animals. I also tried a high pressure paint sprayer, loaded with thrombin solution, to see if it would stop bleeding in surgical wounds, but it doesn't work even with 50 pounds per square inch. A young doctor Poroff is studying adhesions and finding work we did a year & a half ago apparently wrong, so I will probably get into that more next month.

A week ago yesterday, I spent the a.m. in New York with the project committee studying the teaching of social and environmental factors in medicine. There was a wrangle between the lady who wrote the report and some of the medical people who read it. I think we were able to reach a fairly satisfactory compromise. We are also trying to work up a project on the influence of glass on some of the things for which glass containers are used. It seems that a glass company wants to finance it.[32]

Rhoads' condition continued to improve, and he became anxious to return to full-time clinical work. In August 1947, he writes to Ravdin from Kearsarge:

It has been a long time since I have helped a very sick patient get well. It is the most rewarding experience one can have with the possible exception of seeing one of the boys we train turn out well. The latter is less acute but more lasting perhaps.[33]

Rhoads' formal convalescence ended in September, as Ravdin formally discloses to a good number of referring doctors:

I am sure that you will be happy to know that Dr. Jonathan Rhoads has returned and resumed his work with us. He is completely recovered and looks better than I have ever seen him look. I know that you will imagine my personal delight that he is back as a member of the surgical family.[34]

Upon return to full-time work at HUP, Rhoads immediately immersed himself in his characteristic rigorous schedule. As Jack Mackie, Rhoads' colleague and close friend, tells it:

Rounds with Rhoads were sort of a memorable event. Three days a week he would make rounds on the ward service and then go and make rounds on his private service. One of the things he used to do on rounds was to climb up on the roof and get on the ladder and get up on top of the Gates Building and up on the Ravdin Building. Very often he would take the stairway up or down rather than use the elevator. This was purely to take a look at the perspective.[35]

Rhoads liked to operate on Saturdays. For a long time Mackie was the junior staff man on his service. They did a lot of surgery on Saturdays in the White Building, which has windows overlooking Spruce Street. The days were grueling, and Mackie recalls that he lost 30 pounds in one month. Mackie relates:

Many a Saturday in the fall the band would come down Spruce Street to the Stadium and we would hear the crowd cheering and the football going on. Then it would get a little quiet and the band would come back up the street because the game was over, and we were still in the operating room. He loved the Saturday schedule because no one else was in the operating room later in the afternoon. He would take us over to Horn & Hardart's which was over on Woodland. We would go and get something to eat . . . pie or something and then make evening rounds. It was a very full Saturday. He continued that until we couldn't get anyone to work in the operating room on Saturday. I remember one time, it must have been the second year that I was Chief Resident on his service in 1953, and during the summer he had 3 or 4 Whipples [removal of part of the duodenum and part of the pancreas—usually for cancer].[36]

Brooke Roberts, a colleague, had ample opportunity to observe Rhoads in and outside the operating room. In describing an often commented upon aspect of Rhoads' personality, Roberts relates the following story:

Anyone who had known Jonathan for a period of time is impressed with his equanimity. I only once saw Jonathan demonstrate overt annoyance. I think I've known him long enough that I can tell when he's annoyed, whereas somebody who didn't know him might not realize it. I can only recall once. I can't remember the exact condition in the operating room, but everything was going wrong. He had to leave the operating room and put on a new gown or something, and he kicked the operating room door open instead of his quiet shouldering and said, "Oh damn." I think anyone who's ever been in the operating room very much knows the rest of us are not as calm as that.[37]

With his return to full-time academic life, Rhoads resumed his many research projects and collaborations in the Harrison Department. Gibbon developed a heart-lung machine that became a landmark contribution to cardiac surgery. He subsequently returned to Jefferson to become professor of surgery and also became chairman of the editorial board of the *Annals of Surgery*. Rhoads was quite flattered when Gibbon invited him to join the editorial board. In addition, he proposed Rhoads for membership in the Society of Clinical Surgery. Rhoads comments:

When I became a member of it, I must say I almost fell over backwards when I went over the roster of the greats who belonged. So it was a great boost to me.[38]

In the fall of 1947 and into 1948, Rhoads continued to participate actively in numerous research investigations. Studies of adhesion (scar tissue) formation continued with a variety of collaborators, including John Green, then a medical student and later to become chairman of Obstetrics and Gynecology at the University of Kentucky in Lexington. While Green was training in Ob-Gyn, he continued to perform research, and with a colleague Touchstone, they showed the utility of blood estriol measurements in predicting fetal hypoxia.[39] Of note, this important diagnostic test probably saved the life of Rhoads' grandson Thomas, as it was the warning signal that led to an emergency cesarean section. Rhoads writes to Esther:

We are all delighted at the prospect of seeing thee in August. I will be in New Hampshire in July but plan to be here in August. Terry will probably stay at Kearsarge both months with the 4 older children. The twins stay here with Isabella. I have been going to meetings at a rather excessive rate, and I hope to have a relative lull for the next month ending in a great rash of meetings from May 19 to June 12th. It results in getting nothing done—routine plus preparation for meetings. We are trying to raise money for the University, for cancer, for everything else. It is all rather dizzy. So far, my health is supposed to be okay. If I get by one more x-ray, I will have vacation during which I hope to rest.

We are trying to estimate the impact of the new tax laws on our spendable income. I doubt that we are saving as much as we should and no doubt we will regret it someday but we may not. We have tried a few new operations lately which always adds to the interest of life but often to its worry also. Do take care of thyself.[40]

Following the war, both Ravdin and Rhoads became interested in the potential clinical usage of cortisone. Difficult to obtain in large quantities, cortisone was shown to have significant anti-inflammatory effects, especially for arthritis. In an attempt to obtain a potentially abundant source of cortisone for clinical use, Rhoads and Ravdin devised a unique experiment. Archie Fletcher, Rhoads' resident assistant at the time, describes the scene:

It was during my postwar residency years, I believe in '46 or '47. Cortisone had been identified by researchers at the Mayo Clinic as an effective agent in the treatment of arthritis. There was an immediate demand for this substance, which was prepared by a chemical process starting with bile acids obtained from bile in the gall bladders of slaughtered cattle.

THE CHIEF, THE COW, AND THE CORTISONE

Searching for a more constant supply of bile, a pharmaceutical company approached Dr. Ravdin, who was widely known for his contributions to biliary tract surgery and liver function. Dr. Ravdin and Dr. Rhoads speculated that it should be possible to insert a T-tube in the common bile duct of cattle, as was routinely done in the case of human patients, thus obtaining a steady flow of bile.

Dr. Rhoads characteristically took the direct approach to the problem. He arranged with the School of Veterinary Medicine to set up an operation on a cow. He recruited me, a resident on his service at the time, to assist. We gathered some of the largest instruments we could find and headed for the Veterinary School on a blisteringly hot summer day. Our patient was ready, standing calmly beside a large steel table, to which she was then secured while its top was in a vertical position. Intravenous anesthesia was then given and the table top was turned to a horizontal position so that the cow, which now looked very large, was lying on her side ready for the surgeons, though the surgeons weren't quite sure they were ready for her! Already perspiring in the absence of any air conditioning, we stripped off our shirts and got to work.

Dr. Rhoads stood on a stand between the legs of the patient. I climbed up on the table on the opposite side and assumed a kneeling position, reaching across the body of the animal to try to provide some semblance of retraction and exposure. Dr. Rhoads made the incision in what seemed like a reasonable place, but finding the common bile duct amid a huge mass of intestines proved to be a struggle. Sweat was pouring off nose and chin (no masks) into the wound! When we found it, the bile duct seemed remarkably small for such a large animal, but a T-tube was successfully inserted and the wound was closed. We had previously prepared a receptacle for the bile—an inner tube from an auto tire which had been cut across opposite the valve. The open ends were sealed and ropes attached to tie around the body of the cow. The T-tube was then secured to the valve stem to drain the bile into the inner tube.

Amazingly enough the patient survived, but she immediately set about to rid herself of our bile receptacle by rubbing, chewing, kicking or whatever! That was the first problem. The second was that after some analysis of the bile and appropriate calculation, it was apparent that thousands of such operations would be required to provide the quantities of bile needed, not to mention the large ranch which would be needed to maintain all of those T-tube-wearing bovines!

The final blow to the project came a few months later, when chemists came up with a synthesis of cortisone starting with simple chemicals rather than bile acids. Sic transit gloriam! But it was fun while it lasted, and it illustrated Dr. Rhoads' direct approach to the solution of a problem, his willingness to go ahead without waiting for an ideal setup or a lot of fancy equipment, his technical expertise and adaptability, and his sense of humor![41]

Rhoads was acutely aware of the importance of publishing as a prerequisite to advancement in the academic world. Dutch Dyson, reflecting back on his relationship with Rhoads, recounts one such example:

He was great for wanting you to write a paper. When I returned to HUP, Jonathan was all gung ho for me to write a lot of papers and stuff. One of them was on inflammatory bowel disease, Crohn's disease, and he had me look up all of the people at the University Hospital who had Crohn's disease since it was described in 1931 or 32. There were like 22 or something, up to 1948. So I looked them up and Phil Hodes x-rayed them all, got them all back. I thought, well that's nice. I was getting near the end of my residency and I thought that maybe I can get the hell out of here without ever writing the thing.

So anyway we did get the studies done and I went away to Hazleton [Pennsylvania], got busy practicing, and I thought that would be the end of that. No way. Jonathan said, I better come up and see if we can't get something done on that paper. So he came up one Saturday night, and we worked for about an hour or so. My wife was upset because she had prepared a big roast beef dinner. Subsequently, Jonathan and I went through the hospitals in Hazleton, and he looked at what was being done, like he does, and decided that we ought to do some more work on the paper. He said, "You work on it and in a couple of weeks, come down on Sunday and I'll meet you in the hospital and we'll go out to my place and have dinner and finish up on this paper."

So I came down and met him in the Hospital, and I'm to follow him to his house and we're going up West River Drive about 70 miles an hour and a cop stops him and of course me. But somehow he got out of it. I was following in my car, so I don't know exactly what he said and he talked his way out of it, and we finally get to his place in Germantown. It's got a staircase going up with a banister and about half the slots to hold the banister are missing. There must have been thousands of old newspapers stuck under the banister and in the dining room that's sort of separated from the parlor by huge heavy oak doors that you pull across.

So we're working on this paper and once in a while a kid would go zooming through. Jonathan would say, "Boy!" (I always felt he didn't know which one it was.) Anyway, he lived with his two maiden aunts and they must have been about 90 years old and then we all had dinner, roast beef or something. Terry was doing the serving. It was quite an experience, whole day working with him, seeing this house with these huge oak doors that closed off the dining room from the living room. We finally did get the paper done. It was traumatic for me but not Jonathan.[42]

In 1948 Rhoads' mother reached the age of 85 and was living with her two daughters at 43 West Walnut Lane, just a block away from her son's home. The following February, after speaking in San Antonio, Rhoads joined Terry in Mexico City for a brief vacation. Shortly after arriving in Mexico, he received an urgent message that his mother had developed a severe respiratory infection. The Rhoadses flew home immediately, and it was evident that she was terminally ill. Her son was able to tell her that he had been approved for a full professorship. She died on the evening of February 15, 1949, a little over 23 years after the death of his father.

With renewed interest in his alma mater, Haverford College, Rhoads decided to become more involved in the school's administrative activities. The same year, Stanley Yarnall, a member of the Haverford College Board of Managers, invited Rhoads to serve on the Board, an association which continues to the present. His appointment to the board brought Rhoads in contact with Emlen Stokes, chairman of the board, in addition to a succession of remarkable people, many of whom were members of the religious Society of Friends.

In 1963 Rhoads succeeded Stokes as chairman of the board and president of the corporation. He served in this capacity until 1972. During his association with Haverford College (which continues), Rhoads has chaired two major building campaigns, one in the mid-1950s which resulted in the construction of a large field house and a new dormitory. The second campaign chaired by Rhoads raised most of the money for a new science building (Stokes Hall), renovated the old science building to accommodate psychology, and restored a number of buildings to permit a near doubling of student enrollment. As Rhoads explains:

While the Haverford College Board has been rather an expensive club to belong to, I am deeply impressed with the accomplishments of the College. In my judgment, it has a superb faculty, a superb student body, and by and large its alumni have been extremely productive and deeply concerned for human welfare.[43]

Rhoads was able to resume the family custom of spending the month of July in Kearsarge in 1948. During this time considerable political posturing was occurring at HUP, as Ravdin writes to Rhoads:

Nothing much happened at the Medical Board Meeting on July 1st. I merely stuck to our guns saying that we did not have enough space and at the opportune time threw in two or three howitzers and finally succeeded in breaking the meeting up without them doing anything. I went there loaded for I had the number of follow-up patients that we see in the Surgical Out Patient Clinic and reminded Scott and Elsom that they had not counted these. When they were counted, we had the largest outpatient count in the whole hospital, so that was that. . . . Marje tells me that you are building a shack. I can send you a check to have a good carpenter do it if you would like to have a permanent dwelling place. . . . I hope you and Terry are having a good rest.[44]

In 1951 the family moved to 131 West Walnut Lane in Germantown. Caroline writes to Esther of the move:

Well—131 W. Walnut Lane is now inhabited by 8 Rhoadses and Isabella. Mrs. Folin moves in on 2/20. They moved Thursday and Friday—2 huge vans each day. It was very cold. Terry stood in the cold and is tired, but has born up well.[45]

And Jonathan writes to Esther:

131 West Walnut Lane.

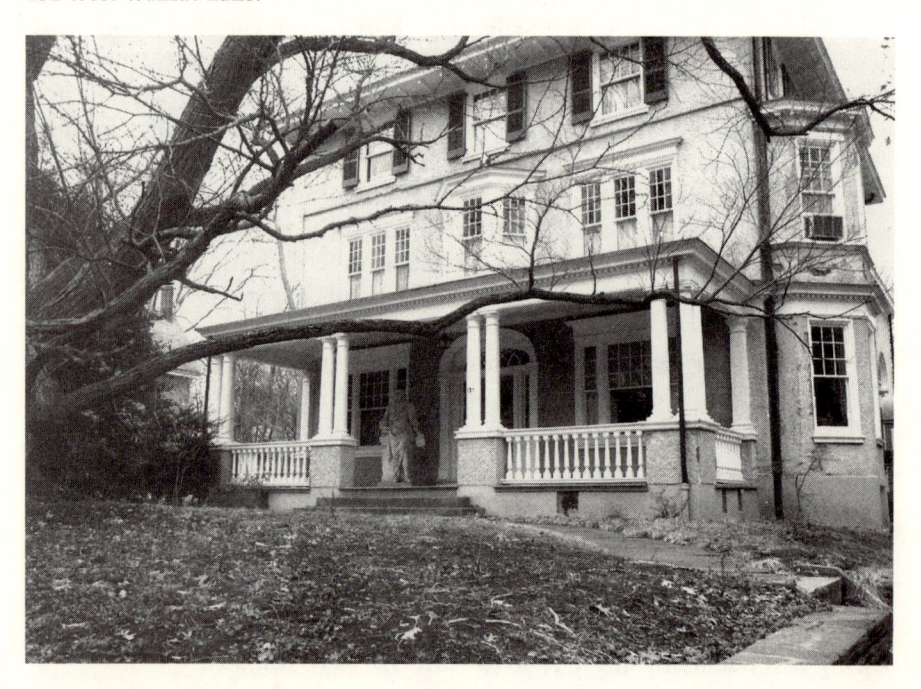

Thank thee for thy letter of 2/22/51. The furniture seems to fit in pretty well, I think. We have M. Ladd's dining table with OWP's chairs (done over) and the Mickle Dresden china in somebody else's china closet— our own buffet and the Folin table for the children and a Japanese telephone table all in the dining room. No doubt other rooms are equally mixed. We left a bed, bedside table, a few chairs, 2 or 3 rugs, a day bed, 3 plants, a desk & clothing bedding and such food as can be stored without refrigeration at 4023 Pine so that I can spend a night there if I have to go back to the hospital late. So far, I have spent one night (in about 3 weeks). We have not taken any definite steps to sell the Pine Street houses but would be open to an offer, I guess.

Speaking of life in general, he continues to write to Esther:

Life is a round of committee & other meetings and arranging for the same. I operate some 3 days week or more and see patients 3 times a week in the office and daily in the hospital. We have the students an average of 4–5 hours per week. This week we entertained some of the research brass from Washington United States Public Health Service, and the National Research Council and Defense Dept. all day Thursday. The week before we staged an all day entertainment for the Detroit Academy of Surgery. Next week we have the College of Surgeons 3 days and the week after 2 days in Washington DC on the burn committee.[46]

At the end of the war, Terry Folin had left her position as a pediatrician at Children's Hospital and devoted all of her time to raising the couple's 6 children. They had agreed that the children would be raised in the Quaker religion and attend Quaker schools and camps in the summer. His daughter Margaret comments on the religious views of her parents:

He [Father] has always gone to meeting. The general pattern of the family was that he would go to meeting if he could. My mother was not a Friend and she did not wish to be. She supported him and she would drive us out to Sunday School, then we would all go to dinner. She was not an atheist. She would always bring up the idea of the wonder of new life being created. I think there was something about the Quaker community that was a little too heavy . . . a little bit too sure of itself, and she just wanted to distance herself from it. I was a birthright member because when the Meeting members came to the house, she agreed that the children should be brought up as birthright Friends.[47]

Reflecting on the Quaker belief that "God is in every man," his son Edward says:

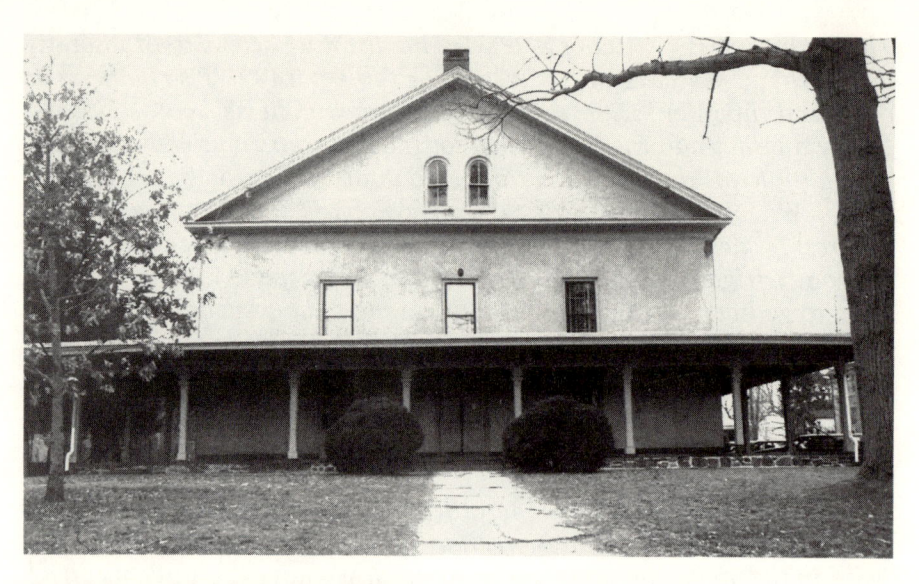

Germantown Friends Meeting House.

It shapes your way of thinking and dealing with people. Father has been very good about dealing with people all of his life.[48]

Although Dr. Rhoads rarely spoke directly to his children regarding religious matters, he did make it clear that he would not bear arms. It was evident early on that the Quaker way of life was an integral part of his existence.

David Stokes, a Quaker and friend, remembers Dr. Rhoads and his family at the meeting house:

My earliest recollections were at Germantown Meeting. As I recall, the Rhoads family entered the meeting house from the west side, and the Stokes from the east. So his imposing figure was an early memory. Later his sons added to the weight of their arrival.[49]

Sunday has always been an important day in the Rhoads family. After Meeting, Jonathan and the children would return home and, along with relatives, friends, and neighbors, would sit down for their traditional Sunday supper. Edward relates:

This was the time to bring everyone together and to share both family stories and outside information. . . . My aunts and my father would occasionally get out the ancestor books and track back who was who.[50]

When he was in town, Rhoads would set aside Sunday especially for his children. He loved to take them to the zoo, local museums, the

Wissahickon Park, and to the airport to watch the airplanes take off. The children didn't see a lot of their father during the week but were able to share a special time with him late in the evening. His son George comments:

People talk about quality time. He was very good at that. He didn't have huge amounts of time, but he spent it well and he enjoyed us and we enjoyed him, and he has always had a wonderful sense of humor which he shared within the family as well as in his professional life.[51]

On a typical weeknight, after the children and their mother had dinner, a full plate of food would be set on a pot of boiling water so that their father could enjoy a hot meal at the end of the day. After he had his dinner, the children and their father would enjoy what came to be known as G-D (general drink) time. They gathered at the dinner table, drank ginger ale, ate cookies or pretzels, and discussed the highlights of the day. They maintained this tradition through their college years. Following G-D time, Jonathan and Terry would go through the day's mail and then turn to one of their mutual interests, the stock market. As Margaret explains,

My mother was very astute at the stock market. She paid a lot of attention to the stocks. When my father would come home they would compare the prices of various things. I think it goes with the game playing and the very sharp mind that she had. My father said recently that she turned in a profit every year.[52]

On some nights, their father would come home, read the newspaper, "attack" the mail, and very often would dictate but more often write his letters in long hand.

The children remember their mother as a generous person, who was a talented musician and juggler. She liked to play the piano and the harmonica. She also was a very talented bridge player. Although a very good athlete, Terry had very little physical stamina through her child-bearing years and indeed for the rest of her life. She had a strong personality and could be very spontaneous. According to her son George,

She was always doling out money to the neighborhood people and children who were less fortunate. Although Jonathan did not overwhelmingly approve of this practice, he tolerated it. . . . She had sort of a spontaneity about helping people without thinking about all of the logistic consequences that he didn't quite share. But he put up with it. As you have probably been told, they are still supporting a homeless man who lives on the porch of the house in Germantown. . . . Jonathan has carried that particular thing along sort of in her memory.[53]

She was never rattled by a crisis, as her son Charles recalls:

My mother could always deal with a crisis. My twin brother and I flew a lot of model airplanes, and we had a test bench on the back porch to put the engines on and run the engines. My brother was out there and he reached over the top to twiddle the carburetor, and as he did the propeller, which was running at better than 800 miles an hour at the tip, snapped off the engine and hit him right in the eyebrow at a distance of a foot or two.

Our house is laid out where the laundry is on one side of the cellar stairs and the kitchen is on the other. . . . It's sort of like a little horseshoe. My brother yelled when the propeller hit him. My mother was standing at the sink out of view and my brother came walking in the back door with his eyebrow cut open an inch or two and he was a sheet of blood coming through the door. My mother was walking up to him coming the other way. "Can you see out of that eye?" she said. He said, "I can see fine." She said, "Well, bleed in the sink."[54]

Life in the Rhoads' household was quite informal. Margaret says that her mother would "vacillate between looking wonderful in fancy dresses and going around the house in a pajama top."[55] Her very good friend and neighbor, Ann Van Gobes, said it was not unusual to walk into the house to find Terry washing the dishes and the maid playing the piano.[56]

The parents, according to the children, had a very good relationship. Margaret describes their interaction:

My mother had a strong personality. . . . Whereas everyone deferred to my father, my father deferred to my mother. She loved him enormously and we always knew that she didn't put up with anything. She would keep him waiting. . . . She would correct how he held his fork. She would tell him to stand up straight.[57]

In addition to sharing an interest in the stock market, they shared another interest. Margaret describes her parents' driving habits:

He was never a slow driver, and he always watched out for the cops. My mother was a fast driver sometimes. When Adam and I were married, she took Adam's mother on a drive and said, "Let's see what this car can do," and took it up to 100 miles an hour. She had a strong sense of playfulness.[58]

Charles remembers talking to his mother about one of the high-performance cars his father got from General Motors:

She responded, "The sooner he gets rid of that car the better." She had ridden in it with him and he had stomped on the gas and the car went from zero to 60 in seven seconds. It would absolutely fly.[59]

Terry and Jonathan did not agree politically—she was a Democrat and he a Republican. He often said that they simply canceled out each other's votes.

Family finances were also important. Jonathan's mother, who lived nearby, kept savings' books for the children and would show them their balances on Sundays. Jack recalls that his father insisted on being careful with money:

He was very clear that if I went out to buy something, I should give him the correct change. If I spent the change on something else, that was a no-no. If something cost $4.50, he would expect 50¢ back.[60]

When the children turned 15, they were given checking accounts and a clothing allowance. Money, according to Margaret, was always adequate, and there was plenty of money for their education. At one point, Jonathan said to one of his sons:

One of the reasons that the family has done so well is that your mother never had any desire to spend money for the sake of spending it.[61]

In addition to their parents, the children were strongly influenced by their grandmothers and aunts. Margaret remembers her paternal grandmother as very nice and kind. Of her maternal grandmother, who was living with the family, she says:

She was a great influence on all of us. She was a very intellectual person and we could go into her room and you could talk about the news. . . . You could talk about interesting things. You had to be quiet when the news was on.[62]

Their Aunt Caroline took a special interest in the children and was a strong influence in their upbringing.

The children were encouraged to do well in school. Their parents supported their decisions regarding their choices of schools and later their careers. Although their father very often did not give them specific advice, he did encourage them to go for the best. According to George,

He said get into the best places. . . . Get to know the best people. He really gave me a sense that you shouldn't sell yourself short, and I think that was a piece of advice which was offered to me in a very nice way.

Reflecting on his father's personality, George says:

He approached everything with apparent equanimity. Like many leaders he had the ability to synthesize what needs to be done quite quickly and enunciating clearly and gets it done . . . like who's going to ride in which car or to arrange a dinner in some meetings that have to be interdigitated. He's quite efficient in pulling those kind of things together without making people angry about it for the most part.[63]

After the war, when gasoline rationing was lifted, the family traditionally spent two months of their summers at their mother's home in Kearsarge. Dr. Rhoads took his vacation in July, and Mrs. Rhoads would stay until the end of August with the children and their babysitter and maid, Isabella. Margaret remembers that her mother wrote to her father almost every day in August. They enjoyed hiking up the nearby mountains, swimming in the local lake, and taking day trips to nearby towns.

The family lived very simply there. The house was small, with a bedroom, sun porch, living room, and dining room. There was only cold water, and they had a wood-burning stove in the kitchen. There was no shower or bath, and the children would take "great pride" in never having to take a bath all summer long. The family would routinely get

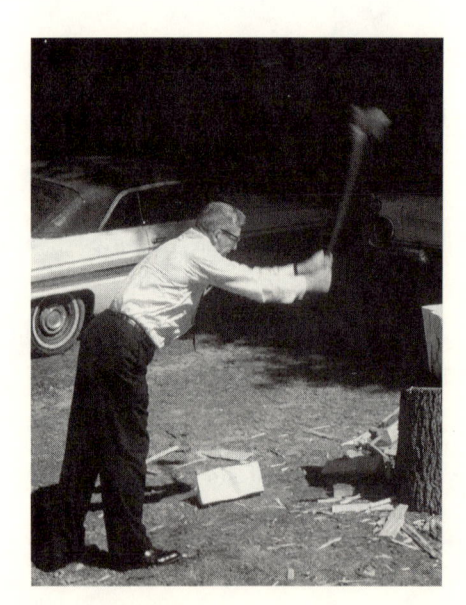

Jonathan Rhoads chopping wood at the summer home in New Hampshire.

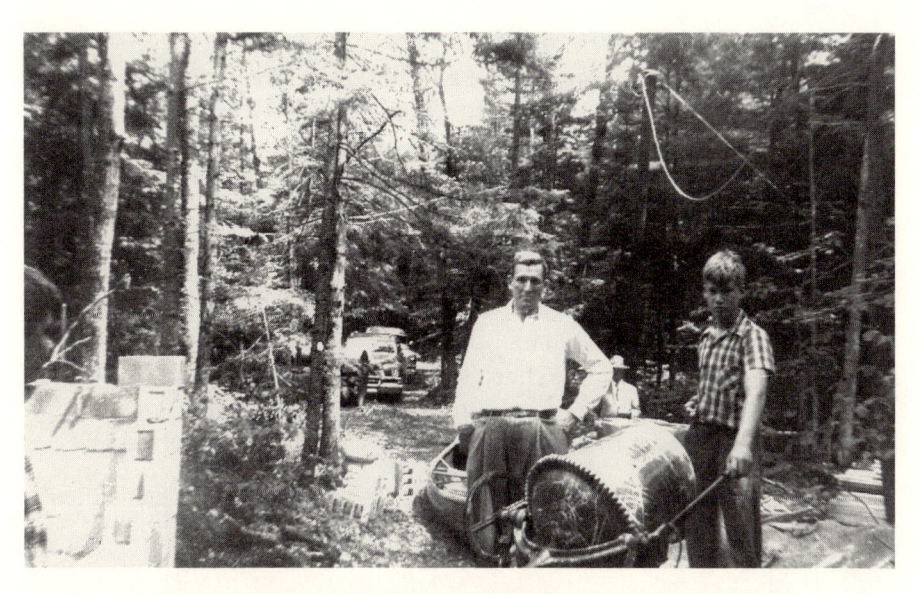

Jonathan Rhoads and his son Jack building the home near Conway Lake.

up in the morning, have breakfast, then go to town to get the day's supplies. They ate their main meal in the middle of the day, after which the children stayed in their beds until 3 o'clock. Later, they went swimming in the nearby lake, and in the evenings they played games.

After a few days, Dr. Rhoads invariably became restless. Margaret observes of her father:

He loves a sense of accomplishment . . . and if he can do something, he will do what he wants to do. He will often say to me, "If something is worth doing, it's worth doing badly. You should not do something because you feel you can't do it to perfection; you should just go ahead.". . . and he has done this. Of course, he is such a talented person that most of the things he does, he does so very well. But he just likes to do things. He combines it with a quiet calm. . . . He always has in his mind what's coming next. Yet he has it very well timed and very well measured, and so he doesn't usually appear to hurry you if he is speaking with you and I think he does that with everybody. He doesn't appear to be in a terrible hurry and yet he is always moving.[64]

To relieve his restiveness, their father planned building projects with his oldest sons. The first summer they built a dog house. In the following summers they built a small house with no plumbing. They later added a porch, and then a few years later, Jonathan bought some lake-front property on nearby Conway Lake and built a concrete block house on it. George describes their time together:

I still remember my brother Jack and I would drive down every day in the morning on the lake front property. . . . I must have been 14 or 15. . . . We suffered the mosquitoes together, and we dug the trenches and laid in the concrete blocks. There was a Pepsi Cola bottling plant on the way, so we bought an old refrigerator and took it down there, and father would buy soft drinks by the case and we would drink them up as we did this work. . . . I have very fond memories of it.[65]

One summer, Jonathan took his younger sons, Edward, Philip and Charles, on a trip out west. The plan was to see all of the national parks in two weeks. Edward and Charles drove in the family station wagon from Philadelphia to Denver, where they met their father and brother Philip, who had flown in the previous day. According to Charles,

We traveled all through the national parks in a clockwise loop, stopping for the model airplane contest in the Los Angeles Naval Air Station. We saw Blue Boy *at the Huntington Museum in Pasadena and we visited Whittier College, and of course we saw all of the national parks without missing any of them. . . . The trip was a great success.*[66]

Edward comments on his father's approach to travel:

We did 13,000 miles in 35 days. We did a lot of windshield driving but we saw a lot. He likes to travel like that. He likes to get overviews. He doesn't like to spend a long time in any one place. Keeps moving all of the time. He still does that.[67]

Although their father was frequently absent during their early years, the children remember the many lasting gifts their father passed on to them—honesty, dealing fairly with people, a good sense of humor, respect for people, and good clear analytical thinking.

In 1954, Rhoads was approached by Dr. Carl Moyer to assist with the preparation and editing of a new and innovative textbook of surgery, *Surgery: Principles and Practice*. This book would ultimately become a major accomplishment in his career and a source of pride and academic recognition for the Department of Surgery at Penn. Moyer was asked to lead this effort as the result of his previous participation in a similar type of multi-edited textbook of medicine.

The timing for the publication of such a book was propitious, inasmuch as many surgeons were completing post-World War II training programs and were eager to learn of the many new advances in surgery. Many of the existing textbooks of surgery were single-authored and somewhat outdated. The relatively new approach of delegating responsibilities within a large text to several individuals to either write or arrange for authorship of their respective sections was an innovative concept. A world-renowned editorial consultant, Morris Fishbein, the editor-in-chief of the *Journal of the American Medical Association*, was obtained as a consultant, and he overwhelmingly approved of the book. Moyer was internationally known for his work on fluid resuscitation, especially in burn patients. A considerable amount of this work was done at the Southwestern Medical School in Dallas, in conjunction with a very young surgeon named Thomas Shires who subsequently became world-renowned in this area in his own right. At the time of Moyer's initiation of the book, he was chairman of the Department of Surgery at Washington University in St. Louis.

Henry Harkins and J. Garrott Allen were selected as co-editors in addition to Rhoads. Harkins was initially on the faculty of the University of Chicago. He wrote a considerable amount on the treatment of burns, and his work was highly regarded. Rhoads recalls a number of Harkins' idiosyncrasies:

Harkins was determined to become a chairman, and he continually carried a card in his pocket on which he listed the Chairmen of the Surgery Departments in the United States due to retire soon. He was named the first Chair at the University of Washington.[68]

J. Garrott Allen was the remaining editor of the book. Allen came from a distinguished academic surgical background at the University of Chicago. Later, he became chairman of the Department of Surgery at Stanford. Rhoads knew Allen for several years prior to the development of this book. Allen was highly regarded for his research on the association between hepatitis and blood transfusions. He was one of the first individuals to demonstrate that the hepatitis virus could be transferred by the sharing of needles among drug addicts. Allen was very knowledgeable about ionizing radiation, and he was one of the initial members of the Manhattan project.[69]

The book was conceived and written in an interesting way. The four editors and their families were invited to the Stead Resort in Colorado at the publisher's expense. The mornings and early evenings were dedicated to writing, and the afternoons were free for family activities.

The book was published in 1957, and it was an immediate success. It included 50 chapters written by 32 contributors and contained 1447 pages. Rhoads singularly authored five chapters and co-authored two others.

The first chapter, titled "Surgical Philosophy" and authored by the co-editors, provided sage advice:

One must spend time in listening to patients and to their relatives, and in trying to perceive and to understand their reactions. Considerable native modesty and a strong liking for people are most helpful. It is also extremely important to know something of one's self. When one's inner hackles rise in irritation or anger, it is time to turn one's attention inward and to try to understand the why and the wherefore before giving vent to such feelings in remarks to the patient.[70]

One of the most important reasons for the enduring success of the book was its emphasis upon the science of surgery. This relatively new concept of surgical science pervaded the contents, including both operative and perioperative topics. The text was perpetuated editorially by James Hardy, a trainee and colleague of Rhoads.

In addition to the monumental task of editing a major surgical textbook, Rhoads actively pursued one of his long goals—of devising a method of feeding patients who could not ingest sufficient nutrients by mouth.

> Jonathan was a man not content with the accoutrements or vestments of honors, achievements and professorship. He took off his suit, donned his scrub clothes, rolled up his sleeves, and delved into the blood and guts, not only of surgical care to alleviate suffering, but of science, to advance knowledge.... The world owes this advance [intravenous feeding] to Jonathan Rhoads. It was one of his several peaks. Just as the loftiness of peaks in a mountain range rise as you recede from the range and can see them in perspective, so also this advance of Jonathan's has become clearly more and more preeminent as the years have passed.
>
> Francis D. Moore[1]

SEVEN

THOUGHT FOR FOOD
NUTRITIONAL RESEARCH AND THE DISCOVERY OF INTRAVENOUS HYPERALIMENTATION

The discovery of intravenous hyperalimentation by Jonathan Rhoads and his colleagues at the University of Pennsylvania has been acknowledged as one of the most important medical contributions of the 20th century. Perhaps this contribution might have been foreshadowed by Rhoads' first publication, co-authored with Ravdin and entitled "The Importance of the Knowledge of Biochemistry to the Surgeon."[2] Intravenous hyperalimentation (I.V.H.), currently known as total parenteral nutrition (T.P.N.), is the method whereby either maintenance nutrients or supranormal (hyperalimentation) amounts of carbohydrate, fat, protein, minerals, and vitamins are administered intravenously through a catheter inserted into a central vein with rapid blood flow. Recalling how the term *intravenous hyperalimentation* evolved, Dr. Rhoads relates:

> We initially called this total parenteral feeding method "intravenous hyperalimentation," stressing the fact that we were not seeking to attain simply nitrogen equilibrium but were trying to give a substantial nutrient surplus to correct preexisting deficits.[3]

For example, more nitrogen must be taken in (i.e., positive nitrogen balance) than excreted for general tissue repair to take place. Today this feeding method is used worldwide in malnourished patients who are unable to take in adequate amounts of nutrients, either by mouth or by tube feeding into the intestine. Patients in need of I.V.H. include those with severe intestinal diseases, critical illness, major trauma, cancer requiring adjuvant treatment, and congenital malformations of the intestine.

The life-saving effect of I.V.H. is perhaps best illustrated in the patient with short bowel syndrome, a condition characterized by significant diarrhea and depletion of body weight due to loss of most of the small intestine. Prior to the discovery of I.V.H. almost every patient with short bowel syndrome would die during the immediate postoperative period if he or she could not absorb sufficient nutrients. Moreover, it was common for surgeons not to remove the extensively damaged or dead intestine because of the uniformly fatal prognosis of short bowel syndrome and the prolonged suffering associated with the malnutrition-induced death. Currently, most patients with this condition can survive with total or partial intravenous feeding, usually administered at home. Many of these patients are weaned from I.V.H. when the remaining intestine grows and increases its absorptive capacity.

The clinical availability of I.V.H. is yet another example of an "overnight" medical discovery following at least 50 years of intensive basic and clinical research. In fact, to identify some of the earliest investigations in intravenous feeding at HUP one has to review the research in the early 1900s. Glucose solutions were sufficiently pure to permit intravenous administration; however, their infusion was frequently associated with high fevers.

One of the earliest uses of intravenous glucose solutions at Penn was for patients with hyperthyroidism. In the 1920s, hyperthyroidism due to Graves disease was of concern to surgeons because of its very high postoperative morbidity and mortality. Dr. Charles Frazier and I.S. Ravdin began to use iodine and continuous intravenous glucose solutions during the operative and postoperative period because they believed that the hyperthyroid patients who received intravenous glucose had an improved outcome and had less tendency to develop thyroid crises than their non-intravenously-fed counterparts. These findings were based more on clinical impressions than scientific measurements.

Rhoads recalls giving intravenous glucose solutions during his internship at HUP in 1932:

My first duty was to give intravenous infusions of glucose solutions each afternoon to a young woman with pernicious vomiting of pregnancy. I

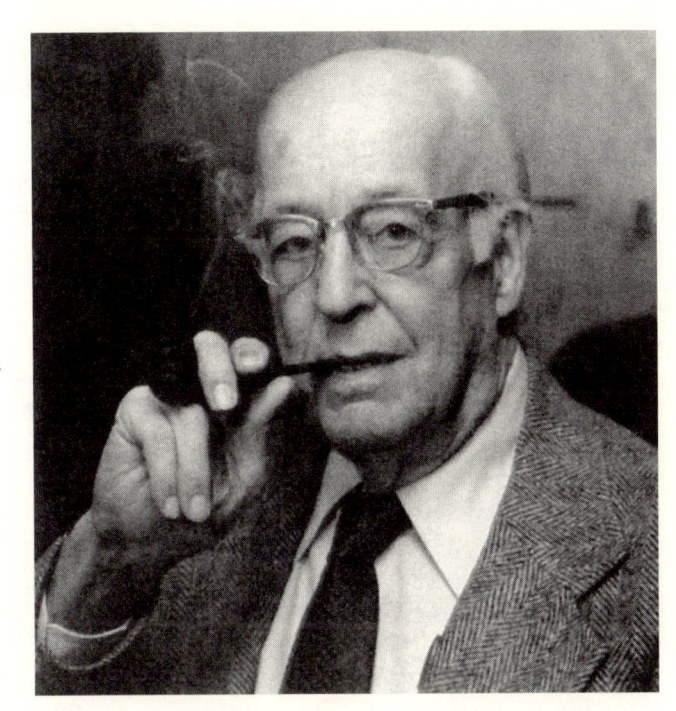

Dr. Harry Vars.

was warned to give the solutions slowly or she might develop "speed shock" and have a chill. This she did on some occasions.

Our practice was to run 1000 cc of 5% or 10% glucose into an arm vein in 45 minutes to an hour. So-called speed shock was probably due to allowing microorganisms to settle in the drops of the flask that we used to hold the solution before they were sterilized. The cause had been identified by Florence Seibert, working at the University of Pennsylvania at the Phipps Institute. She was trying to develop a better tuberculin. She got some unexpected febrile reactions which she tracked back to organisms in the Schuylkill River [the source of water for Philadelphia]. Although the bacteria were dead, their components induced sharp febrile reactions.

It took a number of years for this truth to permeate the medical community, but bit by bit the increased use of intravenous solutions attracted enough interest from the manufacturing pharmaceutical companies so that we could give up making them in our own central dressing room and purchase them from companies that could make them under much better controlled conditions.[4]

With the pyrogenic problem largely solved, the use of intravenous solutions increased rapidly in the late 1920s and early 1930s. Those solutions found suitable in addition to glucose were fructose, sodium chloride, Ringer's solution, and various modifications such as Hartmann's solution.

Ravdin and Rhoads were the dominant forces bringing I.V.H. to its fruition beginning in the 1920s and extending to the mid-1970s. Each of these individuals was keenly aware of the importance of nutrition in the successful management of surgical patients. Every Ravdin-trained resident recalls his pronouncement: "If I can feed the patient and he or she does not have a fatal or terminal illness, I can get them home." While continuing to espouse Ravdin's dictum, Rhoads was determined to devise a way to feed the patient unable to ingest sufficient nutrients by mouth.

Ravdin was one of the first surgeons in the United States to identify the important association between malnutrition and adverse postoperative outcome. In a review article published in the 1950s, he summarizes the important role of nutrition in the overall management of the surgical patient:

The surgeon has some unique opportunities as an applied nutritionist in that his material often comes to him in a depleted condition. He is often presented with, or produces, the stress phenomena in their most pronounced state; many of his patients have gastrointestinal disturbances which complicate their feeding; and he has a unique preoccupation with wound healing. In these situations, nutrition may well make the difference between success and failure.[5]

The logical extension of these observations was to devise a means whereby malnourished surgical patients could be artificially nourished. Despite not having the means to correct preoperative nutritional deficits or administer adequate amounts of nutrients in the postoperative setting, Ravdin and colleagues conducted investigations in the 1920s and 1930s that set the stage for further nutritional interventional studies. Ravdin brought to the attention of surgeons throughout the world several new observations. He identified the adverse effects of nutritional status produced by the preoperative condition and, in some instances, exacerbated by the surgical procedure. Most importantly, he emphasized the importance of specific nutrient deficits, especially protein, on adverse postoperative outcome.

Ravdin also noted that it was important to provide nutrition even after the initial catabolic (operation-induced stress) response had subsided. Ravdin, Rhoads, and their colleagues investigated the effects of malnutrition on liver disease, postoperative gastric emptying, wound healing, cortisone therapy, and the requirements of vitamins D and K.

Ravdin began a series of studies on the physiology and chemistry of bile formation, which has been described by Cooper.[6] Briefly, in collaboration with Cecelia Riegel, a biochemist who worked full-time in the Department of Surgery, and Charles Johnston, a young surgeon on Ravdin's service, Ravdin performed investigations on the effects of anesthesia and surgery on bile formation. These early studies focused on nutrient-induced composition of bile and factors leading to the formation of gallstones.[7]

Commensurate with the work at Penn on nutrition and bile formation, chemists at the Merck Chemical Company synthesized a new anesthetic agent, divinyl ether. Ravdin became very interested in this anesthetic because it was quick acting and easier to administer than ethyl ether. If it was given with ample amounts of oxygen, it could be used for up to 3 hours. If there was insufficient oxygen, liver damage would occur fairly soon after delivery of the anesthetic.

In the early 1930s, a human tragedy had occurred which led to a series of investigations at Penn. The wife of a top executive of Merck died of hepatic failure after being anesthetized with divinyl ether for an elective operation. This prompted Merck to investigate why divinyl ether caused liver damage and whether it was an unsafe anesthetic. To perform these investigations, Merck provided a young investigator-chemist, William Ruigh, to work at Penn in collaboration with Drs. Ravdin, Riegel, Samuel Goldschmidt (professor of physiology), and Bauldin Lucke. This work was performed at Penn because the dean, A.N. Richards, who also served as a member of the board of directors of the Merck Chemical Company, recognized that Ravdin had extensive knowledge of hepatic physiology and pathology in addition to postoperative liver disease.

It became apparent that more nutritional biochemical expertise was needed. After the start of the Penn-Merck investigations, Ravdin approached Samuel Goldschmidt, who contacted his former boss, world-renowned chemist Professor Lafayette Mendel, and mentioned that Ravdin was looking for a nutritional biochemist. Mendel suggested Harry Vars, one of his previous postdoctoral research fellows, who was working at Princeton with Professor Swingle to purify the physiologically active components of adrenalcortical extracts. As the Depression worsened, funds for research salaries decreased, and it became apparent that the research activity of the Princeton group could not continue at the previous level. Vars decided to pursue the position at Penn. At the Federation of the American Societies of Experimental Biology (FASEB) meeting in the spring of 1934, Goldschmidt and Ravdin met Harry Vars at breakfast, and it was agreed that Vars would come to Penn and join their group as soon as he finished his remaining work at Princeton. Vars arrived at Penn in June 1934.

Although not working with Vars directly after his arrival, Rhoads expresses his fond memories of Vars:

Harry Vars came out of the midwest, possibly Illinois, although he was in Colorado for his undergraduate education. He married the niece of the man who saved the earlier President Johnson from being impeached. Harry and his wife had two boys and a girl. Harry went to Yale for his Ph.D. under Mendel. After that he got a job at Princeton with Swingle, who was studying the shock-like syndrome of adrenalectomized animals.

Vars came to Penn as a biochemist in the Surgical Department in the mid-1930's. He had a joint appointment in Biochemistry and Surgery, but he was paid from the Surgical Department. He was a mine of information and a great gadgeteer. He read constantly and retained what he read remarkably well, and he had a small office that was just jammed full of information, and he knew where he could put his hand on it. A very unselfish man, his name appeared on papers but not usually as the first author.

Vars' older boy became a forester and his daughter married a forester. The younger boy, Jonathan, went into the conflict in Vietnam and became a helicopter pilot to pick up casualties. He flew many missions. His helicopter was hit by bullets on two trips and the third time he was killed. His name is on the Vietnam Memorial in Washington, D.C. He left behind a daughter to whom Harry was deeply devoted. Vars did not believe in the War and he was devastated by the death of his son.[8]

Years later, Rhoads operated on Vars' wife, and she subsequently developed a postoperative wound infection. Rhoads recounted that "Vars made the point that it was about time that the hospital get plastic bags to put their dirty linens in instead of tossing them in the wastebasket. It was a few years before that reform came to pass but it did."[9] Vars died of colon cancer at the age of 80. During his recovery from palliative surgery he was given intravenous hyperalimentation. He was honored by the American Society of Parenteral and Enteral Nutrition (A.S.P.E.N.) when their highest research award was created in his name. At a memorial service for Vars on December 1, 1983, Rhoads comments:

Harry had many distinctions and one or two foibles. He became a Fellow of the American Institute of Nutrition of which there are, I believe, only 75 in the United States. He was asked to come back to the University of Colorado to receive their alumni Norlin Award. Another distinction is that he was one of a very small group of people worldwide who was struck by lightning and survived.[10]

The contributions of Harry Vars to the Harrison Department of Surgical Research and subsequently to the discovery of intravenous hyperalimentation are legendary. Similar to researchers today, the investigators were under a considerable amount of pressure, and the investigations did not always proceed smoothly. Moreover, Vars developed somewhat ambiguous feelings concerning Ravdin, as noted in an interview in 1983:

Working with Dr. Ravdin was like working with the weather. It was sweet and lovely one minute and it was the world's worst hurricane the next minute.[11]

Despite these observations and buoyed by their initial findings of nutrient-induced protective effects in the liver, Vars, Goldschmidt, and Ravdin in 1935 began studies on the effects of glucose intake on hepatic glycogen (a form of stored carbohydrate) deposition in the liver. These studies provided the foundation for subsequent nutritional interventions. The investigators noted that both glucose and amino acids were important in the body's response to injury. Moreover, the concomitant provision of these nutrients decreased the anesthetic-induced liver damage and prevented fat infiltration into the liver.[12]

As the result of Ravdin's increasing interest in protein nutrition, investigations were performed in 1938 by Vars and Alfred Stengel to determine the effect of hypoproteinemia (decreased protein levels in the blood) on liver function. An important result of these studies was the discovery of a method to deliver nutrients intravenously to dogs for prolonged periods of time. Vars devised a method (later to be a key component of the early I.V.H. studies) in which infusions could be administered to animals while allowing them to ambulate. To simulate normal conditions, the animals were given as much freedom of movement as possible. Vars created a special swivel carrier to contain the intravenous tubing, and the carrier was connected to a plaster collar to retain the catheter in the internal jugular vein. This permitted the animal to stand, recline, and turn around in the cage without obstructing the intravenous line or creating major difficulties. Throughout the experiments urine was collected to measure nitrogen losses, and dogs were catheterized at suitable intervals without difficulty. Blood samples were taken daily without inconvenience. Intravenous infusions were administered at rates of 25 milliliters per hour to as high as 60 milliliters per hour. The infusion apparatus was easily sterilized, and sterility of the infusions was maintained for the duration of the experiments.

Despite encouraging successes, these early infusion experiments in dogs were not without problems. Infusions were often short-lived because the catheters became dislodged and the plastic collar slipped around the dog's neck, and the rate of fluid administration was variable as the result of inaccurate infusion pumps.

Ravdin was one of the first surgeons in the world to recognize the clinical importance of visceral edema due to protein deficits in patients with gastrointestinal diseases.[13] Edema in prisoners ("prison edema" due to improper feeding and ensuing hypoproteinemia) was known in Europe, and diffuse edema in protein-deficient children (kwashiorkor) had been identified in developing countries before 1900. Ravdin hypothesized that the tissue edema that develops around a bruise, cut, or injury might be the cause for the failure of gastroenterostomies (the surgical connection between the stomach and small intestine, which commonly was performed in the 1930s and 1940s for patients with obstruction of the stomach due to peptic ulcer disease) to open expeditiously.

Ravdin recruited Robert Barden, a resident in radiology, who worked under Eugene Pendergrass, chairman of the Department of Radiology at Penn. He also recruited Paul Mecray, the son of a Camden (New Jersey) surgeon, who was able to work solely in the laboratory for one year. Ravdin and colleagues created "nutritional edema" in the dog by using the technique of George Whipple of Rochester, New York. Whipple subsequently shared the Nobel Prize with Minot and Murphy for the work in pernicious anemia. Whipple and his associates created a model of nutritional edema that consisted of administering a nearly protein-free (1%) diet combined with plasmaphoresis (removal of the major protein component of the blood) for 5 weeks. When the protein level in the blood fell from approximately 6 grams (the normal level in the dog) to 3.5 grams (the level at which tissue edema occurs in the dog), the emptying time of the stomach was prolonged from 1 hour to 6 hours.[14]

With this preparation, animals with either newly created or well-healed gastroenterostomies had very slow gastric emptying as measured by the progress of a barium meal. Surprisingly, not only was this true with a fresh gastroenterostomy, it was also true in the unoperated stomach. Additionally, the time it took barium to leave the stomach and reach the cecum was also prolonged. Indeed, the hypothesis was proven to be correct. The protein depletion-induced edema prolonged transit of contents throughout the intestine and delayed the emptying of contents out of the stomach. When the dogs were placed back on a protein-repleted diet or their plasma protein was reinfused, the intestinal dysfunction returned to normal.

As so often happens in research, an unexpected outcome occurred in these studies. A number of the dogs investigated for the effect of hypoproteinemia on gastric emptying also developed ruptured abdominal wall wounds, presumably due to protein malnutrition. Rhoads remembers these animals:

Some of the animals recently operated upon had wound disruptions. One would come back and find the bowel protruding through the abdominal wound. We had not run into this previously in the laboratory. So we did not believe it was due to a change in surgical technique.[15]

This was indeed a new observation, and it led promptly to studies on wound healing. Ravdin recruited a different team to pursue the wound healing studies. They rendered the dogs hypoproteinemic using Whipple's method and carefully investigated the changes in the histologic composition of the wound. Some of the wounds were almost totally depleted of fibroblasts (the cells which make collagen), a key component of wound healing.

Despite some of the hypoproteinemic animals probably having vitamin C deficiency as well, the mechanism of wound disruption in the hypoproteinemic model appeared to be quite different from the widely publicized vitamin-C-deficient animals investigated by Womack in Boston. Womack identified the defect in wound healing as a failure of fibroblasts to produce collagen. The investigations by Ravdin and coworkers revealed that the decreased protein intake resulted in marked interference with fibroplasia—the process by which the fibrous tissue is actually made.[16]

Rhoads investigated the effects of various stages of hypoproteinemia on the absorption of different types of cat gut sutures.[17] Fortified with the knowledge of Ravdin's studies demonstrating a causative effect between hypoproteinemia and impaired wound healing, Rhoads and William Kasinskas, subsequently known as Dr. Kase, performed similar investigations in another animal model. An ulnar fracture was created in dogs with the use of the Gigli saw, and hypoproteinemia was induced as described previously. Serial x-rays were performed for 69 days. Hypoproteinemia significantly impaired callus (the healing component of the fracture) formation after the experimental fracture.[18] The next year, the dogs were allowed to recover from their hypoproteinemia, and the other ulna was transected. Bone healing was observed for 39 days, and there was considerable callus formation. These studies provided further evidence of the importance of protein intake in the healing process. Rhoads explains subsequent investigations resulting from the fracture studies:

One of the more interesting experiments we did was an effort to see if the impaired healing of the fracture was due to edema or lack of nutritional substrates. The way we did that was to make the animals hypoproteinemic, then give them acacia which had no protein in it. Acacia has a 5-carbon sugar in it and it had been used as a blood substitute. It lost out because a number of people are allergic to it, particularly those who worked in confectionary shops and so forth. The dogs were not allergic to it, and lo and behold they formed fibroblasts very well.[19]

Thus, the restitution of fibroblasts was apparently due to a restoration of blood volume and osmolality produced by the acacia and not solely due to replacement of protein deficits.

Studies of nutritional intervention and liver function continued. Frazier Gurd, who had completed his training in clinical surgery in Canada, came to Penn for a research fellowship with Ravdin, Rhoads, and Vars. He studied the effects of different diets on postoperative liver regeneration. He showed that a 70% hepatectomy could be performed and liver regeneration would occur even on a protein-free diet.[20] The animal would steal protein from other tissues to rebuild its liver, but it did so rather slowly. If animals were given a high-protein diet, the liver would regenerate rapidly and fairly completely.

These studies led to detailed investigations in hospitalized patients performed by research fellow Elizabeth Thoroughgood.[21] She gave jaundiced patients a high-carbohydrate, high-protein diet for 5 to 7 days before their operations. When they came to surgery, liver biopsies were performed and sent to Vars for analysis of fat and glycogen. If the patients were given the diet preoperatively, the liver fat remained within normal range, whereas if they were not pretreated, the fat concentration would often be significantly increased. There was a good deal of evidence around, not extensively confirmed, that people with high fat in the liver were poor operative risks and poorer anesthesia risks. Rhoads commented on the importance of these studies by Gurd and Vars at Vars' memorial service in 1983:

It was this work that persuaded me to question and largely reject the view derived by Cuthbertson in England that it was futile to give additional protein-caloric intake during the period of catabolic loss following injury. Rejection of this view, with the concomitant desire to explore the positive side of nitrogen balance by intravenous techniques, had much to do with the fact that intravenous hyperalimentation was developed here rather than in England or New England.[22]

In his autobiography, Gurd expresses his indebtedness to his mentors at Penn:

During that year [at Penn] I discovered that I could succeed in original research. For this I am forever grateful to my mentors: Jonathan Rhoads, for accepting me on sight and for the support and friendship which continues to this day; to I.S. Ravdin, for persuading me that basic studies were essential to improving patient care; and to Harry Vars, for sharing his vast knowledge, for teaching me the discipline of science and for lifelong friendship.[23]

As the result of the many adverse effects that malnutrition produced on wound healing and other physiologic sequelae important to postoperative outcome, Ravdin, Rhoads, and colleagues directed their investigations to identify the optimal method to feed patients who could not ingest sufficient nutrients, especially protein, by mouth. An early clinical effort to provide some nutritional support was made in the early 1930s when proctoclysis (administration of fluid in the rectum) was a standard method of providing exogenous fluid. There was ample historic precedent at Penn for this approach. Investigations stemmed back to the early work on "nutrient enemas," which were all the rage around 1900. (These were really egg nogs with whiskey added!) Walter Eberlen, a resident of Eliason's, tried to measure the absorption of glucose from the rectum and showed that if the glucose concentration of the rectal infusate was above 2%, water was drawn out of the rectum and glucose absorption was decreased rather than increased. As Rhoads tells it:

Dr. Ravdin conceived the idea of adding some alcohol to the fluid dripping into the rectum, and as house officers we narrowly prevented him from pouring some alcohol from the dressing cart into the reservoir of the proctoclysis. We replaced it with some so-called 100% alcohol which, while very expensive, was pure alcohol without the toxic denaturant. The effect was probably more sedative than nutritional, but it seemed to be well tolerated in small amounts.[24]

Absorption of dietary protein when given into the large and small bowel was investigated by Bill Frazier and the chemist Cecelia Riegel. These investigations were based on some of the early work performed in cats by Otto Folin. According to Rhoads,

There were some dogs with Thiry-Vella loops in the animal house. One was named Irish—he was a mean dog. We used his loop to measure the absorption of hydrolyzed proteins from the small bowel and subsequently created some large bowel loops. That was my part of the project.[25]

Confirming some of the earlier results of Folin, the investigations showed that amino acids, some peptides, and perhaps peptones were absorbed but the amount absorbed was insufficient to significantly replace the protein deficits. Rhoads recalls:

During those days, when I first got here, a great many patients were getting fluid given by rectum at the end of the operation. Dr. Ravdin always used a drip of saline and Dr. Eliason would run a liter into the rectum on the operating table to provide adequate fluid balance.[26]

Ravdin then moved from the rectal administration of nutrients to intravenous feeding. Investigations were designed to identify the optimal source of protein and to discover the ideal method for intravenous administration when the gut could not be used. He persuaded David Drabkin, a professor of biochemistry in the Graduate School of Medicine, to hydrolyze some protein for intravenous administration. Drabkin had prepared the protein hydrolysates that were given into the rectum. Some of the initially prepared hydrolyzed protein was given intravenously to a patient of Rhoads who had been operated on for a colon lesion. Somehow the hydrolysate had gotten infected before administration, and the patient went into septic shock when the hydrolysate was given intravenously with dextrose. This unfortunate event temporarily dampened the enthusiasm for administering intravenous protein to humans at Penn.

Around 1936, Robert Elman, at Washington University in St. Louis, reported successful results with intravenous feeding of a protein product, Amigen, made by the Mead Johnson Company of Evansville, Indiana. The protein product was a relatively crude casein hydrolysate produced by incubation with pork pancreas. Presumably some of the protein derivatives came from the casein and some from the pancreas itself. Interestingly, a protein hydrolysate had been given to a goat in 1913 by Henriques and Andersen with claims of nitrogen equilibrium.[27] After a considerable amount of basic investigation, Elman successfully administered Amigen to patients and demonstrated that protein deficits could be greatly reduced and sometimes even eliminated. In an interview nearly 50 years later, Vars remarks:

Elman did an extensive amount of research on intravenous protein. If he hadn't died, I am sure he would have been the one who had come up with this.[28]

With the emergence of World War II, the emphasis of nutrition research in the Harrison Department shifted to military contracts. Four of these contracts were awarded for studies in physiology and pathology of burns, development of plasma substitutes (later termed plasma expanders), detection and decontamination of poisonous gases in foods, and physiological causes and treatment of surgical shock. Many of these investigations involved the intravenous administration of fluid combined with various nutrients and other substances. New knowledge was gained that would provide the foundation for the investigations and experiments in intravenous nutrition 20 years later.

One of the military contracts deemed vital to the war effort was to identify new and improved plasma expanders. The Penn group decided to study intravenous gelatin. Evidence that gelatin, an incomplete protein lacking four of the essential amino acids, might be an effective plasma expander had been observed as early as 1915. The studies at Penn were performed in conjunction with the Kind and Knox Gelatin Company. Vars, Dee Tourtelotte, a Hopkins-trained nutritional biochemist working for Kind and Knox, and William Parkins, a physiologist, performed these studies. The investigators used gelatin made from bones of Argentinian cattle. Their results showed that gelatin was an effective plasma expander for treatment of dogs subjected to experimental shock.[29] Subsequent evaluations by Bob Dripps confirmed that gelatin was also an effective plasma expander in humans.[30]

Rhoads recounts the early studies with gelatin:

Some of the early work by Henry Shenkin, who later became a neurosurgeon, investigated the effect of gelatin on hemorrhagic shock. Additionally, Shenkin and colleagues examined the influence of body position on the effects of blood loss and hypotension. They discovered that if a person was horizontal, you could bleed them a liter, but if they stood up, only 500 cc's of blood loss was tolerated. The investigators induced blood loss in each other. James Hardy [later to become Chair of Surgery at the University of Mississippi and President of the American College of Surgeons] was bled until his systolic blood pressure dropped to 60. Then, instead of giving him his blood back, he was given intravenous gelatin and his blood pressure went right up.[31]

Rhoads thought this experiment was ill-advised.

One of the undesirable side effects of the intravenous delivery of gelatin was that it remained in the bloodstream only for a short time and was rapidly excreted in the urine. While there were several biochemical attempts to modify the physical-chemical composition of gelatin to prevent rapid excretion in the urine, it could not be significantly improved. An additional untoward effect was that gelatin "jelled" at low temperatures. When the military's final selection was made for plasma expanders to be used in the war effort, gelatin was not included. It was definitely not feasible for the battlefield, and the Penn investigations of gelatin as a plasma expander were discontinued. Ironically these studies provided, in part, important information for the discovery of Dextran, a plasma expander that is used today.

Tourtelotte maintained an interest in gelatin as a means of delivering intravenous protein, even though it did not contain all of the essential amino acids. Studies at Penn were then begun to examine whether the nitrogen in intravenously infused gelatin, often given together with a more complete protein such as hydrolyzed casein, was incorporated into body protein in the dog. These investigations continued to be supported by the Knox Gelatin Company. One of the major difficulties with this research was the aforementioned concern about the rapid urinary excretion of intravenously administered gelatin. This rapid excretion caused large daily fluctuations in levels of blood proteins and interfered with nutritional balance studies. To solve these problems it became evident that not only did the amount of gelatin provided intravenously need to be carefully determined, additional intravenous fluid was required to correct for the excessive fluid losses.

The investigators' interests in pursuing these studies intensified as evidence of preliminary successes from other laboratories "leaked out." This is noted in a letter to Rhoads from his colleague, John Lockwood:

Dr. Tourtelotte was in yesterday and informed me that Alex Brunschwig had combined gelatin, Amigen and glucose with all the precision of a shotgun artist, and apparently with considerable success. He combined equal parts of gelatin, Amigen and glucose solution and finds that in the presence of gelatin the pyrogenic reactions from Amigen do not occur. I thought you might like to give this a preliminary trial.[32]

In order to continue the studies of intravenous feeding it was evident that a feasible method of nutrient delivery needed to be devised. C. Martin Rhode, who was spending a year in the laboratory prior to starting his surgical residency at Penn, joined Parkins, Tourtelotte, and Vars in the development of an improved intravenous infusion system. In a short time they created a system that permitted the infusion of intravenous fluids continuously through a catheter inserted into the jugular vein of the dog. The rapid development of this reliable constant infusion system was facilitated by the availability of improved catheter tubing and large volumes of pyrogen-free intravenous fluids.

The new infusion system consisted of a reservoir for the intravenous solution fitted with a cotton air-intake filter connected to a DeBakey pump, to which was attached polyethylene tubing connected to an indwelling venous catheter. The catheter tubing (containing 6 feet of tubing, which they called the swivel) was connected to the dog's jugular catheter with a sterile needle. All of the dog's turning motions were transferred to the swivel, which often became considerably twisted. Martin Rhode painted a straight line down the swivel tube and estimated the extent of twisting by the closeness of the "barber pole" spirals produced by the dog's movements. The small volume of the infusion tubing and the rapid flow rate reduced bacterial growth to a minimum within the tubing.

The solutions consisted of 50% glucose with Amigen or gelatin. Female dogs were used because their bladders were easier to catheterize than males. The investigators found that 27% of the nitrogen of the infused gelatin was used to form body protein. Moreover, they discovered that infusions could be maintained for as long as 141 days while still producing positive nitrogen balance. Despite these interesting results with continuous intravenous feeding, all investigations in the procedure as a means of administering nitrogen and calories were abandoned by the Harrison Department and were not revived for another 10 years.

These experiments originating from the problems associated with the rapid excretion of gelatin demonstrated that it was possible to keep animals in positive nitrogen balance for prolonged periods of time by intravenous feeding. Following the early investigations at Penn with the administration of protein hydrolysates, both by rectum and vein, and the unsuccessful studies with intravenous gelatin, four major problems were identified. First, many patients could not tolerate more than 3000 milliliters of intravenous fluid per day without developing pulmonary edema. Second, the caloric requirements of patients soon after major operations such as gastrectomy and colectomy seemed to be around one and one-half times the basal metabolic rate. Third, the caloric value of carbohydrate and amino acids was fixed at about four kilocalories per gram. Finally, if the concentration of the infusate increased to 15%, venous thromboses were frequent, which were painful and led to interruption of the infusions.

A series of studies was conducted with albumin to determine if it might be a good source of protein for intravenous feeding. These studies were conducted shortly after World War II when, in 1947 to 1948, the American Red Cross released its stockpile of human serum albumin for clinical studies. This material had been prepared from outdated human blood. Recognizing this was a unique opportunity to study the fate of human albumin infused into normal subjects, Ravdin asked Nicholas Gimbel, one of his residents, to obtain salt-free albumin from the Red Cross and to investigate its metabolic fate. Gimbel, who also served as one of the study subjects, and Cecelia Riegel compared the metabolic fate of albumin administered by infusion with that given orally.[33] Intravenous infusion of albumin increased albumin levels in the plasma, tissue fluid, and lymph and increased blood volume. Some of the infused albumin was incorporated into body protein.

Albumin infusion as a nutritional supplement, however, was seriously hampered by the marked circulatory overloading, especially in patients who were not protein deficient. Several medical students at Penn and Jim Nixon, who later served as the team physician for the Philadelphia Eagles football team, were given exogenous albumin as the sole protein intake for approximately three weeks. Nixon's blood volume rose 85%, and he went into severe congestive heart failure. A mother of one of the medical students was rather upset about the experiment. Rhoads recalls:

The experiment was stopped and a luncheon was held for all the subjects who cared to come. They ate red meat.[34]

Because of these problems there were no further studies at Penn on the intravenous use of human albumin for parenteral nutrition until considerably later. Currently, the value of exogenous infusions of albumin remains controversial.

Concurrent with the albumin studies, C. Everett Koop began studies of preoperative forced feeding by intestinal tube.[35] His study was primarily in neurosurgical patients, most of whom did not have preoperative hypoproteinemia. According to Rhoads,

He did this with much enthusiasm, reaching about 0.8 grams of food nitrogen intake per kilogram of body weight or the equivalent of over 300 grams of protein per day. This was supplemented with a very high caloric intake (up to 6,000 kilocalories per day!) All of the patients except one were in positive nitrogen balance for the 5 days before and 5 days after the operation.[36]

These studies demonstrated that the patient who did not have a significant weight loss before surgery was nevertheless capable of taking in a considerable load of protein and storing it at least temporarily. Rhoads was very impressed with this study:

The rather amazing thing was that you could stuff that much nitrogen into them, and he really stuffed it! If they wouldn't eat he would put a tube down and run it in. Koop's study reminded me of the story of the little boy at Thanksgiving who said he'd like some turkey but he didn't want any of the stuffing. He didn't like it, and, furthermore, he couldn't understand how the turkey could eat all that stuff![37]

Rhoads subsequently received a grant with Isaac Starr to study the effects of increased nitrogen balance on the convalescence of patients after major operations. Convalescence was measured with a newly designed apparatus by Starr known as the *ballistocardiograph*. Nitrogen balance was improved (although not statistically significantly) in the patients receiving I.V.H. when compared with the control group.

The investigations of intravenous infusions resumed in 1948 when Penn surgeons Paul Nemir and Herbert Hawthorne performed a series of studies in dogs with intestinal obstruction.[38] They showed that the duration of survival depended on the ability to replace fluid, electrolytes, and nutrients by the intravenous route. An infusion system similar to that of Parkins, Tourtelotte, and Vars was used to administer fluids into the jugular veins of these dogs.

Preliminary clinical studies were initiated following the success of the experiments in dogs. Nemir, realizing that this would be an effective way to give fluids to patients who were unable to be fed orally, conducted these studies. He surgically inserted catheters into the jugular veins of several patients and administered solutions of 10% glucose, 5% glucose and saline, and protein hydrolysates (Amigen) continuously with the conventional gravitational method (without a pump) used with standard intravenous infusions. He successfully maintained the electrolyte balance and supplied the nutritional requirements of these patients for 30–40 days.

Additionally, B.J. Duffy at the Sloan Kettering Institute in New York used this route of fluid administration to treat 72 patients in 1949.[39] The work of Nemir and Hawthorne, as well as that of Duffy, attempted to jump start the motor of total parenteral nutrition, but to no avail. An additional option was to place a feeding jejunostomy (a tube placed surgically into the small intestine for feeding). The experience with feeding jejunostomies at that time was quite poor. Significant diarrhea occurred, and postoperative complications such as dislodgement of the tube were common.

The next phase of the evolution of intravenous nutrition at Penn addressed the development of a fat-containing emulsion. Because of its high energy content of 9 kilocalories per gram (compared with protein and carbohydrate at 4 kilocalories per gram), intravenous fat was investigated as an energy source during World War II. The initial fat emulsion considered for investigation at Penn was provided by Emmett Holt, Chief of Pediatrics at New York University. Holt was one of Rhoads' teachers at Hopkins. Unfortunately, Holt's emulsion was unstable, and some of the fat separated into visible globules, rendering it unusable.

A number of experimental preparations of homogenized fats derived from soybean oil and cottonseed oil were subsequently made. Early work with emulsions was conducted by Ray Meng at Vanderbilt. Infusions of these emulsions were reasonably well tolerated by dogs. Intravenous fats suitable for use in humans were made and stabilized by Frederick Stare and Robert Geyer at the Harvard School of Public Health. Additionally, their work provided the foundation for the delivery of the intravenous fat-soluble vitamin K which is used today. These emulsions were subsequently manufactured by the Upjohn Company. Merck also was involved in the development of several fat emulsions, but none of these preparations was satisfactory since the emulsion broke down after storage or exposure to varied temperatures.

Upjohn's intravenous fat preparation, Lipomul, a cottonseed oil emulsion, was the most satisfactory American preparation at the time. Ravdin, through his military and industrial contacts, obtained a supply of Lipomul for clinical trials at Penn. These investigations were conducted by a young surgeon, Herndon B. "Bugs" Lehr, who was assigned the task of finding a safe and efficacious emulsion for clinical use. Lehr infused 15% Lipomul in various combinations of carbohydrate, protein, and ethyl alcohol. The 75 grams of fat administered daily provided 675 additional calories. The emulsion was infused into 238 patients. Ten patients received more than 10 units each of intravenous fat. A number of side effects occurred, such as chills and fever, but there were no serious untoward events. Rhoads recalls the difficulties with the initial fat emulsions:

In general, it didn't work very well. There was an awful lot of fever produced and we didn't count fevers of 101 degrees F or 2 degrees above where they started. But exceeding these limits, we had fever in a considerable percentage of patients and thought we had to discontinue. Also some got a curious pain in the back which we never had a clear explanation for, but it sort of worried us as to whether there were little globules getting stuck in the spinal cord. These findings were transient.[40]

Lehr concluded that many of these critically ill patients actually improved after infusions of intravenous fats. When the data from the additional investigational centers throughout the United States and the rest of the world were summarized at an International Fat Emulsion Conference held in Chicago, numerous accounts of "immediate reactions" such as chills, fever, abdominal pain, and depressed hematopoiesis (the formation and development of blood cells) were reported. Additionally, a significant number of late reactions, such as severe coagulation defects and liver failure, were described as well as anaphylactic shock resulting in death. As a result of the many serious side effects associated with Lipomul, the Food and Drug Administration restricted its clinical use. Subsequently, Upjohn discontinued the work on these preparations.

These international experiences with administration of intravenous fat to humans were documented in a summary report that contained more than 1300 references. One of the important outcomes of the fat emulsions conference was that the combined medical and surgical professions recognized the potential clinical importance of intravenous feeding. Additionally, they realized that there were many problems to be solved before it would become clinically feasible.

Concurrent with the investigations at Penn, an intravenous fat preparation made from soybean oil and egg phosphatides was developed in Stockholm by Arvid Wretlind, who had worked with W.C. Rose in Illinois and Oscar Shuberth in Sweden. These soybean oil emulsions were not permitted in the United States for clinical use until they were found to be safe. Following extensive basic and clinical research, these products were eventually deemed satisfactory and were supplied in the United States by a Swedish manufacturer in the 1970s and are currently used throughout the world.

During the early clinical trials it became apparent that there were a number of limiting factors preventing the safe administration of intravenous solutions. One concern was the daily volume of fluid that could be administered safely in addition to providing the required nutrients. This was generally limited to three liters for many patients. This volume limitation was particularly important for elderly patients on fluid-restricted regimens who only tolerated three and a half liters of intravenous fluid for a short period. Pulmonary edema (excessive fluid accumulation in the lungs) occurred when larger volumes of fluid were infused. Another limitation of the intravenous infusions was the high concentration and venous irritation (hypertonicity > 20,000 milliosmoles) of the combined protein and glucose solution. Conventionally, intravenous solutions were administered into peripheral veins on the inner side of the forearm. Glucose, which is isotonic at about 5%, was occasionally tolerated at a 10% concentration. When it was increased to 15%, phlebitis (inflammation of the veins) and thrombosis frequently resulted in obstruction of the vein and stoppage of the infusion.

Rhoads vividly remembers the early frustrations and discouragements associated with attempts to feed patients intravenously:

In combining some of the early work at Penn with that performed in a wider range of patients at Presbyterian Hospital in New York, it became apparent that probably no more than 0.2 grams of nitrogen per kilogram of body weight were needed in a 70-kg individual undergoing a small operation. Approximately 0.3 grams of nitrogen were needed in larger operations such as resection of the stomach or colon.

Efforts to increase these amounts were frustrating. If we increased the volume, we ran into pulmonary edema. If we increased the concentration of the solution, we encountered phlebitis, venous occlusion and obstruction of the infusion. The experiments with intravenous fat emulsions were unsatisfactory because of the toxic reactions. At one point, we concluded that if we confronted patients with severe pyloric stenosis (obstruction of the stomach) and hypoproteinemia, it was just better to load them up by transfusion of blood and plasma and operate upon them rather than to try and improve their nourishment preoperatively.[43]

Rhoads attempted to solve the problem of volume limitation of intravenous feedings. An idea came to him while he was serving on the Board of Associated Universities. In that role, he dutifully made a site visit to the National Radio Astronomy Laboratory at Greenbank, West Virginia, which was under the aegis of the Board of Associated Universities along with the Brookhaven Laboratories. During one visit in 1960, his mind turned to the volume limitations of intravenous feeding:

I made one trip down to see the National Radio Astronomy Laboratory and spent a night down there. . . . They had these dishes; the more accurate one was about 110 feet in diameter and it was poised so that it could be timed to follow the heavens and correct for the rotation of the earth, like an astronomical telescope. . . . Anyhow, I listened to the astronomers or astrophysicists without much understanding, went to bed, woke up early the next morning around 5 o'clock and looked out the window in this lodging they had there, and way across the field was this big thing sort of turning around getting poised. . . . It was eerie. . . . It just got me out of my usual tracks. . . . Then I got to thinking about our intravenous problems and it came over me that our medical colleagues were giving diuretics on a chronic basis.[44]

More specifically, physicians were administering the newer diuretics, such as Diuril, for prolonged periods to treat high blood pressure. These drugs were not as toxic as the earlier mercurial diuretics used in the 1930s; therefore, Rhoads reasoned that these drugs might prevent the fluid restrictions of the intravenous feeding regimen. He postulated that if the excess water was removed by administering diuretics, it might be possible to increase the volume of intravenous fluid from 3 liters per day to 5–7 liters per day.

The technique was deemed the "5-liter program." It was thought that the added volume of infusion would in turn increase daily caloric administration by increasing the glucose concentration from 5% to 10% and that the excess fluid could be driven out with diuretics. Rhoads proposed that the 5-liter program would increase the calories administered each day from the usual 1200 to 2500–3000. To administer the 5-liter infusions, very small diameter sterile ureteral catheters were inserted into a vein in the forearm with advancement into the superior vena cava in patients with diffuse cancer. To determine the effect of the indwelling catheter on the vein, autopsies were performed in these patients after the fatal disease had completed its course. There was considerable clot formation about the catheters, and the ureteral catheter technique was thus abandoned for the fear that it would induce a pulmonary embolus.

The opportunity arose to study the effects of intravenous feeding with diuretics in patients under more favorable conditions in the Clinical Research Center, where accurate calorie and nitrogen balance studies could be performed. Investigations were begun in normal human volunteers, many of whom were strapping young men who worked as orderlies in the hospital. They could be recruited for financial consideration inasmuch as all they had to do was to lie around the Research Center, give up all oral foods, and receive continuous intravenous feedings.

The experiment was largely unsuccessful because these very fit young men became bed-ridden patients. They developed marked protein catabolism and went into negative nitrogen balance. These results prompted recollection of earlier studies performed at Cornell during World War II, when volunteers were placed in body casts and were unable to move. They all went into negative nitrogen balance. As the result of these observations, Rhoads reasoned that it was important to study patients with preexisting nutritional deficits rather than healthy volunteers. Rhoads comments on the next development:

Subsequently, a man was investigated who was dying of cancer of the stomach. His wife worked as a cashier in the hospital. I remember her well. She was a Boston woman with a strong accent. She'd say, '"This fellow came in and wanted a reduction on his bill. I told him he couldn't have one. He reached into his pocket and took out a roll of bills big enough to choke a cow and paid it off."

It was difficult for her to take care of her husband at home, and she could see him frequently if he was hospitalized in the Clinical Research Center. He agreed to the experiments, and he lay there for a full month receiving intravenous feedings of 5 liters a day combined with 4 different types of diuretics. While given three of the diuretics concurrently, he emerged into positive nitrogen balance. It was then concluded that at long last a method had been developed, albeit awkward, of getting patients into positive nitrogen balance.[45]

To perform accurate studies of the concurrent use of intravenous feeding with diuretics, highly controlled investigations in animals were needed. Rhoads' son Jack, then a medical student at Harvard, agreed to spend the summer working with Vars to see which diuretic would cause the least disturbance of plasma electrolyte levels. One of the problems of the early investigations with diuretics was the marked depletion of various minerals in the blood, notably sodium and potassium. To perform these chronic infusion studies, Vars and Jack Rhoads "resurrected" and restored the access apparatus used on the earlier gelatin studies with dogs. Surprisingly, the dogs tolerated extremely high volumes of intravenous fluids without the need for diuretics. The equivalent of 19 liters daily for a human could be infused into the dog without untoward effects. Careful studies were performed with the diuretics and detailed measurements of losses of sodium and chloride were made. One of the remarkable observations of that summer's experience was the excellent physical condition of the animals after nearly 2 months of intravenous feeding and nothing by mouth except water. The animals were well nourished, their coats were in good condition, and they were quite active. They were exercised regularly, which undoubtedly contributed to their well-being; however, this was difficult because intravenous lines had to be disconnected, and there was always the risk of loss of access.

Based on preliminary successes in the studies of adult dogs, Rhoads and Vars decided to conduct studies in growing animals. They reasoned that if a puppy could grow to adulthood, this single experiment would prove that all of the essential nutrients for life could be given intravenously. Furthermore, this continuous-infusion growth experiment was chosen because its progress could be reasonably well assessed by one simple measurement, the dog's weight. Moreover, the proposed studies seemed feasible because of the absence of the complicated analytical procedures and the elimination of the cumbersome data accumulation associated with the previous nutritional balance studies, as well as the paucity of funds and technical support. Additionally, they decided to study growing animals because if there was a nutritionally-induced weight gain in adult animals, it might be attributed to an increase in body water and not lean body mass.

Lessons learned from the early works of Ravdin and Rhoads were major factors contributing to the design of the proposed investigations in puppies. J. Garrott Allen, a close friend of Rhoads, had given intravenous albumin as the sole source of protein to puppies who consumed their caloric intake by mouth. The puppies grew and the Penn group was very impressed with these studies.

Based on the work performed in adult dogs by his son and colleagues, Rhoads deduced that the most weight gain they could expect in the adult dog was 10%. Rhoads explained his thoughts concerning measurements of body weight:

The naysayers would say that this was just retained water. We were also quite cognizant of the fact that Francis Moore in Boston had been doing a lot of body fluid determinations with isotopes. It was evident to everyone that at least he knew more about measuring body fluid than we did. It would therefore be a good deal better to study growing puppies. Pat Spagna started the studies, but he didn't have very good luck. He did establish that if you waited until the dogs were weaned at 12 weeks, they tolerated the feedings better than right after birth. We also borrowed an idea from Garrott Allen, who had performed protein studies in growing dogs. Allen sequentially photographed his growing dogs against a tile wall with a grid. This provided visual evidence of the comparable rates of growth in the chow fed and intravenously fed dogs.[46]

Two major problems needed to be solved in order to begin these experiments. A suitable intravenous diet for the puppies had to be devised, and the old infusion system needed to be improved. The elemental liquid diet, successfully used to raise rats for three generations, was the basis for designing the intravenous diet for the puppies. Special care was given to estimating the requirement for each nutrient because of concern for potentially toxic overdoses due to the direct infusion into the bloodstream. Inorganic phosphate was supplemented to prevent hypophosphatemia, mental abnormalities, muscle weakness, and possible death associated with refeeding. Approximations of nutrient needs were based on collected data of the National Research Council in discussions with Paul Gyorgy, Lew Barness, and Jim Jones, each of whom made important contributions to the final composition of the diet.

Puppies on oral diets regularly require 2% to 4% of their total calories as essential fatty acids. The investigators realized that feeding would be simplified if the required fatty acids could be supplied with intravenous fat preparations, but there was no intravenous fat commercially available at the time. Vars collected all of the leftover cottonseed oil emulsion at HUP, Graduate Hospital, Harrison Department of Surgical Research, and the Children's Hospital. When this fat supply became exhausted, only the small amount of fat required to supply the essential fatty acid linoleic acid was administered each day. Calcium and phosphorus were bound to organic molecules to prevent precipitation in the infusion mixture. The composition of a supplement containing all of the available trace elements—cobalt, copper, iodine, manganese, molybdenum, and zinc—evolved by trial and error.

Providing the vitamins required for the puppy's growth was a problem, as there were no known intravenous vitamin preparations available to meet these needs. Puppies require biotin, choline, and *para*-amino benzoic acid. These substances were obtained in crystalline form, dissolved in water, and added directly to the infusion fluid. Commercial mixtures of the B-complex vitamins and vitamins A and D were added separately. Vitamin B_{12}, folic acid, vitamin K, and iron were also added.

It became evident that if the technical problems of infusion delivery were going to be solved, someone had to be relieved of his or her clinical duties for a prolonged period. Stan Dudrick, a surgical resident, was asked to work with Vars to solve these technical problems. Rhoads has vivid recollections of his early interactions with Dudrick:

Stan was the oldest child in his family, and he had Polish ancestors on one side of the family and German American on the other. Stan's father was in the insurance business. His family lived in Nanticoke, Pa., which is down the Susquehanna, 10 or 20 miles from Wilkes Barre, the home of mining people. He went to Franklin and Marshall College and played football and got his nose broken. He was typified by enormous energy, a very bright mind, and a very outgoing personality. He was a very hardworking, industrious, and perceptive person.

His faults were perhaps to be too trusting of people, too enthusiastic, and perhaps not careful enough about making more commitments than he could fulfill. By the time that Stan was an intern he had 6 children. I saw he had to have more money, and instead of the hospital, we were providing the money for interns and residents in those days. He was interested in everything that was going on, and he was acknowledged as a superior intern. Fran Wood wanted him in medicine and I wanted him in surgery. So I offered him an annual salary of I think $6000, at a time when $3500 would have been standard. I don't know whether or not it was the money, but he came to surgery.[47]

For 11 months Dudrick and Vars tested, modified, and retested the continuous intravenous infusion apparatus. They initially used the same pumps used by Tourtelotte in the late 1940s. The work started on a shoestring budget, as indicated by their first task, which was to "sequester" the required dog cages in the Harrison Department as well as to borrow others from the Cox Foundation. All of the cages were old and rusty and required extensive cleaning and repair. The sterile infusions were prepared by Dudrick and Vars, and the nutrient components were obtained from various sources at the medical school and hospital. It was not until the first paper was published from the "new" Penn group that an actual budget was available for these experiments. Funding was obtained through the efforts of Robert Kark, a consultant to Abbott Laboratories, and from the Army Liver Commission, which was greatly impressed by this work. Rhoads comments on Vars' seminal role in these studies:

In all of these studies Dr. Vars was a participant and a tremendous resource, as he had an encyclopedic knowledge of the biochemical and nutritional literature, which permitted him to develop mineral and vitamin supplements without which these experiments might have failed. In short, most of the people who worked in the Harrison Department of Surgical Research between 1936 and the present have direct or indirect

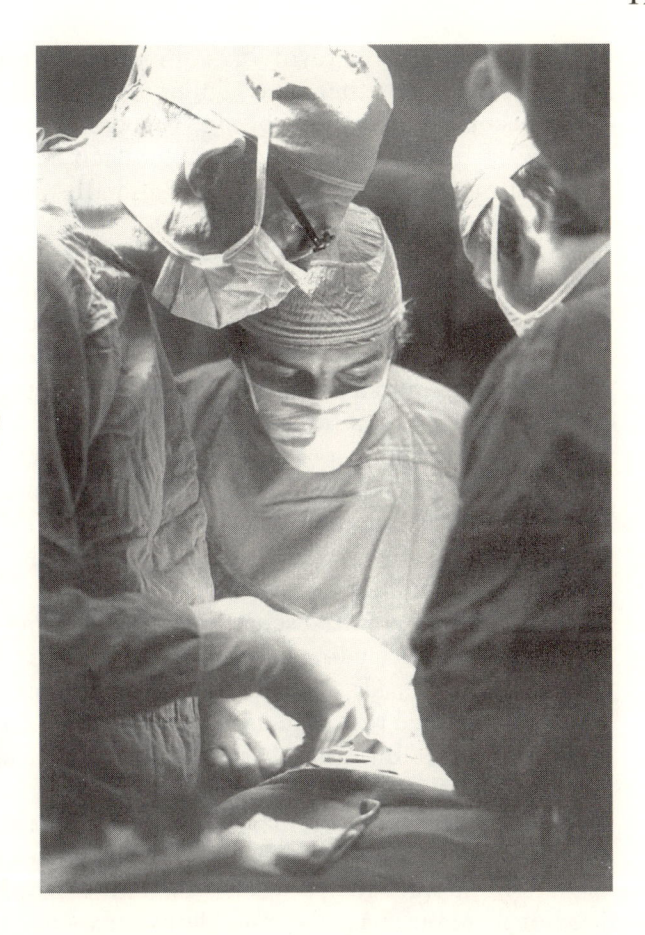

Jonathan Rhoads (left) in the operating room with Stan Dudrick (center)— University of Texas, 1975.

debts to Harry Vars for his selfless cooperation, and his endless devotion to science.[48]

Catheters were inserted into the jugular vein and advanced to a point just above the dog's right atrium. The other end of the catheter was threaded through a tunnel under the skin to a point between the scapulae and then brought out through a small incision in the skin. A custom-made soft canvas harness-jacket, fitted with an aluminum or stainless steel supporting apparatus (the pagoda), was used to secure the catheter. The first of these canvas jackets was made by Dudrick. Subsequently, his colleagues at the Veteran's Hospital helped to make the different-sized jackets as the dogs grew. (A vest based upon this principle was used to hold the pump and solutions in the first ambulatory patients to receive home intravenous feeding.)

A major improvement in the new infusion system used with the puppies, when compared with Vars' initial apparatus, was the elimination of the twisting of the swivel tube. In the "puppy-proofed" system the entire segment between the revolving component of the infusion system and the dog turned together. The jugular venous catheter was connected to the infusion tube at the top of the "pagoda," and the revolving connector was covered with speedometer cable. Each day the puppy was disconnected from the infusion apparatus and allowed to exercise freely in a closed area.

Of the substances tested for use as the intravenous catheter, polyvinyl chloride was found most suitable, for it could be autoclaved. Teflon was too stiff, and Silastic was too soft, hard to repair, and not readily available when the experiments started. Finally, polyethylene kinked, clogged, and required cold sterilization. Constant attention and improvisations were required to maintain a continuous and uniform infusion in the system concocted of speedometer cable covering, electrical connectors, Luer-lok fittings, and other laboratory "junk." The first long-lived beagle earned the name "Sticky Bun" as proof of the effort required to overcome the catheter leaks and obstructions that occurred with active, freely mobile puppies.[49]

Similar to many initial scientific investigations, the early experiments with intravenous feeding of the puppies were unsuccessful, and several animals died. Rhoads and Vars requested the consultation of a veterinarian. He examined the animals and in about 5 minutes extracted numerous mites out of the animals' ears with an applicator stick. The animals fared much better after these treatments.

Dudrick worked extremely hard and monitored the animals every 8 hours for 8 months. The initial experiments were designed to support growth of puppies for 10 weeks. Two four-member litters of purebred beagles were purchased at considerable expense to help control for the generalized health of the animals. In each litter, two of the animals were fed by mouth and two were fed intravenously and received only water by mouth. Each of the animals grew well. Surprisingly, those fed intravenously grew a little faster than their isocaloric chow-fed siblings. Growth was assessed by measurements of body weight, and the general health of the animals was monitored by vital signs and a physical examination. Measurements of minerals in the blood, bone x-rays, and photographs of the animals were performed at regular intervals.

The experiment ended after 72 days, and the animals were examined at postmortem. The intestinal tracts of the intravenous animals were shortened and narrowed, but had no other gross abnormalities. There was no clot formation or other damage associated with the catheter in the superior vena cava, and there were no infarcts or evidence of emboli in the lung. The acinar cells of the pancreas were atrophic, but the islet cells were prominent. The liver contained some lipid deposits that presumably resulted from the intravenous fat or excess carbohydrate. Iron breakdown products were observed in the liver as well. Such deposits of iron in the tissues were eliminated in subsequent experiments by reducing the amount of iron administered.

Three animals were fed with continuous intravenous feeding for a hundred days. The longest periods of feeding were 235 and 255 days. These animals tripled their body weights and had growth patterns identical to their litter mates receiving dog chow. In both intravenously fed and control puppies (animals ingesting normal chow), the deciduous teeth were shed and replaced with permanent teeth at a similar time in their growth. The intravenously fed animals were just as active as their control litter mates, and there were no obvious abnormalities of their skin, coat, or bone development.

A review of the early patient studies of I.V.H. at Penn revealed that it was possible to administer as many as 2500 calories per day.[50] However, the troublesome complications of phlebitis, thrombosis, and fluid and electrolyte imbalances made this approach clinically unacceptable.

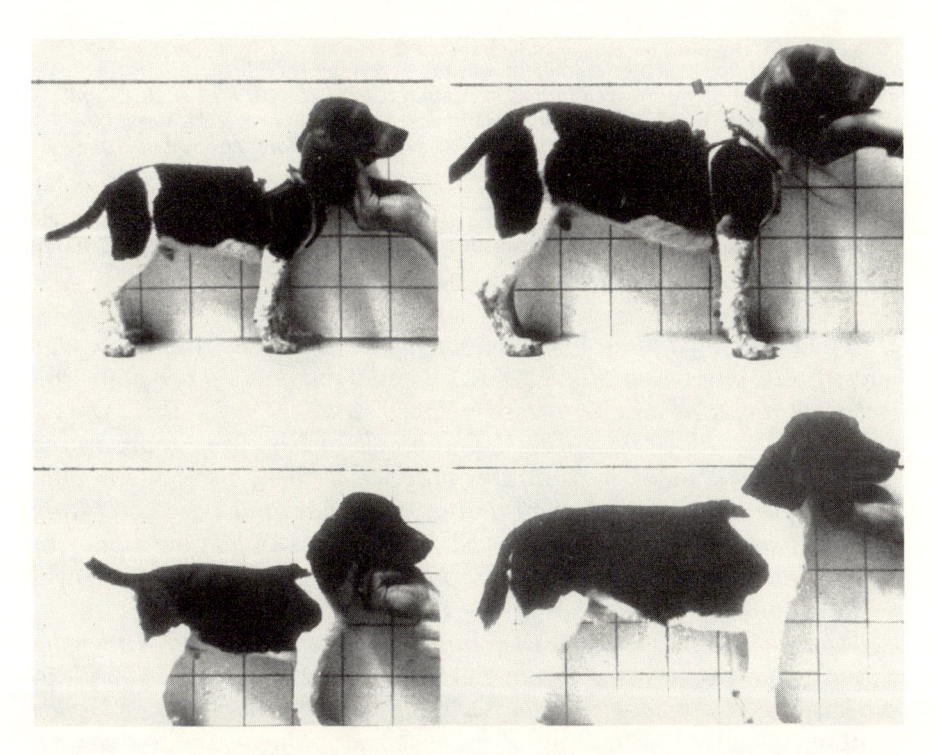

Beagle pup at 12 weeks and following total intravenous nutrition for 235 days (top). Isocaloric oral fed control litter mate (bottom). (Reproduced with permission from S.J. Dudrick, D.W. Wilmore, H.M. Vars, J.E. Rhoads: Long-term parenteral nutrition with growth development and positive nitrogen. Surgery 64: 134–142, 1968.[51])

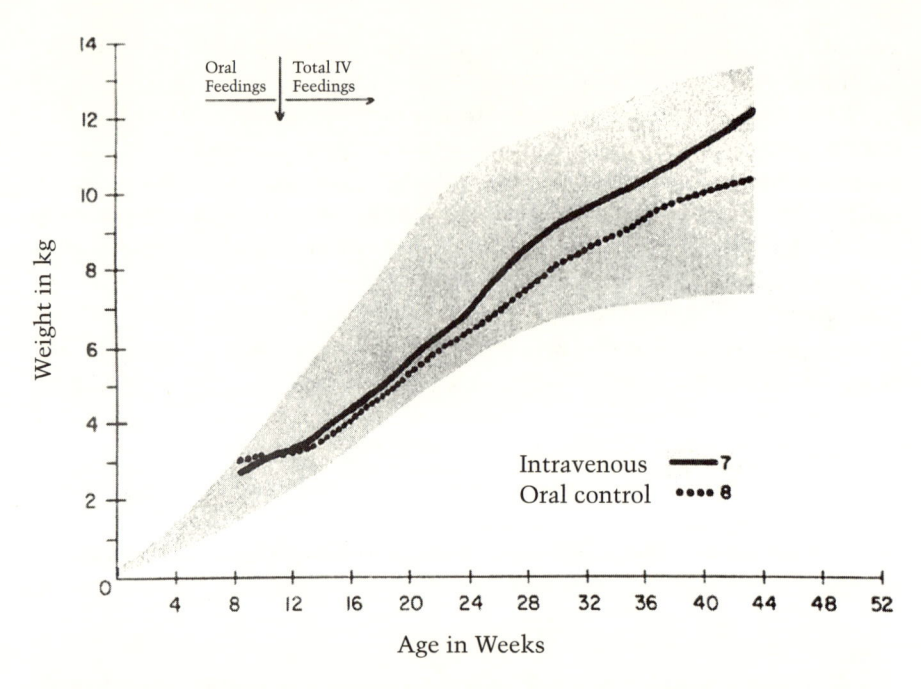

Comparison of body weight change in animals receiving total intravenous feeding and oral controls. Shaded area indicates normal rate of growth for beagle puppies. (Reproduced with permission from S.J. Dudrick, D.W. Wilmore, H.M. Vars, J.E. Rhoads: Long-term parenteral nutrition with growth development and positive nitrogen. Surgery 64: 137, 1968.[52])

Douglas Wilmore, a surgical resident and coinvestigator of the early work with both the puppies and the patients, recalls:

Stan [Dudrick] had done 4 pairs of puppies when I came to the lab. One puppy of the pair was orally fed, one I.V. fed. I did another 4–6 pairs, collected all the urine and performed balance studies. During this time we were making solutions in the Vars lab or another small room in the Harrison Department. This mixing practice resulted in frequent solution contamination. The hospital obtained a Laminar flow hood from Abbott. I spoke with the pharmacist, Stan Serlick (who now works for Abbott), and we moved the preparation of the formula admixture over to the hospital.

Because Stan was now on the clinical service, he started to identify patients who would benefit from T.P.N. The solutions could be made in the hospital pharmacy—we had just trained a pharmacist to make dog solutions. The I.V.'s were inserted via the external jugular vein—we used the old intra caths—and threaded down into the superior vena cava. A woman named Helen Smits had performed a study as a medical student on the use of topical antibiotics applied to the catheter entrance site, and it was published in The New England Journal of Medicine. *She became a medical resident at Penn. That is how we got started with the catheter care protocol.*

One night a urology resident, Bob Mogel from Temple, saw us either inserting or caring for an external jugular catheter. He asked why we weren't using subclavian catheters! He inserted a subclavian catheter in one of our patients, then subsequently taught Stan and me how to perform the technique. As you can see, we became converts.[53]

Dudrick also found a percutaneous subclavian vein puncture technique initially described by Aubaniac, a French military surgeon serving in Vietnam during the French Indochina War in 1952.[54] This technique had also been used by Dominic DeLaurentis and colleagues, Robert Mogil, and George Rosemond at Temple University for measurements of central venous pressure.[55] The percutaneous technique avoided a cutdown on a large vein, and there was a shorter length of indwelling catheter that might become infected.

Additionally, the catheter was positioned in a very large vein (innominate–superior vena cava) with a rapid flow rate. The rationale for using this technique for intravenous feeding is that the very rapid flow of blood in the vena cava dilutes the concentrated nutrient infusions almost immediately, thereby preventing injury to the vein. Indeed, Vars had observed this experimentally by placing two catheters in the superior vena cava in the dog with one above the other. When the concentrated glucose solution was introduced in the higher catheter and blood was withdrawn from the lower catheter, the measurements of glucose were within the normal range, even though the catheters were quite close together. According to Wilmore:

The central venous catheter technique with intravenous feeding was being used before it was developed at Penn. When I first started, I was given the Acta Chirurgica Scandinavica Supplement #325. *This was from a symposium held in 1962. The authors suggested using the external jugular vein for introduction to the superior vena cava, and this may be where we got the idea to use the external jugular.*

There was another interesting incident. We were at an International Symposium in Nashville. I presented a few cases, and Stan presented the adult cases and the baby material. This guy got up (I think from New Orleans) and presented this large clinical series. No one knew him or had talked with him. I copied his statements, for he was clearly ahead of us at the time.

You may know of another surgeon, the Chief of Downstate from Minnesota in the 40's and 50's, who also used central vein infusions in patients with extensive bowel disease.[56]

For the first time, the new infusion technique made it possible to safely infuse highly concentrated solutions of glucose and amino acids because of the high velocity of flow in the large central veins and the rapid dilution of the infusion. Dudrick played an important role in describing and teaching the technique of percutaneous insertion of subclavian venous catheters. He visited many major medical institutions throughout the world and inserted catheters into patients and initiated infusions.

The new infusion technique was subsequently used in a number of hospitalized patients at Penn with intestinal fistulas (abnormal connection between the intestine and either the skin or other organs). The fistulas were due to breakdown of surgical anastomoses or primary disease of the intestine, such as inflammatory bowel disease. The patients were restricted to nothing by mouth, and they were nourished solely by vein. They responded quite well, and to the pleasant surprise of the investigators and the patients, some of the fistulas closed spontaneously and completely. This was quite serendipitous in that the reason for giving the intravenous feeding was to prepare the patients for operative closure of the fistulas. One of the first patients with a fistula who was treated with I.V.H. is fresh in Rhoads' memory:

There was one woman who had a ruptured esophagus and had survived with chest drainage, and she continued to have a fistula out through the chest wall and had a chest tube inserted. Her nutritional status had deteriorated and the granulations [tissue on top of a wound] were sort of gray and unhealthy looking. She was put on I.V.H., and within a week or two, these had pinked up, and pretty soon the tube was removed and the tract closed. After this was "noised about" a bit, a lot of fistulas were sent in so that in a year's time, 78 patients were treated. Approximately, 70% closed spontaneously. Those that did not close often had distal tumors.[57]

Despite these initial successes, I.V.H. was not widely accepted by the medical community until the birth of a child with an intestinal defect in July 1967. Harry Bishop, a pediatric surgeon at the Children's Hospital of Philadelphia (CHOP), asked Rhoads, Dudrick, and Wilmore to see a newborn girl on whom Bishop had operated for a near-total atresia (failure of in-utero development) of the small bowel. Following massive resection of the obstructed, nonfunctional atretic intestine, the short length of jejunum was anastomosed (sewn) to the minimal (3 cm) remaining segment of ileum. Part of the poorly developed segment of colon was bypassed by performing a left-sided colostomy above the site of the strictured colon.

The baby then had bowel movements through the colostomy, but these were severely diarrheal in nature because there was such a short segment of small bowel in intestinal continuity. The operation, performed on July 19, 1967, was extremely difficult, and she suffered a cardiac arrest during the surgery but survived. In an interview nearly 25 years later, Bishop comments on the operation:

When we had a child with a very short intestinal tract, there was really nothing that could be done for the patient except for keeping them barely alive for almost a month. They all died. I'm amazed we hooked her together.... Why I decided to hook her up I don't remember, but she only had 3 cm of ileum hooked on to her duodenum and then two atresias of the colon.[58]

The child continued to lose weight. Efforts to nourish her both by mouth and scalp vein did not succeed. By 19 days of age, her weight had fallen to 4 pounds from a birth weight of 5.5 pounds. It was obvious she was dying of starvation. After carefully examining the patient and evaluating the clinical problems and potential moral/ethical issues, Dudrick and Wilmore decided to feed the infant intravenously through a central venous catheter. Additionally, this unfortunate infant provided an opportunity to determine if human growth and development could be obtained with I.V.H. similar to the results in the puppies. Bishop reflects further upon the decision making:

I remember Stan [Dudrick] and Doug Wilmore were called down to Children's. Wilmore had been there as a resident and so he knew people. Stan had been down there for a bit. Stan was older by a couple of years. I vividly remember both of them looking over the little crib and asking if this was possible and whether the family would really go along with it. I talked to the family, and they obviously were agreeable to everything.[59]

Due to the lack of precedent for the proposed nutritional regimen, the feeding evolved through trial and error in some instances. Certain nutrients were added individually as the course of the infusion progressed, and other nutrients were withdrawn if they caused adverse reactions. The formula was pumped into the infant with a Harvard infusion pump, which had been used in the animal experiments and subsequently cleaned. A Millipore filter was placed into the delivery system to remove any bacteria that might gain entry into the bloodstream.

Working with Dale Johnson, the chief resident in pediatric surgery, the surgeons made a cutdown over a vein in the neck, threaded a polyethylene catheter into the internal jugular vein into the superior vena

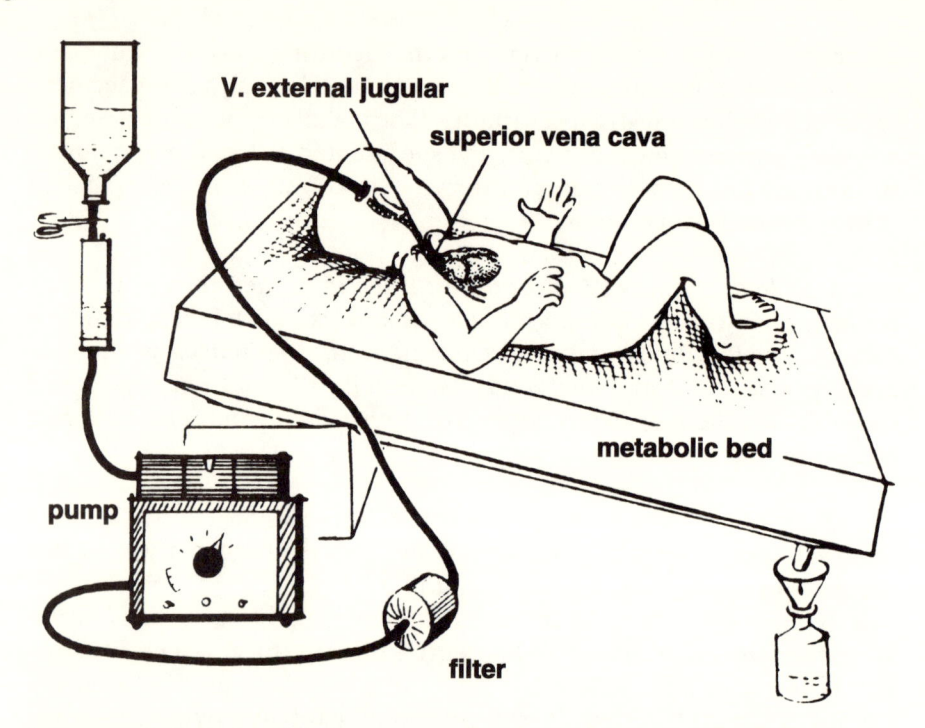

Infant metabolic bed and delivery system for total intravenous nutrition. (Reproduced with permission from D.W. Wilmore, S.J. Dudrick: Growth and development of an infant receiving all nutrients exclusively by vein. JAMA 203: 140–144, 1968.[60])

cava, and also tunneled under the skin to exit just above the ear. There had been previous neurosurgical successes with the use of polyethylene catheter for decompression shunts in the brains of hydrocephalic children. It was reasoned that if the exit site of the catheter was a considerable distance from the entrance site into the vein, the risk of infections from skin organisms would be decreased. Although the investigators feared that the indwelling venous catheter would become infected after a short time, they were pleased to find that the catheter remained free from infection for 40 days. To maintain the infusion, the surgeons catheterized the jugular vein 6 times, the saphenous vein once, the cephalic vein in one instance, and the subclavian vein 8 times. The feedings were carefully calculated to meet the child's needs, and the ration was increased in proportion to body weight as the child grew. The results were indeed dramatic. The baby was fed for 22 months and reached a weight of 18.5 pounds. The head circumference increased by 6.5 cm, and her chest enlarged by 8.5 cm. The child's behavior pattern was observed by child psychologists who felt that her emotional development was also satisfactory. Wilmore reflects on the early nutrient infusions:

We just did it. It's interesting if you don't let things get in your way, you can just get things done. There was a small treatment room in the nursery at the Children's Hospital, which was in South Philadelphia at 17th and Bainbridge. We simply took her back to the treatment room, used equipment and catheters that we used with the puppy dogs, and did a little cutdown on the external jugular vein and inserted the catheter. Bishop had modified some knitting needles. We could hook the catheters onto the end of the knitting needles, and we used this apparatus to create a long subcutaneous tunnel for the catheter. We mixed the solutions in the treatment room. Dale Johnson, the Chief Resident, inserted a Millipore filter, which was used to keep foreign material out of arterial lines. She was placed in a special bed with a mesh net covering which had been used in other metabolic studies at Children's. We were able to collect all of her urine. I saw the child 2 or 3 times a day for 6 to 8 months. We just did it.[61]

Rhoads was carefully apprised of the child's progress. Wilmore recalls an early visit by Rhoads:

He called me, I guess at home, and his wife was a pediatrician and she was curious. So the two of them met me on a Saturday or Sunday afternoon

Infant at start of total intravenous feeding. (Reproduced with permission from D.W. Wilmore, S.J. Dudrick: Growth and development of an infant receiving all nutrients exclusively by vein. JAMA 203: 142, 1968.[62])

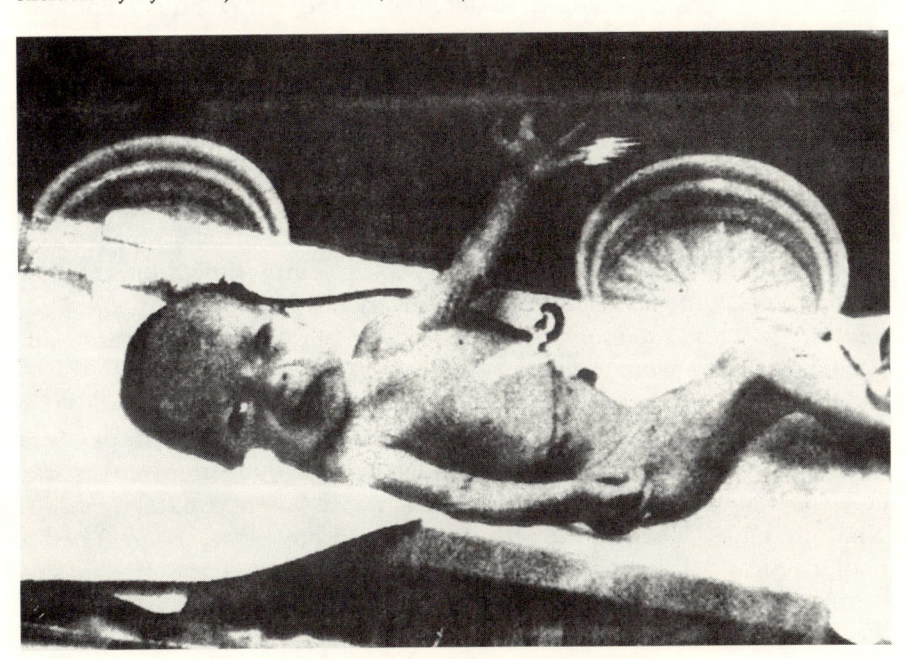

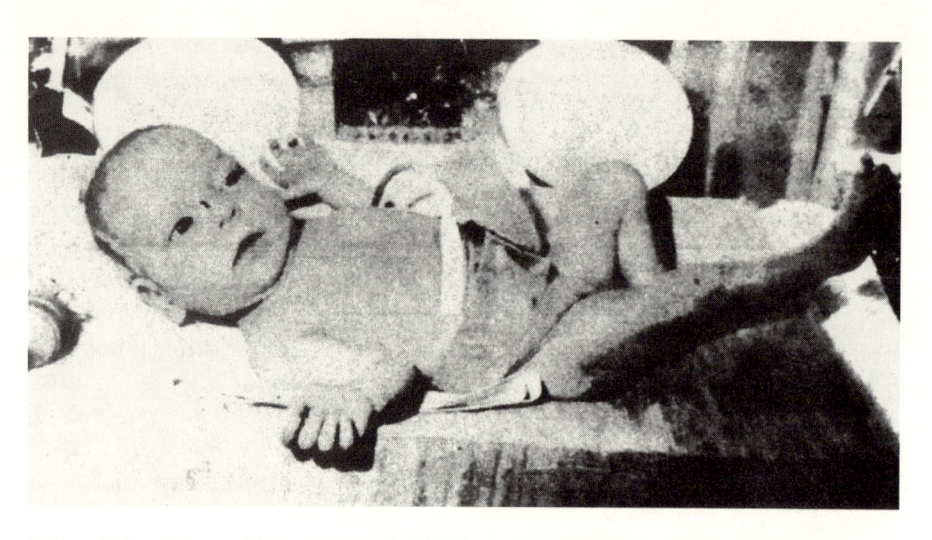

Infant following total intravenous for 44 days. (Reproduced with permission from D.W. Wilmore, S.J. Dudrick: Growth and development of an infant receiving all nutrients exclusively by vein. JAMA 203: 142, 1968.[63])

at CHOP. We all gowned and went into the nursery and saw the baby and played with her. Rhoads was amazed. Here was this baby growing and, for all intents and purposes, looked normal.[64]

Even with these early demonstrable nutritional benefits, there were many unforeseen problems associated with the intravenous feeding of the child. Wilmore recounts:

The problems became evident fairly early on. We didn't have to wait until the end of the baby's life. Someone picked up the child maybe 4 to 6 months into the feeding period and broke the baby's humerus. It was quite clear that the baby had rickets. We had just not appreciated the requirements of vitamins, calcium and phosphorus. Catheter sepsis was a repeated problem. And very gradually, candidemia [fungal infection in the blood] became an issue. We worked very hard in terms of behavioral development and the like. But at the end of 6 or 8 months, it became apparent that there were problems with behavioral development.[65]

The infant died on May 25, 1969. Permission for the autopsy was granted only for the abdominal examination. The duodenum was markedly shortened (9 cm) and significantly dilated (approximately 8 cm in circumference). The total length of the small bowel was 6 cm. The remaining terminal ileum was about 4.5 cm. in circumference. The anastomoses were well healed without evidence of obstruction. The body weight at death was 1500 grams, and there was diffuse edema. Some of the terminal findings included acute interstitial pneumonia, nephritis (inflammation of the kidney), and acute inflammation of the small intestine with dilatation.[66]

This case, published in the *Journal of the American Medical Association*, was a landmark contribution demonstrating the feasibility of the method, particularly for newborn children with serious defects of the gastrointestinal tract. Members of the pediatric surgical community were among the first to recognize the importance of this feeding technique. Shortly following Dudrick's presentation to the Society of University Surgeons, Judah Folkman, the newly appointed chief of surgery at Boston Children's Hospital, approached Dudrick as he was walking off the podium and said, "We've got to learn this technique so that we can use it at Boston Children's Hospital." Bob Filler, the second in command at Boston Children's and later to become the chief of surgery at Toronto's Hospital for Sick Children, came to Philadelphia to learn the technique. He returned to Boston and investigated a series of patients and published the results.[67]

Despite the death of the patient, this courageous family and patient gave the Penn nutrition group the experience and needed confidence to extend these clinical studies to adult patients. Additional studies of intravenous feeding were performed in patients with abnormalities of the gastrointestinal tract that precluded the ingestion of sufficient nutrients by mouth. The results were remarkable. The wounds healed, granulation tissue (an important tissue in healing wounds) significantly increased, and the patients went into a strongly positive nitrogen balance and gained weight. One of the early patients who received I.V.H. was a woman who was operated on 26 times by Rhoads for small bowel obstruction.

Early investigations with I.V.H. revealed it to be particularly efficacious in the patient with multiple catastrophic complications (critically ill patient). Interestingly, critically ill patients comprise the most important treatment category for the current use of T.P.N. Each of the complications could be approached with appropriate surgical aggressiveness aided by the ability to maintain adequate perioperative nutrition by vein.

I.V.H. was life-saving in another critically ill patient with superior mesenteric venous thrombosis, massive small bowel resection, anastomotic rupture, multiple episodes of sepsis, thrombophlebitis, pulmonary embolism, and gastrointestinal hemorrhage. The patient underwent five emergency operations during a 5-month period. During much of the prolonged hospitalization, the patient's intestinal tract was maintained at rest, allowing resolution of the underlying infection, healing of the anastomosis and various wounds, and gradual adaptation of the markedly shortened small bowel to its enormously increased absorptive task. The surgeons concluded that the man's life would not have been saved and that the decisions which resulted in his complete recovery would not have been possible without total intravenous feeding. The successful

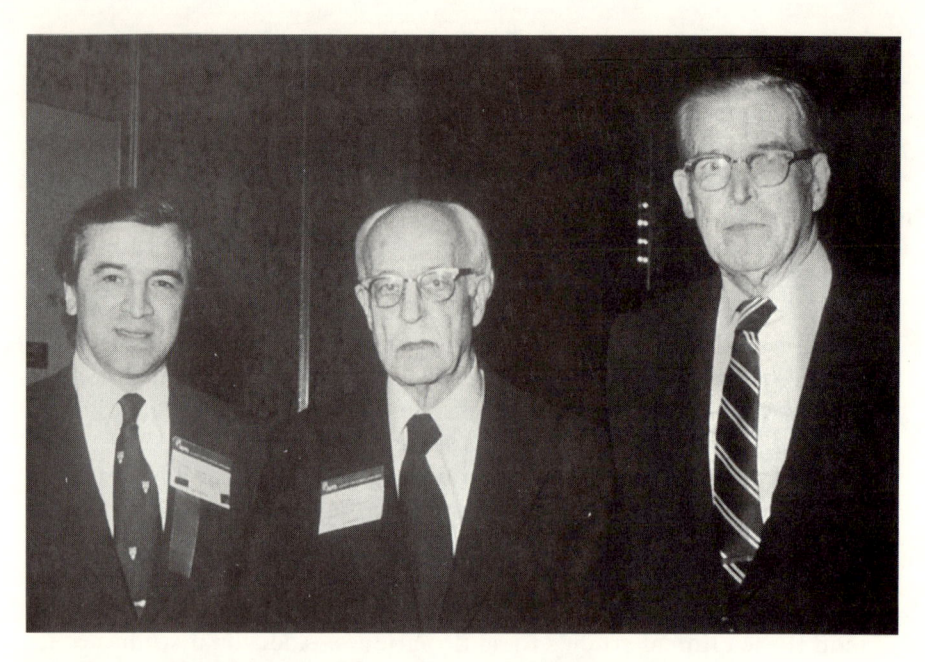

Dr. Rhoads (right) in 1982 with his colleagues in the development of hyperalimentation—Drs. Harry Vars (center) and Stan Dudrick (left).

outcome of this patient resulted from several treatment strategies that were not possible prior to the availability of I.V.H: (1) delaying reoperation to improve nutritional status; (2) creating an end jejunostomy (an ostomy with an opening in the skin emptying the intestinal contents into a plastic bag) without fear of uncontrolled fluid and nutrient losses; (3) allowing adequate time for adaptive absorptive function of the remaining short bowel; and (4) performing a complex operative procedure after 4 months of critical illness and many complications.

Following the investigations in the puppies and the patient at Children's Hospital, additional individuals made major contributions to the nutritional research efforts at Penn. Robert Ruberg, who became a professor of plastic surgery at Ohio State, studied fistula patients who received pure amino acid formulations by vein. Ezra Steiger, who became an attending surgeon at the Cleveland Clinic, developed a method for giving rats continuous intravenous feeding. This development was an especially important contribution because of the reduced cost of the rats, when compared with the cost of dogs. Moreover, the rat model made it possible to study large numbers of animals. Steiger showed that intestinal wounds gained strength due to intravenous feeding.[68]

The early studies of intravenous feeding at Penn were summarized in a landmark publication in the *Journal of the American Medical Association*.[69] Dudrick and Rhoads received the prestigious Joseph Goldberger

Award of the American Medical Association, which is given each year for contributions in the field of nutrition. It was the first time that this award had been given to surgeons.

The clinical importance of I.V.H. is placed in perspective when intravenous feeding in the late 1940s is compared with that of today. Fifty years ago patients who could not take nourishment by mouth could only be kept alive a short time by intravenous feeding.

To order T.P.N. in the 1990s, one simply consults the multidisciplinary nutrition support service composed of a physician, dietitian, nurse, and pharmacist. A subclavian venous catheter is inserted percutaneously with reasonable ease, and it can be left in place for prolonged periods in lieu of the daily starting of peripheral venous lines. The intravenous solutions are carefully formulated in the pharmacy, and they are infused into the circulation with a microprocessor-controlled pump with many safety devices. Glucose concentrations as high as 25% are infused with 5% concentrations of amino acids. This formula meets maintenance and, in some instances, repletion needs for both protein and calories. All of the required vitamins and trace metals are added to the mixtures, and fat is frequently added directly to the protein and carbohydrate mixture as a "3-in-1" infusion. Pyrogenic reactions and infection of the catheter are infrequent because of the use of carefully standardized and sterilized disposable infusion sets. As the result of these advances, patients are fed intravenously for indefinite periods with minimal discomfort and reasonable mobility.

Nearing the end of his years of active research, Vars reflects on the progress that had been made:

When you consider how far we have come in nutrition research in just 50 years, the future looks very promising indeed. Over each decade in science there is a returning to the "soil" of the same topics and more "diamonds" are picked up each time. Each order has a different terminology and thinking, but each adds much more to the body of knowledge. This is equally true in the field of nutrition research.[70]

Indeed, Rhoads has said that intravenous feeding is "one of the rare things in medicine that has turned out to be better than its sponsors anticipated."[71]

There have been many important sequelae resulting from the discovery of intravenous feeding. The multidisciplinary American Society for Parenteral and Enteral Nutrition (A.S.P.E.N.) was founded in 1976. Its functions include providing continuing education courses, presenting research studies, and discussing clinical problems to advance this important science. Fittingly, A.S.P.E.N. has established annual awards named in honor of Rhoads, Vars, Wilmore, and Dudrick. Moreover, a Rhoads

Research Foundation has been endowed to perpetuate the growth of young investigators in this field. Dudrick was named the first President of A.S.P.E.N., and Wilmore has remained active in the research support of this society.

The discovery of I.V.H./T.P.N. has increased the awareness among physicians and surgeons throughout the world of the importance of nutrition in the clinical care of hospitalized and home patients. Nutritional diagnoses, such as protein-calorie malnutrition, are now listed along with the patient's primary diagnosis at the time of hospital admission. Nutritional treatments are prescribed similar to the prescription of drugs and other therapies. Nutritional therapy is now considered to be a mandatory component of the care of the critically ill patient.

The discovery of T.P.N. has given a new identity to the hospital-based dietitian. In the pre-T.P.N. era the dietitian was largely confined to the hospital kitchen, and her clinical responsibilities were relegated to remedial tasks. With the emergence of T.P.N., the dietitian became acknowledged as the only person, in most hospital settings, with formal training in nutrition. To better apply this training, dietitians are now closely involved in the daily administration of both intravenous nutrition and enteral feeding. These duties include daily consultations with physicians and patients, in addition to dietary recommendations based upon careful daily monitoring of nutrient intakes and losses.

A further outcome of the discovery of T.P.N. is the recognition that more extensive nutritional education is needed in medical school curricula than in previous eras. Departments of Gastroenterology are now named Gastroenterology and Nutrition. In many medical schools basic scientists are actively involved in teaching the scientific basis of clinical nutrition. Nutrition-metabolic questions are now included on the qualifying examinations of the National Board of Medical Examiners, and standard surgical and medical textbooks contain considerable information on nutrition. The availability of a potent nutritional therapy such as T.P.N. has led to the discovery of objective measures of assessing nutritional status. New methods of body composition measurements, calculation and estimation of nutrient requirements, and accurate determinations of nutrient losses are now clinically available. Interestingly, the discovery of T.P.N. has led to the "rediscovery" of enteral nutrition—the administration of liquid formula diets by tube or mouth into the gastrointestinal tract. More recently, it has become apparent that T.P.N. and enteral feeding are complementary and not competitive. To meet nutrient requirements, critically ill patients are usually fed concurrently with both of these delivery methods.

The discovery of T.P.N. has led to the birth of a new clinical science—nutritional pharmacotherapy—defined as the use of nutrients that have more pharmacologic effects than nutrient effects per se.

Finally, the discovery of T.P.N. has led to the development of a new industry for home infusions. Home T.P.N. is largely administered by private companies that provide experienced nutrition support professionals to monitor the patients. Permanent feeding catheters are placed via a surgical technique and are monitored carefully at home. In the 1990s a system of managed health care has emerged that has wholeheartedly embraced the concept of home health care, and nutritional support companies are at the vanguard of delivery of health care in the home setting.

The discovery of I.V.H./T.P.N. has led to the emergence of a billion dollar a year industry. It is tempting to wonder retrospectively why the Penn surgeons did not patent these important discoveries or pursue these financial issues in a more aggressive manner. Rhoads responds:

When I was brought up, I remember my father telling me that you didn't patent things in the medical field. If you made a discovery, the ethics of the profession called for it to be made available to every doctor who was taking care of patients. The idea of physicians or departments making money came along somewhat later. I also thought it would be difficult to be totally ethical about further research in which one holds patents. I never had any regrets about not attempting to get patents. I think it could only have held the field back. As soon as you begin to get patents, it disqualifies you as a witness in the future. Whether it is true or not, people think that your interest is commercial.[72]

Despite the many proven benefits of T.P.N., it is important to acknowledge that it is not risk-free. The placement of the subclavian venous catheter requires technical expertise, and its malposition may result in considerable morbidity and, in some instances, death. The long-term presence of a foreign body, such as the catheter, directly in the bloodstream provides a nidus for infection. Catheter sepsis is often severely debilitating, especially when it is due to fungal organisms. Moreover, the long-term administration of T.P.N. produces bone destruction (similar to osteoporosis) and occasionally leads to severe liver damage.

T.P.N. is contraindicated in the patient with metastatic cancer who is not a candidate for adjuvant chemotherapy or radiotherapy. Concerning these unfortunate patients, Rhoads reflects:

I often think of the advice of an early preceptor, Dr. Eldridge Eliason, who was Chairman of our Department before Ravdin. He was not an experimentalist but quite strictly a clinician. However, he was a very keen observer. He counselled against placing a feeding gastrostomy in the patient with severe esophageal cancer. [Esophagectomies were not performed at that time.] He stated that his experience was that without a gastrostomy they died painlessly of inanition. When a gastrostomy was performed, they lived until their tumors invaded their nerve pathways and gave them a lot of pain.[73]

Despite these concerns, most clinicians believe that the benefits of I.V.H./T.P.N. strongly exceed its risks. This is especially evident in the critically ill patient with significant weight loss. The impact of the discovery of I.V.H. is best expressed in Rhoads' comments on success in his Roswell Park Memorial Lecture in 1982:

Perhaps the most satisfactory definition of success in scholarship for me is one given by the Nobel Prize winning economist, Milton Friedman, of the University of Chicago. After receiving the Nobel Prize, he said that he felt success did not lie in what one's colleagues said about one nor about prizes or awards, but rather in the degree to which one's ideas and contributions became imbedded in the body of knowledge that comprised one's discipline.[74]

If one thinks of good as encompassing life, liberty and the pursuit of happiness, one comes upon the question—Is this furthered most by focusing on the group or by focusing on the individual? Since the individual cannot develop fully in solitary confinement and since the group cannot exist without individuals that compose it, I suspect this question is more inflammatory than constructive. Nevertheless, I am steeped in the tradition of focusing on the individual—believing that society will derive greatest strength from the fullest possible development of the individuals that compose it. I do not defend these biases, I admit them—but with pride.

Jonathan Rhoads[1]

EIGHT

A HAPPY FACULTY
PROVOST

Jonathan Rhoads expressed these thoughts in his report to President Harnwell and the university community in the last year of his tenure as provost of the University of Pennsylvania. When he resigned in April 1959, his accomplishments as provost were widely recognized by the administration, faculty, students and staff alike. Harnwell remarked of Dr. Rhoads:

> ... *[his] incumbency as provost has been marked by a most distinguished advance in every phase of the academic life of the University. His leadership has stimulated all of the schools of the University, his personal distinction has been an inspiration to his colleagues, and his warm human understanding has won the hearts of the entire University family.*[2]

The student body expressed its gratefulness in an editorial entitled "Rare Combination" in the student newspaper:

> *One of Dr. Rhoads' most outstanding achievements as provost has been the establishment of smooth relations between faculty and administrative personnel, two distinct intra-University groups that are often wont to conflict with one another in matters of policy. This faculty-administrative*

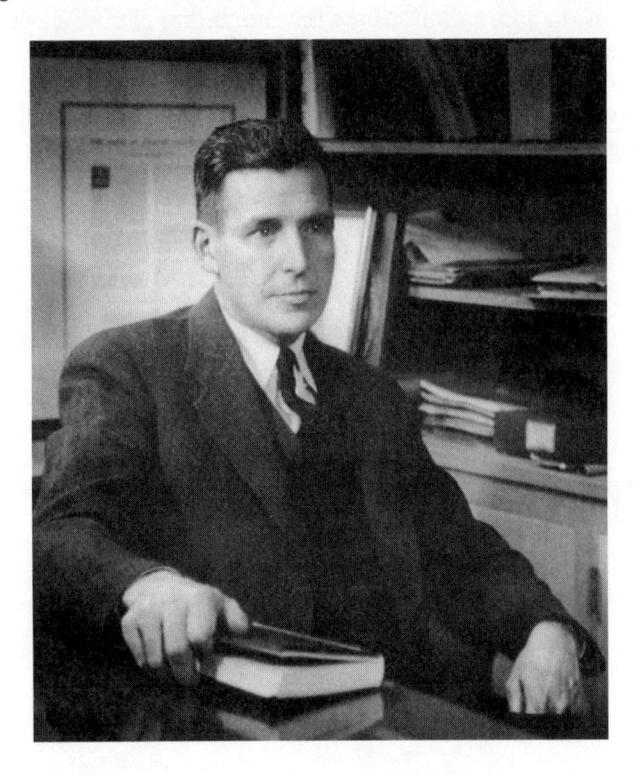

Jonathan Rhoads, Provost, 1956.

liaison works especially well at Pennsylvania, whose president, provost and vice provosts are all both teaching scholars and practicing administrators who can reconcile the two varying points of view. . . . He can step down as Provost leaving a job well done.[3]

The ability to seek and achieve consensus between contentious groups or individuals figures prominently in the Quaker ethic. Quakers hold the belief that consensus must be reached, and if not, no decision is made until it is. Howard Brinton, a Quaker educator and historian, distinguishes this from compromise:

The final result is in general not compromise. Often it is a new and unexpected result brought about by a synthesis of different points of view.[4]

There is no doubt that Jonathan Rhoads has successfully brought this skill to bear in his many activities in and outside the world of surgery. Whether this is the product of uncanny intelligence, inheritance, or both is not clear, but his mother, recognizing this talent in her husband, Edward, writes:

Father has a happy faculty of formulating the discussion, especially when there is much divergence of thought, and hitting upon something, upon which the meeting agrees or tolerates.[5]

This "happy faculty" possessed by Jonathan Rhoads as well was in dire need by a very unhappy faculty at the University of Pennsylvania in 1954. They were demoralized by salary levels well below those at their sister institutions in the Ivy League and by a very unresponsive administration that turned a deaf ear to their many concerns. Fueling this contentious atmosphere, the trustees had recently appointed Harold Stassen as president of the university without consulting the faculty. The thinking was that a national political figure would be far more instrumental in fund raising than the man who currently held the position. Stassen became known as the "boy wonder" when he was elected governor of Minnesota at the young age of 30 and had just run unsuccessfully for president of the United States in 1948.

The appointment of Stassen came as a surprise not only to the faculty but also to the man who currently occupied the position. He learned of the new appointment one Sunday morning when he opened the newspaper. President McClelland, a professor of English and former provost, was highly regarded by the faculty. "Highhanded business," Rhoads said later.[6]

Already active with the Haverford College board of managers, Rhoads had become interested in faculty issues at Penn when he learned that they intended to form a faculty senate. It would have the authority to elect its own officers, to meet and pass resolutions, and to forward these to the president and the trustees. Its rationale was to create a formal avenue of communication. Leading this movement were Alex Fry of the Law School and Reavis Cox of the Wharton School of Business. As a "believer in democracy and the dignity of the faculty," Rhoads cut short a stay in Chicago and returned to Philadelphia to attend one of the senate's initial meetings. In time he became very active in this movement and after two years was elected chair or president of the senate.

When Stassen resigned as president of the University of Pennsylvania in 1953 after another unsuccessful run for president of the United States, the trustees appointed Gaylord Harnwell as his successor. Harnwell, a graduate of Haverford College, was a Phi Beta Kappa and a member of the same class as Rhoads' cousin Philip. Later, Harnwell became chairman of the Department of Physics at Pennsylvania, where he created a first-rate department and proved to be an able fundraiser. As chair of the senate, Rhoads met frequently with Harnwell, and they worked well together.

In 1955, Rhoads was approached by the nominating committee of the senate to serve another term. He initially turned down the offer because no previous chairman had sought reelection, and he thought it was taking too much time from his surgical practice. Learning of his decision, his very able secretary of the time, Jinny Mager (later Balsham), was saddened by the news. She evidently felt that he was passing up a great opportunity. Rhoads spent a restless night thinking it over and in the morning approached the chairman of the nominating committee to ask if they had any other nominees. On learning they had none, he agreed to stand for reelection and was unanimously elected to a second term.

During this time, Provost Edwin Williams decided to return to teaching and research, and he asked to be removed from his administrative duties. A faculty search committee for a new provost was formed, which consisted of individuals named by the president and suggested by the faculty senate. Among the latter was I.S. Ravdin. Rhoads describes the result of their deliberations:

I know nothing of the deliberations of the committee, but apparently they submitted a list of possible nominees for provost to Dr. Harnwell which included my name. I received word that he wanted to come see me. Realizing that my cluttered office did not suggest much efficiency as an administrator, my secretary and I got most of the loose papers out of the room before he arrived. He asked me if I would be willing to serve as Provost if elected, and I indicated that it would be an uncertain venture for me and that I would hate to cut off all of my ties to surgery because if I wanted to return to surgery, I wanted to have something to come back to. He agreed that I might be able to continue some work in the hospital. It turned out that on Saturday mornings the university offices were closed, and it was finally agreed that I could reserve Tuesday mornings for surgery and thus operate on Tuesdays and Saturdays. My duties as Chief of one of the Surgical Services were transferred to Dr. Fitts, and after being duly elected I took office about the first of February 1956.[7]

Rhoads, the 18th provost of the university, was only the second member of the medical profession to hold the post—the other was Dr. William Pepper, provost from 1881–1894. The provost is the chief educational officer under the president. He is responsible for the undergraduate, graduate, and professional schools as well as the libraries, museums, and institutes of the university. Understandably, Rhoads' appointment was enthusiastically greeted by the faculty since he had fought hard as chair of the senate for salary raises—not an unpopular cause.

One of Rhoads' first duties was to appoint two vice provosts. He decided early on that the work of the provost would be broadly shared with these men. Ravdin advised Rhoads that Scully Bradley, who had been very loyal

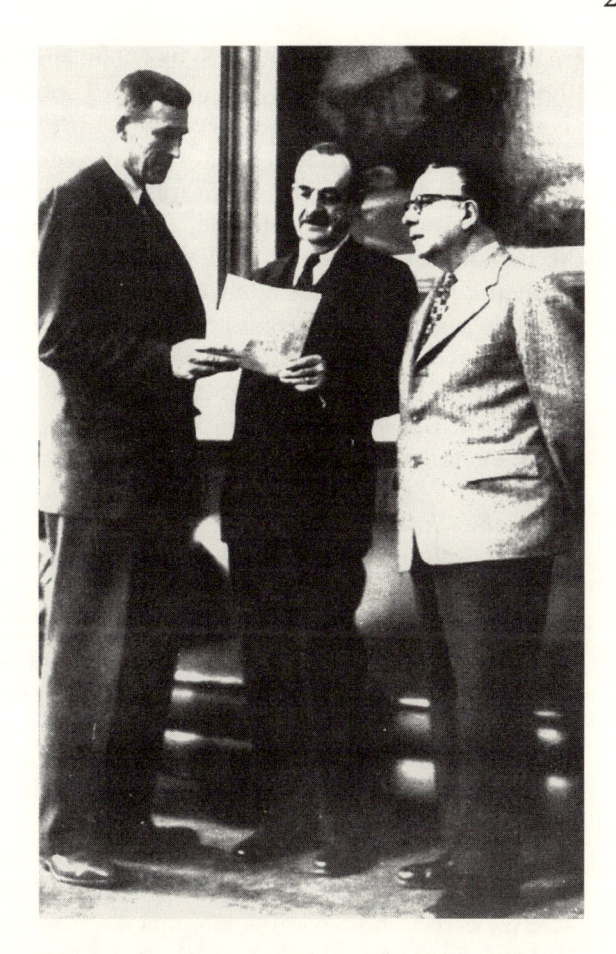

Jonathan Rhoads with Vice Provosts Roy Nichols (center) and E. Sculley Bradley (right).

to Rhoads while he was active in the senate, would make an outstanding vice provost. Bradley, a professor in the English department, had authored the variorum edition of Whitman's *Leaves of Grass*. As one of the vice provosts, he was appointed to oversee undergraduate education.

The other appointee, Roy Nichols, was already serving as vice provost and had performed very ably in that position. Nichols, the dean of the Graduate School of Arts and Sciences, was enormously respected, and he had won a Pulitzer Prize for one of his history books and had an honorary degree from Oxford University. He was instrumental in the establishment of a study program in American civilization at Penn and was considered a pioneer in the field. He continued to assume responsibility for all aspects of graduate education.

A third very important figure during this time was Joseph Willits. A former director of social sciences of the Rockefeller Foundation and former dean of the Wharton School, he had been appointed in 1954 to oversee Penn's "Educational Survey," which was the largest academic study of its kind in the United States. The survey was still ongoing when Rhoads was appointed. Its purpose was to study systematically, in detail, all of the functions of the university. This enormous undertaking drew upon the best talent from within the university and from the best academic centers in the United States. All aspects of undergraduate and graduate schools were evaluated, and recommendations were made with the goal of making the University of Pennsylvania one of the leading academic institutions in the country.

Balancing a surgical practice with the tremendous responsibilities of provost was no easy task. As Rhoads tells it, "The change of emphasis was quite an extraordinary experience."[8] Marion Carbone, who had been working at the university and later became one of his very able secretaries, experienced this move in reverse:

I thought I knew the University well, but south of Spruce Street [the hospital and medical school] was entirely different.[9]

Just before becoming provost, Rhoads, in addition to his private practice, was co-chief of half of the general surgery ward service. The university offices were closed in the early morning hours when Rhoads operated on Tuesday and Saturday. Rhoads gave up his operating time on Thursdays. Rounds were conducted before 9 a.m. and after 5 p.m. With the able help of Clete Schwegman, his surgical and administrative burdens were more easily handled.

The provost staff conference was held on Wednesday mornings. Typically, faculty appointments from the level of assistant professor and up were reviewed, and recommendations were forwarded to the president and the trustees or were sent back to their respective faculties if not approved. Particular attention was paid to those faculty up for tenure. Provost staff conferences were usually attended by the president and the academic vice presidents for engineering and medicine, and deans could be invited to attend on a necessary basis. Thursday mornings were reserved for the president's weekly staff conference, at which the provost and the various vice presidents provided information and advice. There were also meetings with the board of trustees. Eight schools reported to Rhoads: the College, College for Women, Wharton (business), Education, Social Work, Fine Arts-Architecture, City Planning, Law, the Library System, and in his last year the Annenberg School of Communications. The provost had budgetary authority over all of these schools at Penn with the exception of engineering and the medical group. With respect to monetary problems Rhoads reflects:

In general, I noticed that the University had multiple constituencies and that they were not transferable. There was the constituency at the Museum which would only give for archeology, especially expeditions.

Most of these donors wouldn't think at all of giving to fine arts or the college or anything in medicine. They were interested in archeology period. The medical constituencies were even more clearly defined. They would give to the Department of Medicine, but would not give to Surgery or some other discipline so that I had the feeling that you really didn't gain much by pushing something ahead of the donor's interest.[10]

Rhoads was confronted with a broad variety of administrative challenges in the 1950s. In addition to a low-paid and somewhat disaffected faculty, the deanships of the Wharton School of Business and School of Education became vacant. The School of Social Work, then located at 2410 Pine Street, ten blocks from Penn's main campus, was in need of an overhaul. There was a good deal of fragmentation on the undergraduate level. There was an acute shortage of dormitory space for female students. A centralized facility was needed for the faculty.[11] Additionally, there were the problems of student riots, controversial speakers, disappointed parents whose children had not been admitted to Penn, and unhappy trustees. Against this background, the effects of Senator Joseph McCarthy's smear campaign still lingered on at Penn and at many other universities in the United States.

The most important challenge facing Rhoads was the problem of faculty salaries, which were deplorably low—in terms of purchasing power, they were substantially below 1935–39 levels. In his first year, with the vital support of Harnwell, Rhoads increased faculty salaries by $850.[12] Communication between administration and faculty was greatly improved. Rhoads, writing to a trustee, relates:

We have tried to improve communications this year by successively getting one or another member of the Administration to speak at each of the Dean's meetings to brief them on the University's problems as viewed centrally. . . . I do not believe in keeping things secret around the University, and I think periodically Committees of Deans or of Faculty members ought to have a frank look at these matters and address themselves to the correction of inequities. The Senate has assumed this function to some extent and the reports of the Educational Survey will have an important bearing on it also.[13]

Willis Winn, acting dean of the Wharton School in 1956, says that Rhoads approach to the problems confronting the university was "ground breaking and innovative." He had full confidence in the faculty.[14] By the time he resigned to return to full-time surgical practice, there had been a dramatic change not only in faculty salaries but also in the general atmosphere at the university.

Penn's School of Social Work was different from nearly all the schools of social work in the country in adopting a "Rankian" philosophy as opposed to a Freudian-based philosophy. As Rhoads explains:

I think the Rankians believed that you can't help persons unless they can frame the questions that needed to be answered, whereas Freud was interpreting the personality using dreams as avenues to pierce the subconscious and so forth, e.g., to dig back and see what was eating you.[15]

The dean of the school was considered rather ineffectual and often gave in to the wishes of two very strong professors who were solid Rankians. Rhoads felt that new leadership was in order. The faculty, not anxious to have the dean replaced, believed that any outsider would not share their beliefs. Provost Rhoads found one faculty member, Ruth Smalley, who was both acceptable to him and the faculty. She was ultimately appointed as the new dean of the School of Social Work.[16]

The law school faculty presented yet another challenge to Rhoads. Composed of only 18 law professors, it taught between 400 and 500 students in the three-year course. Most of the 18 were full professors. They had recommended the promotion of a man who had been serving as assistant dean of the Law School. Noting that most of this man's work was administrative and not academic, Rhoads felt this experience was not an adequate basis upon which to promote someone academically, and he blocked the appointment. "This was a very sticky problem," Rhoads said later. He met with the law faculty about this problem and felt that he had probably not won them over to his position, but he noted that the man later came to him as a patient and probably felt Rhoads was justified in his decision.[17]

Because of the emphasis on research as a basis for appointing faculty, there was a concern that the undergraduate schools were not being well served. Additionally, the quality of teaching varied among the schools. With the help of Vice Provost Bradley, Rhoads organized an all-day faculty conference on undergraduate education. The program provided a forum within which the faculties of the several schools teaching undergraduate students could discuss the problems confronting them. Outside speakers also were invited to address problems of undergraduate education. This type of forum was a first at Penn, and it contributed greatly to the cohesiveness of the undergraduate faculty. Rhoads and his staff received a good deal of favorable comment for the success of the meeting.[18]

In August 1956, Loren Eiseley, stepping down as president of the faculty senate, wrote to Rhoads:

We did have a rough time this year, didn't we? . . . I shall follow the further activities of the Senate with interest and perhaps a little wistfully now that I am through with it all. I think I am the person who should be thanking you for your generous and cooperative help during a time when you must have been confronted with many new and unforeseen problems.[19]

On January 12, 1957, Rhoads was invited to give the Founder's Day Address at the mid-year graduation ceremonies. He began:

This is the time of year for messages on the State of the Union, and since the University is a union of 19 schools and colleges, I thought you might like to hear a brief synopsis on the State of the University.[20]

He reported that the main campus was composed of 123 acres and 170 buildings. There was a 4–5% increase in the student body, which was the equivalent of a small college. There were 1,118 full-time faculty compared with the previous year's level of 987. He addressed the subject of faculty salaries and reiterated again his belief in the importance of reasonable compensation:

Important as additions to our plant have become, I am convinced that it is in the field of faculty resources that this University will succeed or fail to make the sort of contribution we expect of it.[21]

The research program was productive—with 1500 separate reports having been published in a single year. Research grants exceeded $6 million in the academic year 1956–57. The University Press was reorganized: 21 new books were completed, 3 were reprinted, 16 were approved for publication, and 24 old titles had been restored. The library, which contained 1.5 million volumes, was the 10th largest library in the country. Plans for a faculty club and more dormitory space for women were under consideration. On the medical and hospital front, the I.S. Ravdin Institute was in the fundraising and planning stages.[22] Like Ravdin and Harnwell, Rhoads was an able fundraiser. Isaac Roberts, head of the Ravdin campaign, wrote to Rhoads and expressed his appreciation for the money he raised for the Ravdin Institute:

You are a grand solicitor as the report on the six cards you had shows—I wish I had your ability. Many thanks for what you did.[23]

There were perennial problems with the student body. A student riot on May 3, 1956, drew strong community criticism of the university. The riot began when 4 students who were playing stickball began to throw small pieces of piled debris onto the road. More students joined in, and within a short time a crowd had gathered to watch them build a barricade on Locust Street. The Police arrived and the students began to throw eggs and rocks at the patrolmen. One hundred fifty students were arrested, and the riot made the headlines in the local papers.[24] Concerned alumni wrote to the provost. Rhoads responds to one of them:

We all regretted the student riots this Spring very much. I thought you would like to know that a total of twenty of our students were suspended for varying lengths of time. It is always difficult for me to see these things in perspective, particularly when I read about them at a distance. One has the feeling that the students of a particular university are repeaters in almost every sense of the word; whereas in most instances this is not the case, and the new riots represent the activity of a new class of students. We all hope that our extracurricular program may develop to the point in which the loose energies of students are better absorbed and directed. From the newspaper reports this Spring, it was evident that Penn students were not alone in their activities, as you point out in your letter. We will do our best to insist that our students be good citizens. I hope our efforts will be more successful in the future, but the long history of the past does seem to indicate that most of the boys involved in such activities do end up as useful citizens as they mature.[25]

While Joseph McCarthy had been censured by the U.S. Senate in 1954, academic communities throughout the United States were still smarting from his outrageous smear campaign. He had accused many of them of communist leanings and of being traitors to their country. During Rhoads' first year as provost, Alger Hiss, who had just been convicted of perjury, was invited to speak by the student political union at the university. While this visit was controversial, it did not compare to the uproar generated by the invitation extended to John Henry Gates, a self-declared Communist and editor of the *Daily Worker*. Gates had been charged by the U.S. Attorney General's Office with contempt of the Smith Act of 1941, i.e., "being a member of the Communist Party and knowing while being a member of the party that it advocated the overthrowing of the United States by violence and force."[26] Rhoads writes to Harnwell regarding Gates and the impact of his visit on the university community:

No doubt there will be fairly heavy criticism of having Mr. Gates here to speak. Some will feel that in allowing this the University is in some way endorsing Communism, or lending its resources to the cause of Communism. I have never felt that this is the issue. . . .
   The issue here seems to be whether the administration of the University is willing to tell a recognized and established student organization

that they may not listen to an exponent or a set of beliefs which we do not share. I do not believe that we can represent ourselves to our students, our colleagues in other Universities and not in the long run the general public, as advocates of freedom of inquiry, freedom of thought, freedom of speech, not as custodians of the academic traditions of Western civilization were we to apply this sort of censorship. . . .

It should be pointed out that his remarks do not constitute the sole program but that he is to be followed, on the invitation of the students, by one of the professors in the Department of Political Science, who has indicated that he will endeavor to point out the weakness of the case for Communism. In arranging the program in this way, I would be prepared to agree that the students have shown a disposition to seek the truth. I think our students are well able to evaluate a doctrine when presented in this manner. Another personal opinion is that an exhibition of abnormal fear of Communist propaganda is more likely to interest the students in it than an open opportunity for them to hear a Communist speaker. . . .

We realize the great practical disadvantages to the University to have criticism leveled at it in this field. There is always danger that such criticism will decrease its public support, particularly support from conservative and successful businessmen and financiers. In the long run, however, I am sure it is wiser for us to maintain the academic traditions of those institutions with which we would like to compare ourselves despite these practical disadvantages.[27]

Willis Winn, whom Rhoads had appointed as dean of the Wharton School of Business, credits him with "supportive experimentation" and novel appointments to the faculty. Rhoads, according to Winn, had the courage to approve appointments of several of the faculty who were former members of the Communist Party. One later won the Nobel Prize for Economics.[28] Witness this exchange between the president of Armstrong Cork Company, a trustee, and Provost Rhoads in July 1959:

On a number of occasions I have expressed myself as being pretty vigorously opposed to what might be generally termed the drift toward collectivism in this country as influenced by education and in other areas of American life as well.[29]

Rhoads responds:

I suppose conservatism is in some sense a spectrum. I know that I am regarded as much too conservative by many of the people I meet, including some of my own children and their friends. Very probably you are further on the conservative side than I am. As I have accumulated more age and more property, I note that I tend to be more conservative. I am not sure that there is a cause and effect here but it just seems to have happened. Even my most leftish acquaintances, however, seem to want nothing like the communist pattern. . . .

Certainly the United States has adopted a great many things on a bipartisan basis which would have been so far to the left in the year that I was born as to have made most citizens of that era shudder. The income tax alone, under which many of us work several months of the year for the government and without remuneration, is a simple example. On the other hand, we enjoy driving our cars over a new expressway and both the car and the expressway are in many ways manifestations of collectivism, or at least of collective effort. The car more through the private enterprise type of collective effort and the expressway more through the government type of collective effort. . . . While I share Mr. Root's fear of Communism, I am not sure that I can define collectivism in a way in which it is all bad and none of it good.[30]

There were many social obligations attendant to the office of provost. Rhoads, true to form, attended as many as possible. His days and nights were replete with meetings, university events, office hours, patient calls, hospital rounds, and hours in the operating room. With all of this he had time to help a patient, not his own, one evening. The man had been diagnosed with cellulitis and had great difficulty contacting his physician. Finally, the doctor responded and informed the patient that he had tried unsuccessfully to get a bed for him at Northeast, Nazareth, and Frankford Hospitals in Philadelphia. The patient, probably knowing of Rhoads' reputation throughout the city, decided to call him. The grateful patient writes to Rhoads:

You must understand how grateful I am to you, Dr. Rhoads, for seeing that I got care. . . . It seems odd that a physician would make himself very inaccessible to his patients (he has no phone listed under his name only an exchange number) while Dr. Rhoads could be reached even at a party![31]

There was always time to write to a disappointed parent whose child had not been admitted to Penn. To one such parent, Rhoads writes:

We are all so ambitious for our young people that we tend to "force them a bit," to use a horticultural term. While nobody claims infallibility in judging what people can do, our Admissions Department does have a lot of experience to go on. At my request they have reviewed the record and credentials of your daughter with extra care, and they give the most serious warning signs of impending academic disaster were she to be admitted here. Having just been through some very sad negotiations with families whose children were admitted in the face of such signals, and who proceeded to have a very unsatisfactory time, ending in academic failure and dismissal from the various schools of the University, I have no real belief that one does any favor in disregarding these signals. It seems a good deal better to allow the student to seek his or her own academic level. I have reluctantly done so in the cases of two of my own children who were having academic difficulties, with full confidence that if the ability is there they will use it when they are ready. It may cheer you to know that my general observation has been that students flower best where they are not under excessive academic pressure, and we all know that the chief factors in making for success in life are outside the academic field.[32]

He made time to interview young men who were interested in becoming doctors. A grateful parent thanks him:

I wish to again thank you for giving your valuable time and wisdom, especially at this time of year, to my son and myself. You made a

Jonathan Rhoads with unidentified woman, Milton Eisenhower, and Gaylord Harnwell.

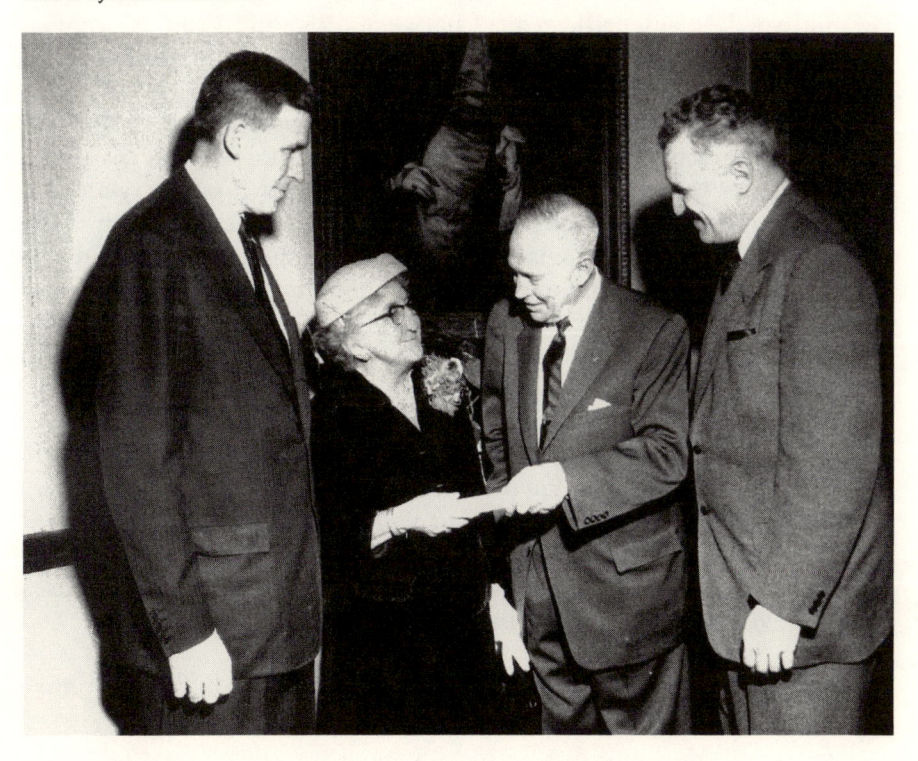

wonderful impression on Jim and I'm sure a lifetime admirer. It is association with men such as you and not myself that has inspired him to become a physician.[33]

Rhoads' tenure as provost brought with it many rewards other than the obvious intellectual ones. He became a member of the Rittenhouse Club, which had exchange arrangements with the Union Club of Boston, the Traveler's in London, and the Interallie in Paris. He also became a member of the Sunday Breakfast Club, which numbered among its members many of Philadelphia's key people in business and communications. Finally, and most important, he was elected to the American Philosophical Society, the oldest of the country's learned societies, founded by Benjamin Franklin and his friends in 1743. This exclusive society, numbering some 650 members throughout the world, was founded "to promote useful knowledge." In his later years, Rhoads became a prominent and very important leader in this organization. During these three years as provost, Rhoads was president of the College of Physicians of Philadelphia, the International Surgical Group, the Society of Clinical Surgery, and the Philadelphia division of the American Cancer Society. In addition, he served as governor in the American College of Surgeons and continued to serve on the board of managers of Haverford College. He published 14 scientific papers between 1956 and 1959. Moreover, *Surgery Principles and Practice*, the textbook he coauthored with Garrott Allen, Carl Moyer, and Henry Harkins was published in 1957.

Former Dean Winn describes Rhoads' years as provost as "ground breaking." He credits him with reapportioning the university's resources, raising faculty salaries to competitive levels, improving faculty and administration communications, and overseeing the implementation of the Educational Survey which changed the course of the university and prepared it for what was then projected to be a doubling of the student population.[34] One of the trustees wrote to Rhoads on his departure as provost to express his thanks:

I want to take this opportunity to say that, in common with all who have had any opportunity to know the great contribution you have made to the University as Provost, I feel our institution will be eternally in your debt. I have been amazed at your ability to keep as fully informed on all of the many areas of university activity, and have been impressed, too, with your manner of working with people, in many cases involving very delicate situations.[35]

Dr. Rhoads conveyed an incredible grasp of each patient's problems, special details of the case, unusual characteristics of the patients' wives, and what had been and should have been done for them. As he was gracious and knowledgeable on rounds, he was fearless but not flamboyant in the operating room. Rather he was cautious, fastidious, and technically correct, and I cannot recall a single mishap in the hundreds of times I worked with him.

Hilary Timmis[1]

NINE

I WONDER WHERE THAT PLANE IS GOING?

SURGICAL STATESMAN

At the age of 52, Rhoads became the John Rhea Barton Chairman of Surgery in 1959. His selection resulted from one of the shortest deliberations of a search committee on record. Clearly, Rhoads possessed the important prerequisites to become a successful chairman, namely proven clinical expertise, an international reputation in surgical education, and a research experience held in high regard by his colleagues. Rhoads' appointment was auspicious, for it was a great honor to succeed his beloved mentor, I.S. Ravdin, who had built the department into one of the leading programs in the country. Leonard Miller contrasts the personalities of Ravdin and Rhoads:

They were 180 degrees apart in appearance and personality. Ravdin was very short and Jonathan towered over him. Dr. Ravdin was very portly and excitable and garrulous . . . always chewing the residents out for this and that, and after you got to know him you realized that it really wasn't serious . . . constantly badgering people in the operating room and so forth. After a while you sort of laughed it off. Dr. Rhoads was just the opposite, very quiet . . . seemed to be introverted. It's remarkable they got along so well.[2]

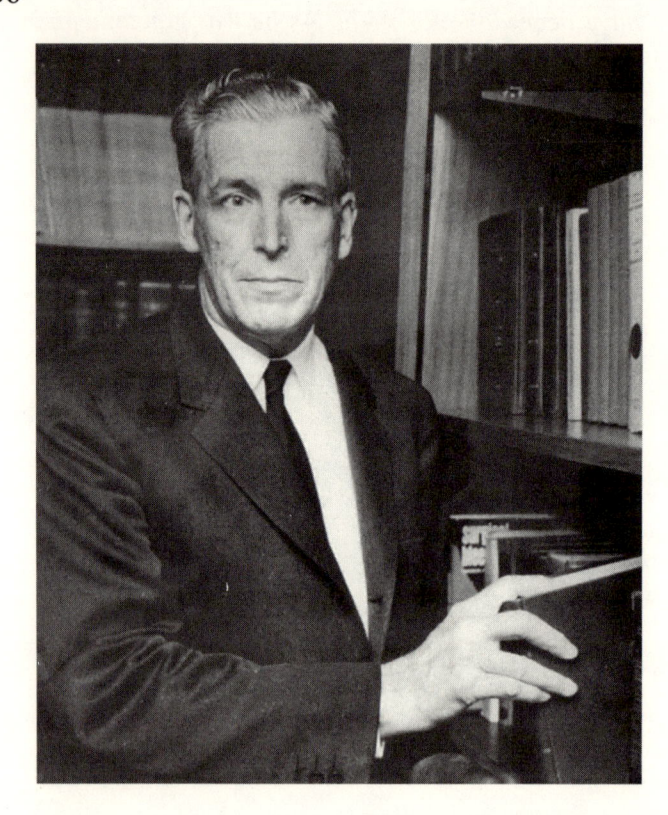

John Rhea Barton Professor of Surgery and Chairman, HUP, 1969.

James Thompson, former chairman of surgery at the University of Texas Galveston, once confided in Jack Mackie what he thought were the differences between Rhoads and Ravdin:

Rav knew how to use power and didn't hesitate to do it. Dr. Rhoads recognized power but was more discreet about how he used it. He would go out of his way to look on the other side of the coin. He would exercise it in ways that were out in the open and obvious.[3]

According to Jack Mackie,

They were very different people. They had great respect for each other. From a resident's standpoint Ravdin was a predictable surgeon and chief. He wanted things done the same way all of the time. It was easy to anticipate what he wanted, and you knew if you didn't get it done the way he wanted it done what the consequences would be. He would let you know about it. In a sense it was easy to work for him because you really had a routine and it didn't vary much.
Dr. Rhoads, on the other hand, was different. I always said that the most predictable thing about him when I was a resident was that he was

unpredictable. This in no way affected the relationship with him because he was always very gracious and agreeable and pleasant to be with no matter how badly you goofed up or whether you thought that you knew what he wanted you to do and it turned out that it was something else; but he was always very much a gentleman and very easy to get along with . . . unpredictable in terms of how he might want patients managed.[4]

There were many ongoing changes in American surgery when Rhoads became the Barton Professor. Private practice was flourishing for many surgeons, and there was increased government funding for research from post-World War II reapportionment of federal spending. Rapid advances were occurring in diagnostic technology such as angiography, leading to the development of a very important new subspecialty—vascular surgery. Exciting and technically demanding new operations such as the portal-caval shunt for hepatic cirrhosis were evolving. Kidney transplantation was acknowledged as the beginning of a new therapeutic era in surgery. Of great interest to Rhoads was the emerging emphasis upon pre- and postoperative care to improve outcome.

Despite these advances, there were challenging problems and new concerns. In inheriting a department that was at the top of the ladder of academic and clinical excellence, Rhoads needed to maintain this position and still allow for his own imprimatur. He reasoned that it would be difficult to improve a program that was already functioning extremely well. Competition for residency positions in surgical training programs was intensifying because of the aforementioned advances and the large number of new medical school graduates interested in surgery. There was a new emphasis upon subspecialization, which in turn led to the need for compartmentalization and decentralization of many surgical departments. In addition to responding to these changes, Rhoads was determined to increase the scope of his private practice and the overall clinical activity of the department. His involvement in surgical care returned almost immediately in a very busy way.

Many residents have fond memories of starting or finishing rounds in front of the Coca-Cola machine with him and imbibing their first "meal" of the day, or of being treated to a late afternoon lunch consisting of a couple of slices of American cheese between two slices of white bread. Barry Ellman shares his recollections:

Dr. Rhoads impressed everyone with his unlimited depth of knowledge of surgery and other scientific matters. In particular I remember him quoting from the periodic table and commenting on the new elements that he had recently read about. He seemed to have a photographic memory for all details of his patient care and was always a supreme gentleman.

We were making rounds with Dr. Rhoads and he mentioned he had a favorite resident. He would not say who that resident was, but the reason he was his favorite resident was that he never wasted a step on rounds. He said the resident had sequentially timed all of the elevators in the hospital and knew exactly which elevators to take at which moment in time to make the circuitous voyage through the Hospital of the University of Pennsylvania. . . .

In one instance we were on rounds in the Ravdin Building, where there were big picture windows in the patient rooms. Dr. Rhoads was a notorious lecturer and traveled all over the world, and he was patiently listening to a very, very long presentation of a patient's problem. As the junior finished with the history and physical and assessment of the surgical problem, he looked up to Dr. Rhoads for a comment. After a long silence, Dr. Rhoads, who had been gazing out the picture window, said in his very soft voice, "I wonder where that plane is going?" Most of us had a hard time keeping from breaking out in laughter.[5]

Former residents Arthur Brown and Marc Wallack recall rounding with Rhoads. According to Brown,

Over the years I have been most impressed with Dr. Rhoads' memory. I can remember as a resident on one occasion he called me at about 2:30 in the morning from the airport desiring to make rounds. I met him at the front door of the Ravdin Pavilion and proceeded to take him to see his patients. He knew everyone's name, their room number, and more impressive to me at that time, he knew all of their lab data from the time he left.[6]

Wallack adds:

A particular patient whom Dr. Rhoads knew very well was complaining from the minute we entered the room to the time we left, about the nurses, the residents, the operation, the hospital, her incision, her bill and her life. Dr. Rhoads patiently listened and looked down at her and said, "My dear, you are one of the world's great sufferers!" This obviously went over her head and I chuckled internally as she continued to complain. Finally he got up from his chair and walked to the window, all the time listening to the patient. As he looked out the window he saw a plane in the sky, and said, "Oh, there's a plane; I wish I were on it."[7]

Rhoads became increasingly involved in the surgical treatment of cancer. In the late 1930s he had worked with Ravdin and Pendergrass in devising an innovative approach to the treatment of breast cancer. Dr. Rhoads explains:

Dr. Pendergrass thought he could take care of the axillary nodes. He persuaded us to do simple mastectomies and irradiate the axilla. We did that for a year or two as Dr. Ravdin was running the service. Then some nodes came back and we cleaned out the axilla secondarily and found cancer cells that had not been killed by the radiation. So we backed away and went to the Halsted mastectomy [removing the complete breast and underlying muscles of the chest wall] with axillary dissection.[8]

Ironically, nearly 50 years later, conservative resection of the breast tissue with axillary irradiation would become the standard treatment for many types of breast cancer.

Rhoads was also interested in thyroid cancer and especially solitary thyroid nodules. In collaboration with Bob Horn and Ted Enterline, he determined that the risk of a solitary nodule becoming malignant was 12–15%. The risk of malignancy decreased to 3–5% when multiple thyroid nodules were present.

Rhoads subsequently pursued the association of colonic polyps and colorectal cancer. In conjunction with Leonard Miller, he noted that the size of the polyps and the presence of multiple polyps were important determinants of malignancy. The investigators also showed that while the prognosis for patients with a perforated colon cancer was worse than that for a nonperforated lesion, there still were a number of survivors 5 years postoperatively.[9]

Rhoads' determination to persevere with the surgical treatment of cancer despite formidable odds is recalled by Hilary Timmis:

It was said that he hated cancer and there was no anatomic barrier too complex or boundary too forbidding to prevent him from doing a "complete" resection. The stomata produced in such a battle were legendary in their variety, and I'm sure many a patient would have been considerably short lived with a lesser, more timid surgeon.[10]

Rhoads also pursued the surgical treatment of pancreatic cancer. He describes these early experiences:

After Dr. Whipple wrote up his 2-stage removal of the head of the pancreas and the duodenum, we were, of course, dying to get on that bandwagon. I got a case in 1941 and Dr. Ravdin let me do it. We got it out all right. I don't know if the patient would have lived any great length of time, but anyhow he died suddenly of a pulmonary embolus on the 10th postoperative day. At autopsy, there was a little collection that was kind of right up against the vena cava. So it was a failure but it was good experience. . . .

I was then 33 or 34 years of age, and was perhaps an example of what old Dr. Deaver used to emphasize at his Saturday operating sessions. He would speak to his long-time theater nurse and say, '"Miss Brown, what is it every young surgeon feels he has to do?" The stock answer was '"Fill 3 cemeteries, Dr. Deaver." And I did, in point of fact, fill one cemetery lot with this unfortunate man, though we had rather a good go at it. The next time I tried the operation was 2 or 3 years later.[11]

Despite his increasing experience with the surgical treatment of pancreatic cancer (Whipple operation), the postoperative morbidity and mortality were considerable. This was in part due to the high rate of leakage associated with the anastomoses (surgical connection) of the pancreatic duct. One of Rhoads' residents, Dick Park, found an article by Milbourne in *Acta Chirurgica Scandinavica* that described the sewing of the pancreatic duct to the stomach.[12] Rhoads and Mackie began to use this technique, which in turn led to an improved postoperative outcome.

Rhoads became known for his ability to devise new operations and to modify established procedures based upon the needs of the patient. One particular operation stands out in the mind of a resident, Harvey Sugerman:

After two years in the research laboratory I started as a third-year resident on the Rhoads Service. The first patient was, believe it or not, his aunt, who had a large colonic polyp at 35 cm from the anal verge. She was given a spinal anesthetic and sedated, prepped and draped for surgery in the dorsal lithotomy [legs in stirrups] position. The plan was for Dr. Rhoads to use an extra long sigmoidoscope to see if he could reach the polyp. Should that be unsuccessful, I was to make a left lower quadrant muscle splitting incision and thread his aunt's colon over the sigmoidoscope for him to reach the polyp.

And so there we were, my Professor and Chairman underneath the drapes between his aunt's legs with an extra long sigmoidoscope and myself, nervous, standing on her left side with the scrub nurse opposite me. When Dr. Rhoads was unable to visualize the polyp, I heard from below the drapes, "Harvey, go ahead with the muscle splitting incision." I began with the incision, but, as it was obviously too small, the scrub nurse spread her hands suggesting that I make it bigger. Anxious and tense I slowly proceeded to enter her abdomen when I heard from beneath the drapes, "Harvey, how are you coming?" Clearly I was not working fast enough, and I was sure Dr. Rhoads had an important appointment with the University Board of Trustees or the Philadelphia School Board or the PennWalt Corporation. So I knew I had to work faster.

Eventually we got into the abdomen and I could see his scope. I threaded the sigmoid colon over his scope and he saw the polyp, but I saw another lesion which was more threatening and suggested that there might be a carcinoma higher. Finally, Dr. Rhoads came from beneath the drapes, scrubbed, and finally joined me at the operating table where we performed a partial sigmoid resection for what turned out to be partially obstructing, fibrotic diverticulitis. This was one heck of a welcome back to surgery.[13]

William Pierce remembers the famous "Hicks operation" named after the operation that Dr. Rhoads performed on Mr. Hicks:

This patient had some type of bile duct anastomosis that kept narrowing, thereby causing jaundice and ascending cholangitis [inflammation of the bile ducts]. Dr. Rhoads developed an operation whereby some type of wire with an attached bougie was left in the patient. To the best of my understanding, one end came out the front and one end came out the back of the patient. At prescribed intervals the physician (and possibly the patient) could simply move the wire to and fro and dilate the offending stricture of the bile duct.[14]

Armistead Talman shares Rhoads' unique approach to perioperative care:

Unusual memories of Dr. Rhoads range from his late Saturday night tuxedo rounds to his innovation of retrieval of a long-entrenched Miller-Abbott tube. By standing on a chair he was able to tower even more upright over the standing yet unsuspecting young patient as she guzzled mineral oil. Incidentally, it worked![15]

Similar to the frenetic pace during his years as provost, Chairman Rhoads dove into many new challenges in his remarkable administrative style. Office activities were balanced among patient concerns, research projects, educational commitments, travel, and numerous other demands. Rhoads committed two hours a week to Marion Carbone, the secretary who was responsible for academic affairs. Irene Brown, one of his personal secretaries at the time, recalls an amusing incident:

It seemed that he was always late in his appointment with her and Marion would take a back seat. One afternoon he wanted to talk to Marion. I dialed her before I told him to pick up the phone and tell him *that Marion was on the phone. Not knowing that Dr. Rhoads was on the phone, I said, "Here's Jonny!" He laughed louder than I did and I almost went through the floor.*[16]

Marion Carbone comments on one of Rhoads' notable qualities:

He had a way of detaching himself from his position as Chairman or Professor of Surgery and sort of focus on the problem of the individual—one of his greatest strengths.[17]

Irene Brown explains:

He was sensitive about interviewing or helping people get into medical school. He would meet with them and would never write a letter for someone he had not met.[18]

During his 13-year tenure as chairman Rhoads took 624 trips. Rhoads' exhaustive travel schedule was a "challenge" for his secretary. "I'm sure I wrote a thousand plane tickets for him," says Brown. She remembers one trip in particular:

When he was Chairman of the Board of Regents of the American College of Surgeons and really active in the College of Surgeons, he would frequently fly to Chicago. There was a United #143 that left at 8:00 in the morning here and got into Chicago at 8:45 Chicago time. One morning he called me at home and he said, "Irene, I'm in Chicago and there doesn't seem to be a meeting. Where should I be?" I thought, Oh my God, I gave him the wrong tickets, and indeed I gave him the incorrect folder. He turned around and came right back home without remorse.[19]

Barrett Noone garnered an important lesson from Dr. Rhoads' travels:

Dr. Rhoads' travels at the time I was a resident were legendary. It was not unusual for him to travel to the West Coast following a brief morning of surgery, attend a dinner meeting in San Francisco, and return to Philadelphia on the red-eye in time for rounds the next morning. Late one night (or early one morning) when I was a junior resident I received a telephone call from Dr. Rhoads inquiring about one of his postoperative patients. This seemed a bit unusual since we knew Dr. Rhoads was at a medical convention in Europe. He told me on the telephone that he was between planes in Reykjavik, Iceland, and that he simply wanted to keep in touch with some of the data on his patients. Whenever I am in an airport, productively getting some work done between planes, I remember Dr. Rhoads' Iceland story.[20]

One of Rhoads' most memorable patients was his colleague, Julian Johnson. According to William Pierce,

Perhaps the most famous operation that took place during my training at Penn was the one that Dr. Rhoads did on his colleague. Julian Johnson was a world-renowned cardiac surgeon and had worked with Rhoads since the early 40's. He had enjoyed particularly good health. Sometime in 1968, Dr. Johnson began to experience crampy abdominal pain and suspected that something might be going on. He apparently called one of his friends in radiology and suggested that he might swallow a little barium to see what the problem could be.

By the next day, not only had the diagnosis of a left colon lesion been made but a partial large bowel obstruction had become a complete obstruction. Dr. Johnson was in trouble. He was admitted to the finest bed on Eisenlohr, and Rhoads was called. After multiple deliberations a plan was made. The Miller-Abbott tube was ordered. With luck the tube would pass into the large bowel and decompress the colon and an elective procedure could be performed under favorable circumstances.

Rhoads had a meeting in Washington that afternoon, and as soon as Dr. Johnson was "squared away," Rhoads was off to the airport. On his arrival in Washington, his first thoughts were about Johnson. He called back to the University and things were clearly worse. The Miller-Abbott tube remained in the stomach and Dr. Johnson's colonic distention was marked. Urgent surgery was required. Dr. Rhoads remained at the airport, caught the next plane back to Philadelphia. Dr. Mackie was to be the first assistant and Dr. Schwegman and I were to help.

The timing all had to be precise. Dr. Johnson was moved to the operating room, and Dr. Rhoads was to call when he reached the Philadelphia International Airport. Anesthesia would begin at that time. Dr. Mackie wanted to be sure to have the patient prepped and the skin incision underway when Dr. Rhoads arrived in the operating suite. Moreover, he knew right where Dr. Rhoads parked his car. As soon as the car was sighted, prepping would begin and things would be underway.

He and I were to watch the parking spot and give the signal to anesthesia. After what seemed like an interminable time no automobile arrived. Where possibly could Dr. Rhoads be? All the possibilities were discussed, and finally one of us had the brilliant idea of checking back in the operating room. There was Dr. Rhoads gowned, gloved and completing the abdominal incision alone. That evening he had been in a hurry and had not parked in his usual spot.

As you might imagine, on that day the ten-minute scrub by the first assistant was magically condensed into 60 seconds. Within a very short period of time the full team was assembled, including the chief of surgical pathology awaiting the specimen. I am pleased to report that the

results of the operation were impeccable. Dr. Johnson was among the first to receive parenteral hyperalimentation to insure a strong bowel suture line and sound wound closure.[21]

Despite his increasing clinical responsibilities, Rhoads made time for community activities. In 1965 he was interviewed for a position on the Philadelphia School Board. He explains:

I received a letter from a group of people that were reforming the Board of Education under the new city charter, asking if I wanted to be considered for that board. I really didn't want to go on the board, but I didn't want to take the position that I wouldn't be willing to. So these people called me after a while and asked me to come down for an interview. I did and they asked me my views on busing. Well, I really didn't quite know what busing was at the time, but I had the impression that it was a process by which children were picked up in an area and plunked down somewhere else. I said that I wasn't very much in favor of busing and that I thought it was not entirely appropriate to use the educational system for purposes of integration. I thought that if they would integrate housing, this would be preferable to the educational system and then it would automatically be integrated. I thought that that would end it. It didn't. Somewhere in the mix Mayor Tate chose me for the Board.[22]

Richardson Dilworth, former mayor of Philadelphia, was appointed president of the board and his inaugural comments were indeed prophetic: "I don't think anyone on this Board is going to be very popular."[23]

Rhoads says of Dilworth:

I came to like him and admire him a great deal. He was a fascinating sort of guy. He would talk without having prepared his remarks—one of his best remarks was that he was born with a silver foot in his mouth. He had run for governor and had been defeated and terminated his political career partly because he talked too freely.[24]

Dilworth was very good at informing the public of the problems of the school system. Meetings were broadcast on radio and television and were held in various schools throughout the city. According to Rhoads,

We went to various schools and we were not paid to be on the Board, but we had a car and driver assigned to us for school business. I didn't want a car and driver, I wanted to be able to leave the meeting and come back to the hospital when I got called. So I drove my own car, and

it got to be known that Dr. Rhoads drives his own car. Dilworth was afraid that I might be set upon between where I parked my car and the school—he would get somebody to meet me at the car.[25]

The major issues confronting the board were inadequate salaries for teachers, busing, and the need for new primary and secondary schools. Dilworth was successful in getting appropriations from the state and city for these activities. Salaries were made commensurate for teachers in similar urban settings. Rhoads was appointed to the subcommittee overseeing the selection of names for the new primary and secondary schools:

The guidelines were that whomever you named the schools for had to be dead. I got one named for Clarence Pickett, the man who was the head of the American Friends Service Committee who went over to get the Nobel Prize for the Committee. One school was named for John Webster, who was the great great grandfather of my Westtown roommate John Webster.[26]

Busing was initiated, although it was not entirely successful. According to Rhoads,

We ended up doing some busing, and interestingly it was opposed by many of the black parents who didn't want their children to go far away from home.[27]

Rhoads' ability to devote extensive amounts of time to the activities of the school board in addition to his responsibilities as chairman was a constant source of amazement to his colleagues and residents. Mackie explains:

I thought when he was on the school board I would lose my mind listening to the arguments and the fuss that was going on. They had meetings every night. He would be traveling, he would be operating, and he's doing all of this. At any rate, we were making rounds early one morning after a particularly heated discussion about something; they had T.V. cameras outside where they met, and I said, "How in the world can you do all of the things that you do and go down and put up with that kind of meeting every night." He looked at me and said, "Jack, I never thought I would be having so much fun at this time in my life." I think that this says something about him. He doesn't fear anything, and he does not let things bother him, particularly if there's nothing you can do. I don't mean he doesn't consider things or think about them. But he doesn't let things get to him.[28]

Horace MacVaugh III remembers Rhoads' frequent participation in various administrative boards:

He told me that he thoroughly enjoyed his board meetings of Bryn Mawr College and Haverford College, which were normally held on Saturday afternoons, and he thought it was much more worthwhile to do that than, to use his example, "play golf."[29]

As the United States became increasingly involved in the Vietnam conflict in the mid-1960s, the Department of Surgery at Penn was significantly affected, as were other departments throughout the country. In 1969 Rhoads accepted an invitation from the American Friends Service Committee (A.F.S.C.) to help with the rehabilitation of civilian casualties in Vietnam. The A.F.S.C. had become internationally prominent because of post-World War I relief work in France and Russia performed by Rufus Jones. Moreover, there was ample precedent for Rhoads' involvement in the A.F.S.C. activities. His parents had strongly supported their work, and his sister Esther worked for the A.F.S.C. to relocate interned Japanese-Americans in California during World War II.

Rhoads' first involvement with the organization was in 1952 during the Korean War. He was asked to visit South Korea to select a site for their directed medical care for the civilian population because nearly all of the South Korean physicians had been drafted into the Army. Rhoads' group visited 6 of the 8 sections of South Korea and recommended a site on the south coast, not far from where MacArthur made his famous landing. Additionally, he visited a Presbyterian Missionary Hospital, which honored an important Korean custom:

I remember they had a special room for the patient's family next to the operating room. There was a little cubicle where you could look out and see what was going on. It was a Korean custom for the family to be present for the operation.[30]

In 1965 the United States started bombing North Vietnam, and the war intensified with the Tet offensive in 1968. There were thousands of civilian casualties on both sides. In July 1969 Rhoads left for a 3-week trip to Vietnam under the auspices of the A.F.S.C. A press announcement was released:

In Quang Ngai, Dr. Rhoads will visit the Quaker rehabilitation center run by the A.F.S.C. in conjunction with the Quang Ngai Provincial Hospital, observing and advising the work of the staff in providing physical therapy and making and fitting of artificial limbs for civilian war victims. It is estimated that there are as many as 60,000 amputees among civilians in South Vietnam alone. The A.F.S.C. program in Quang Ngai was begun in October of 1966 and included a child day care center for approximately 100 children of widowed refugee women. Quaker organizations also sent penicillin to civilian war sufferers, and the A.F.S.C. was currently arranging for delivery of instruments for open heart surgery to the North Vietnamese.[31]

The main objectives of the trip were to rehabilitate the civilian casualties and to deliver parts to repair the broken heart-lung machines in Hanoi. With a fellow Quaker, Professor David Elder from the University of Wisconsin, Rhoads spent several days at the service committee office in Hong Kong and then flew to Saigon to visit the Rusk Rehabilitation Center. Howard Rusk, the leading U.S. expert in physical medicine, was a graduate of Penn and an internationally renowned expert in the new subspecialty of rehabilitation medicine. Additionally, he was a gifted speaker and writer and was a correspondent for the *New York Times*. Rusk coined the phrase "third phase of medicine"—the first being diagnosis; the second, treatment; and the third, rehabilitation. After visiting the rehabilitation operation in Saigon, Rhoads and Elder traveled to the A.F.S.C. rehabilitation facility in Quang Ngai. It was under the control of U.S. forces during the day, but at night the Viet Cong (North Vietnamese sympathizers) had it well surrounded.

It wasn't safe to go out there. I arrived at this place not knowing where the heck I was going. I had a little button with the emblem of the American Friends Service Committee on it, and I showed it to some non-English speaking Vietnamese, and they had seen this at the headquarters.[32]

While in Quang Ngai, Rhoads received permission to operate on Vietnamese patients in the civilian hospital. He remembers revising stumps from amputations where the muscles were cut too long and floppy and they couldn't fit against a prosthesis. Additionally, Rhoads has a vivid memory of one of the A.F.S.C. staff physicians:

I thought she was one of the most extraordinary people I've met. She had been captured the year before further north in Vietnam and marched off as a prisoner for hours and hours and miles and miles on foot, and she eventually got sick. The North Vietnamese who had her in tow thought enough of her and sent for a doctor who had traveled about 24 hours to see her. I think she had dysentery. Undeterred by this she continued to work there. They let her enter into some sort of prisoner exchange and she got back on the American side and became a general practitioner.[33]

She took Rhoads to a nearby camp for political prisoners. Rhoads recalls:

This was a compound, I suppose, which was 400 yards by 200 yards with a certain amount of housing around it. A lot of wire fences and so forth. You entered by going up a path about a hundred yards with barbed wire on this side and that side and a machine gun nest trained on you. She went apparently two or three times a week to attend the sick, including pregnant women and women with newborn children. I went and saw some of these. I remember one woman who had been quite politically active along with the Viet Cong and had been in prison. She looked at you with an intensity of gaze that you knew that if she had the means she would be glad to kill you. Then I found out that there were a lot of nasty things going on there, beating pregnant women and so forth.[34]

Because of his concern for the poor treatment of the civilian prisoners, he heeded the advice of his colleagues and returned to Saigon to meet with the U.S. ambassador.

They asked me to go see the American Ambassador. So when I got back to Saigon I had only one suit, and it was pretty badly out of press. There was an A.F.S.C. representative there, and they had a house where you could sleep, and so he went with me and we went to a tailor shop and let the tailor take my pants, and he stood by to make sure the tailor didn't send me out without them. Then I went to see the Ambassador. He lived in what was relative splendor and was air conditioned, and had a lovely big room with American type furniture with beautiful scenes of New England along the wall. I told him what I had seen and had been reported. He assured me that this sort of thing had been going on in the Far East for centuries. It was not likely to stop. He didn't like it but he felt he was powerless to stop this.[35]

The second objective of the trip was to deliver equipment for open-heart surgery in Hanoi. At the time there were certain branches of the U.S. Government that were tired of the war. They thought that it was futile and wanted to establish some unofficial relationships with the North. The State Department approved Rhoads taking parts for the heart-lung machine into North Vietnam. According to Rhoads, "They thought the parts had no military value and anybody needing cardiac surgery was not going to be a soldier."[36] Despite the initial approval, the A.F.S.C. ran into numerous bureaucratic snags because many of the international regulations were not under the authority of the State Department. Because of continuing problems securing the appropriate visae and licenses for export of equipment, Rhoads acquired the parts in Hong

Kong en route to Vietnam. Bureaucratic obstructions continued, and he and Elder decided to go to Hanoi by way of Cambodia.

We went to the capitol Phnom Penh. The reason we went to Phnom Penh was that we thought that I could get a visa there. There was a weekly flight from Phnom Penh to Hanoi. The plane was flown by an international commission and Canada was one of the four or five nations operating the plane once a week.[37]

While Rhoads was unsuccessful in obtaining a visa, Elder did procure one and was able to venture as far as Laos before the plane was detained. Eventually the mission had to be aborted.

Almost 20 years after his trip to Vietnam, Rhoads received a letter from Lady Borton, a previous member of the A.F.S.C., asking him to sponsor several North Vietnamese surgeons for membership in the International Surgical Society. She remembers Rhoads' visit to Quang Ngai in her letter to him:

I'm not sure you would remember me, but I have a clear memory of your visit to the A.F.S.C. Quang Ngai project. I was taking you to the airport at the last minute when our Citroen deux chevaux broke down. There was nothing to do but plunk you on the back of a motor scooter, which I had only driven solo. I was impressed with the ease with which you rode off into the unknown, a black bag in your lap.[38]

The Vietnam conflict had a significant effect on many of the Penn surgical residents. James Finnegan remarks about his residency during this time:

As I began my third year of residency in July of 1967, the war in Vietnam was reaching a fever pitch. . . . I have a very long family tradition in the military and in our country's war efforts. In contradistinction to that history, Dr. Rhoads stood as a leading exponent of the Quaker movement in Philadelphia. He was clearly but quietly opposed to what was happening in Vietnam.

In September of 1967 I went to him and told him I was voluntarily relinquishing my Berry deferment (for completion of a medical or surgical residency) in order to accept an appointment with the Third Marine Division in Vietnam. I was driven by my own need to do so, and probably not fully cognizant of the havoc I would wreak on the residency schedule, and certainly not paying significant attention to Dr. Rhoads' position, vis à vis his own beliefs.

After I explained to him what I felt I had to do, he did two things in his usual quiet but definitive way. First, he said that it was the long-standing tradition of the University of Pennsylvania's Department of Surgery that if a man left to serve in the military that his place would be reserved, and he wanted me to know that when my commitment was concluded that I would be welcomed back to the surgical residency. And then in what has to be one of the most magnanimous gestures that I have ever experienced, he wrote on a piece of paper his name, his home address and home telephone number and said, "Give this to your wife, and tell her that if she has any problem or special need whatsoever, she is to call me immediately."[39]

There were also issues to be dealt with concerning surgeons who were returning to their residencies following their time in Vietnam. Gary Nicholas reminisces about his interactions with Dr. Rhoads:

I had been drafted from the residency after my first year of training, and upon returning I met with Dr. Rhoads to discuss my reentry into the surgical residency. He inquired as to my family and two sons, and I indicated that we were struggling to find housing in the suburbs in order that my children could receive a good education in the public school system. He asked of me my financial status regarding the down payment for a home, and I indicated the small sum that we had been able to save. He turned and picked up his phone and called the University financial office and provided for me a $2000 supplement for the down payment we would need to obtain a satisfactory house so that my family could live comfortably and safely during my surgical residency. I had no time to object to his course of action, although I really was not sure I was ready to incur more debt. His concern and direct response to my needs have been forever appreciated.[40]

Perhaps Rhoads' greatest contribution as a surgical chairman has been his ability to nurture the careers of his many trainees. He derived great satisfaction from seeing the department thrive in an environment conducive to constant promotion and fostering of ideas rather than aggressive competition. Rhoads labored to help every Penn-trained surgeon succeed. In his 13 years as chairman he trained 62 surgeons who have served as faculty members in 34 different medical schools, with 28 serving as full professors and 11 as chairmen. In the words of Francis "Frank" Rosato, a former resident and now chairman of surgery at Jefferson Medical College:

His major strength as a Chairman of Surgery was his involvement at every level of organized surgery—local, regional and national—and then his ability to place his colleagues in positions of responsibility in such societies so that they had the opportunity to play a leadership role in American surgery.⁴¹

Rhoads' accomplishments and extraordinary personal qualities are perhaps best illustrated in the many comments and anecdotes of his trainees. His indefatigable work ethic was highly respected by his residents, among them Raleigh White, IV:

As I look back to those days, the impression that is most strongly dominating my remembrance is the fact that the whole environment was positive. Everyone respected Dr. Rhoads immensely, and yet no one feared him. He was a man who led by example and by role model, demonstrating a work ethic and a concern for patient care that established a very high standard for all of us to shoot for. He also was a man who facilitated the careers of those within his department.⁴²

Resident Joseph Diaco was affected by Rhoads' humility and inner strength:

What impressed me most about Dr. Rhoads was his compassion both for his patients and even more importantly for his residents and students. He went out of his way to make a student, intern and resident feel comfortable around him. He never did try to impress anybody with his knowledge. I think that's what impresses me the most about him—his quiet strength and inner peace that translated into someone who made you feel at ease around him at all times. . . . I attribute the reasons for his success to his constant need for knowledge and his constant need to know the reasons for any failures that he had. He wouldn't be satisfied with a patient dying—he had to know why and what he could have done differently to save them. I think this again translated into an inner strength from which we all learn so much.⁴³

Despite his formidable travel schedule, extensive administrative duties, and clinical commitments, Dr. Rhoads was usually available to provide advice and counsel to his current house staff and former trainees. Gene Cayten remembers:

Once when I felt a surgeon from another hospital had slandered me in a public meeting, I went to Dr. Rhoads for advice on how to confront this surgeon. Dr. Rhoads counseled me to avoid the confrontation and indicated that I should continue my efforts. He stated that there are little people in the world who attempt to build power by putting others down while the real power comes from accomplishments. He felt that this individual would be long gone by his own devices.⁴⁴

Rhoads' inimitable involvement in many areas outside clinical surgery was a source of inspiration to his residents. Barrett Noone recalls:

Dr. Rhoads served as a role model for me in many areas. I still rely on lessons indirectly learned from him, and in my career I have attempted to emulate his abilities to participate in many areas of organized medicine, as well as providing patient care and contributing to scientific progress. In other words, I feel that I have modeled my activities to extend myself in other areas of medicine in addition to surgery and patient care. I doubt that I would have had the interest or knowledge of the pursuit of these avenues without the direct exposure I had to Dr. Rhoads.[45]

Many current chairmen of surgery in the United States were trained under Rhoads, and they recall invaluable lessons learned under his tutelage. Frank Rosato remembers:

When I left Penn in 1974 to assume my first Chair in Surgery at the brand new Eastern Virginia Medical School, the only advice he gave me was, as chairman to try to put myself in the place of those who would be coming into my office with questions, problems, requests or other matters. His advice was something to the effect of, "Put yourself in their place. Ask how you would like to be treated in a similar circumstance and then with the university's interest in mind make the best and fairest decision you can." I think Dr. Rhoads' openness and willingness to hear all sides before making a decision have always impressed me greatly.[46]

William Curreri, another former resident and now chairman at the University of South Alabama, finds Rhoads' stamina remarkable:

Probably the single thing that impressed me about Dr. Rhoads was his amazing stamina. He had the capability of not only working very long hours, but also the stamina to combine a very busy surgical practice with administrative responsibilities and extensive travel associated with his responsibilities with various surgical associations.[47]

The opportunity to publish a paper with the chairman is a major honor for a resident. Frank Rosato relates one such occasion:

I remember as a resident writing my very first paper in conjunction with Jack Mackie, which was a retrospective review on 40 patients with pancreatic pseudocysts. When we had completed the paper and had it in typed form, we gave it to Dr. Rhoads for his review and within 4 to 5 days I had it back in my hands, very carefully red penciled by him. He had done a very precise editorial review on the paper, suggested some changes, some additions and even had gotten down to correcting grammar and punctuation. He obviously had spent some time on this. I thanked him and asked his permission to add his name to the list of authors, which Jack and I had agreed to; Dr. Rhoads refused. He said that he had not been involved in anything but some finishing touches, and that as he had not recommended the study to me nor been involved in any of the data collection or analysis or the writing of the paper, he thought it unfair to put his name among the authors. . . . It was a great lesson for me in honesty of authorship.[48]

Edward "Ted" Copeland III, chairman of surgery at the University of Florida, comments on Rhoads' influence:

Dr. Rhoads' greatest influence nationwide has come through the multiple successful surgical residents trained at the Hospital of the University of Pennsylvania. Each of us who is a chairman has established a residency program that reflects the one in which we trained. Our residents are well-schooled in the art of pre- and postoperative care, are gentlemen and ladies, are helpful to their peers, are appreciative of their elders, and are concerned for their patients' well-being 24-hours-a-day, seven-days-a-week. As each of us trains our residents and these residents in turn join surgical faculties or practice in the community, they influence others. Consequently, the pyramid of influence begun by Dr. Rhoads via the training program he established is, possibly, the most influential one in existence in the United States today, as measured by the number of chairmen the program produced and by the influential positions Dr. Rhoads' trainees have held.[49]

In addition to the many strengths of Rhoads' chairmanship, there were inherent weaknesses. Almost all of his faculty recruits were selected from among those who had trained at Penn. He reasoned that this approach provided ample opportunity (5–7 years) to observe and evaluate the performance of a potential faculty recruit; however, the "inbreeding" reduced the residents' exposure to different approaches to clinical problems that occur when faculty are recruited from outside institutions.

It is not known what the appropriate amount of time is that a chairman should devote to travel. Clearly the national and international exposure results in enhanced departmental prestige and leads to important friendships and political posturing. Rhoads' extensive traveling resulted in unparalleled benefits; however, it also led to disruptions in attendance at teaching rounds and decreased participation in research at Penn. During one protracted travel period the residents referred to him as the "Pan American Chair of Surgery."[50]

Perhaps Rhoads' influence on his residents is best characterized by Hilary Timmis:

Words and phrases fill my mind . . . mentor, friend, seldom wrong, humble but self-assured, unhurried but wasting no time . . . wonderful surgical role model, courageous, bold, dignified, noble in bearing, phenomenal memory for personal details, respectful and respected, solemn with a twinkle in his eye, motivating, and inquisitive in science. He was filled with goodness and no detectable rancor. He is of splendid proportions in his knowledge, his family, his civic and academic and surgical prestige, and his consideration for those with whom he associated. He has given me reason to pause and reflect on my own life relative to his, and in this sense he seems larger than life. But his character is one to aspire to, and his touching my life has left it more enriched.[51]

In 1972 Rhoads stepped down as chairman with a resolve to "slow down" and spend more time with family and friends. Those closest to him knew the resolution to slow down would never be reconciled with Rhoads' lifelong work ethic.

> *I guess it was Woody Allen who said that 88% or 90% of life is showing up. Jonathan certainly illustrates that. He shows up at everything.*
>
> Leonard Miller[1]

TEN

WISE COUNSELOR, FIRM FRIEND

REMARRIAGE AND A DEDICATION

Shortly after Rhoads' retirement, Clyde Barker, John Rhea Barton Professor and Chairman of Surgery at HUP, observed a change in his demeanor:

> *In 1972, Dr. Rhoads stepped down as Chairman. We knew that this would not by any means relax him, but one might say that after this, he seemed to attack life with a slightly more casual intensity. . . . He seemed different and more approachable. . . . He became a more relaxed and skillful after-dinner speaker.*[2]

The chairmen who succeeded Rhoads continued to ask him for advice. Former Chairman Leonard Miller remembers:

> *I did go to him on several occasions, mainly for advice to see how he would react to something. I was never disappointed. I think many more prominent people than I would go to him for advice. I don't think they ever came away unsatisfied.*[3]

In the decade from 1972 to 1982, Jonathan Rhoads saw the birth of 4 of his grandchildren and sadly the deaths of I.S. Ravdin, his sister Esther, and his colleagues "Bugs" Lehr and Bill Fitts. In that same period of time he took 436 trips and visited 28 foreign countries. He was the recipient of honorary degrees from Duke University, Jefferson Medical College, and Georgetown University.

In the 1970s Rhoads became, through a series of appointments, deeply involved in cancer research and funding. It was Eugene Pendergrass, one of the early presidents of the American Cancer Society, who first got Rhoads involved with that organization. Serving first at the local level and then nationally, Rhoads was elected president of the American Cancer Society in 1969. Art Holleb, former senior vice president for Medical Affairs at the society, said of Dr. Rhoads:

He is one of the very great leaders of the American Cancer Society. He had a great wisdom and patience about solving problems, and his solutions were always in the best interest of the American Cancer Society. No task for Dr. Rhoads was too small or too large. He always seemed to have time to do whatever had to be done.[4]

Around 1970, Mary Lasker, the philanthropist and one of the founders of the American Cancer Society, persuaded Ralph Yarborough, senator from Texas, to form a special committee to look into the possibility of doing for cancer what had been done for space exploration. Dr. Rhoads appeared as a citizen witness before the Appropriation Committee of the House of Representatives. He suggested that the National Cancer Institute ask that their funding be increased from 2 cents per citizen to 2.5 cents per citizen per week, with the idea that the time might come when it would be worthwhile to spend up to 5 or 10 cents per person per week. Senator Yarborough asked the Senate for a small appropriation to assemble a civilian committee to answer two questions: was it probable that a sharply increased expenditure for cancer research would significantly accelerate progress in the field of cancer, and if so, how could it best be applied?[5]

Jonathan Rhoads (first row, center) was chairman of the National Cancer Advisory Board, appointed by President Nixon. Also pictured: back row, first on the left, James Watson, Nobel Prize winner (DNA), and seated next to Dr. Rhoads on the right, Frank Rauscher, then head of the NIH, 1972.

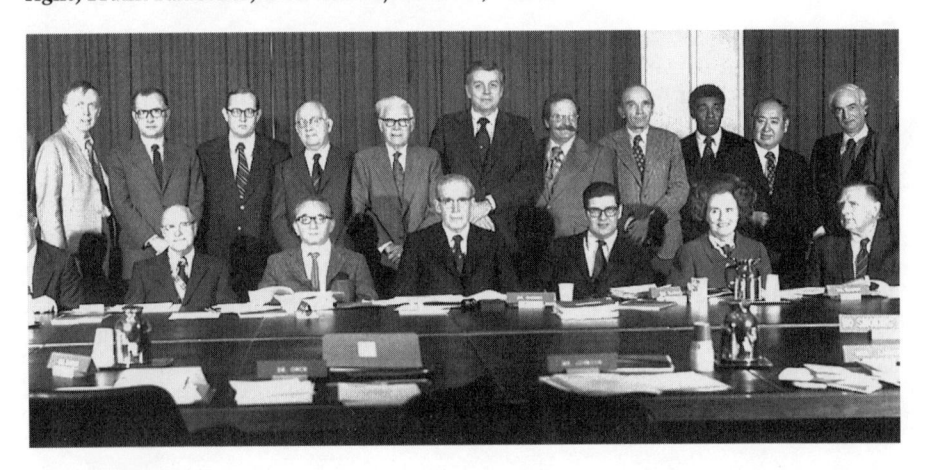

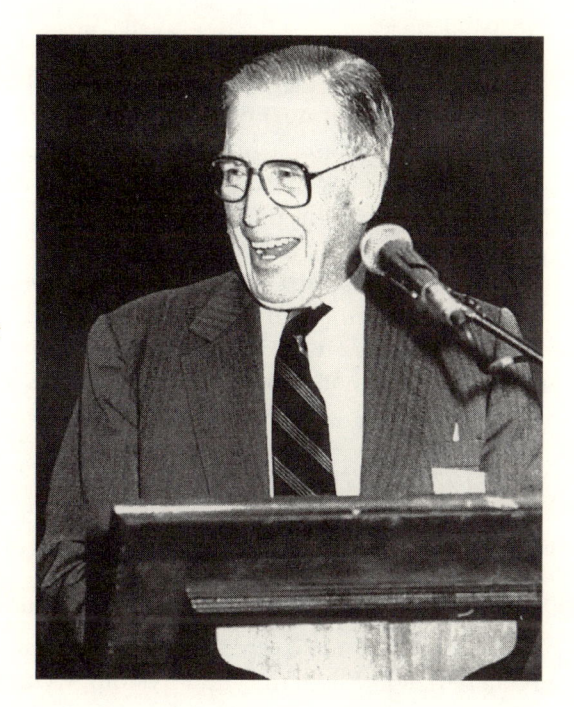

Dr. Rhoads in a lighter moment at the National Institutes of Health.

Dr. Rhoads served on this committee under the chairmanship of Benno Schmidt and the co-chairmanship of Sydney Farber, until Dr. Farber had a heart attack, and then of Dr. R. Lee Clark, who was head of M.D. Anderson Hospital in Texas. The citizen committee made their recommendations, which resulted in the National Cancer Act of 1971, with two notable exceptions: they were denied the freedom to prescribe drugs without having them cleared through the Food and Drug Administration, and they were unable to get the National Cancer Institute (N.C.I.) moved out from the larger National Institutes of Health. The committee had direct access to the president of the United States and had the authority to investigate all aspects of the operation of the N.C.I. According to Rhoads,

We were advisory and didn't have authority to change things, but the advice of such a body comes down pretty heavily on the Director. Elmer Bobst may have seen that I got put on the Board, and Mary Lasker and Benno Schmidt threw a party for the Board the night before it was to meet for the first time. . . . During the cocktail hour Benno came around and said we want you to chair it. It was an impressive group of people. Among them was James Watson, who shared the Nobel prize for the discovery of the structure of DNA.[6]

Rhoads was appointed 3 times for a total of 7 years. Said Rhoads, "It was really a ringside seat to what was going on around the country in cancer research."[7] Rhoads was present at the signing of the Act by President Richard Nixon. The Act provided for the formation of at least 15 new comprehensive clinical cancer centers, each having capabilities roughly comparable to those at Memorial Sloan Kettering Hospital in New York City, Roswell Park in Buffalo, and M.D. Anderson in Houston.

On the strength of his involvement with the National Cancer Advisory Board and his association with the American Cancer Society, Rhoads was chosen to edit the journal *Cancer*. He concurrently served as editor of the *Annals of Surgery* and *Cancer* for one year, stepping down from the *Annals* in 1973. During his tenure as editor-in-chief, *Cancer*'s circulation ballooned to nearly 23,000 subscribers.

In 1973, Joe Fortner, a senior surgeon at Memorial Sloan Kettering Hospital, and Roger Smith, an executive vice president of General Motors, approached Rhoads to help oversee a group of prizes, similar to the Nobel Prize, to be awarded for research in cancer. General Motors had already expressed a deep interest in cancer research, having contributed heavily to Memorial Sloan Kettering. Smith and Fortner pointed out that the Nobel Prize in Medicine and Physiology was given by the faculty of medicine at the Karolinska Institute in Stockholm, and that they had given few awards to researchers in cancer. They thought the field would be better recognized if there were prizes every year.

They decided to set up three prizes. Selection committees were appointed for each award: diagnosis and treatment, basic research, and cause and prevention. Fortner was appointed president and Rhoads chairman of the Awards Assembly. They were sent to Sweden and conferred with the secretary of the Nobel Committee. They decided to set up the prize structure very much like the one in Sweden.

The General Motors Cancer Research Assembly met three times a year, and the three selection committees each met three times in most years. This opportunity allowed Rhoads to come into contact with prominent researchers in cancer throughout the world. The rotating committees were composed of prominent cancer researchers, and professors and associate professors from universities throughout the world who were asked for nominations.[8] In connection with his role on the board, Dr. Rhoads met Presidents Jimmy Carter and Ronald Reagan.

There was another benefit—Rhoads and Fortner were rewarded with General Motors demonstrator cars. This fit in splendidly with Rhoads' love of the automobile. In his late 70s he drove a Fiero, a Corvette, and a truck, and has had a succession of Cadillacs, Buicks, Pontiacs, and Chevrolets. Every three months a new car of his choice was delivered to the front of the hospital. Rhoads would meet the driver, pick up his car, and zoom off.

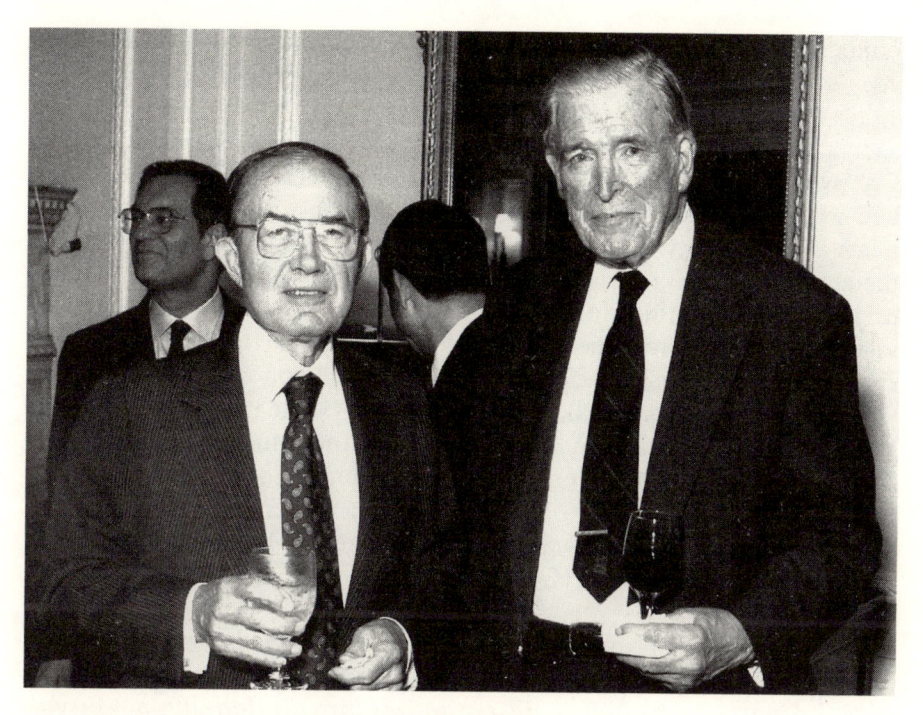

Joseph Fortner (left) and Jonathan Rhoads (right).

In May 1973, when he was 66 years old, Rhoads was admitted to HUP with a presumed diagnosis of a heart attack. His son Charles recalls his mother calmly gathering the children and taking them to the intensive care unit. Later, he noted that his father "looked like a trapped rat."[9] He had taken 37 trips out of town that year and visited Denmark, Germany, and Italy.

In 1976, the year of the nation's bicentennial celebration held in Philadelphia, Jonathan Rhoads was honored with the highest award its citizens could confer on one of its own—the prestigious Philadelphia Award. Established in 1921 by publisher Edward W. Bok, it carries a cash prize of $15,000. Past recipients include conductors Leopold Stokowski and Eugene Ormandy, former mayors Joseph Clark and Richardson Dilworth, physicians Robert Austrian, Hilary Koproski, and in 1956, Rhoads' mentor, I.S. Ravdin. In presenting the award to Rhoads, Marvin Wachman, the president of Temple University, said:

Each year the Philadelphia Award is presented to someone who has advanced the largest and best interests of the general community . . . with almost half a century of outstanding service in medicine education and civic affairs, Dr. Rhoads more than amply meets that requirement.[10]

In accepting the award, Rhoads began by telling the story about a man who won $200,000 in the lottery. His wife received the message that he had won and was very reluctant to tell him because he had a known heart condition and she was afraid he would keel over. Therefore, she made arrangements for the minister to pay them a visit, and at the appropriate time he would inform the man of his good fortune. The minister visited, and the conversation proceeded, and at a particularly opportune time the minister asked the man, "What would you do if someone told you that you had won $200,000 in the lottery?" The man replied, "Well, I'd give half of it to the church," whereupon the minister dropped dead. Dr. Rhoads continued, "I don't want Dr. Wachman to drop dead here this evening so I am not giving half of this money to Temple."[11] He went on to honor his wife Terry, his children, friend James Magill, and colleagues I.S. Ravdin, Harry Vars, and Stan Dudrick. He concluded by saying:

I want to express my thanks not only for this Award, which comes as the culmination of a remarkably happy career, but to thank all of you and the institutions you represent for making Philadelphia a city of opportunity for me. Some years ago when the late William Wistar Comfort, then President of Haverford, gave the William Penn Lecture, he was reported to have started off by explaining to the audience that Quakers believe in the fatherhood of God, the brotherhood of man, and the neighborhood of Philadelphia.[12]

Robert Austrian, writing about Rhoads' service to the community said:

His influence rested not only on his recognized talents as a surgeon and investigator who had made notable contributions to parenteral alimentation, but also on his extensive knowledge of his native community, its power structure and its institutions. I have encountered no one in my 30 years in Philadelphia better informed about the community.[13]

And Robert Cathcart, a past chief executive officer of the Pennsylvania Hospital, relates this about Rhoads and his native city:

I arrived in Philadelphia when I was 25 years old after spending 19 years in Iowa, 3 years in the armed services and 3 years in postgraduate educational activities in Toronto and Michigan. I knew very little of Philadelphia, its power and social structure, its strengths and weaknesses. He helped me learn that the Philadelphia community I would work in and serve placed great value on quality performances, that big is not necessarily better, to value the past of the community and to learn from this history, and to try to exceed the performance of those who preceded me.[14]

According to two of his surgical residents, Dr. Rhoads once spent a summer driving around Philadelphia so that he could learn the name and location of every street in the city.[15] In his late 70s local and state officials called on him to investigate corruption in the Traffic Court and the feasibility of placing a trash-to-steam plant within the city limits.

In the same year that he was honored with the Philadelphia Award, Dr. Rhoads was elected president of the American Philosophical Society, the oldest and most distinguished learned society in the United States. He served in that position until 1984. Founded by Benjamin Franklin in 1743 "for the promotion of useful knowledge," the society was patterned on the Royal Society of London, which had made Franklin a member for his work in electricity. Members are divided into 5 classes: mathematics and the physical sciences, biological sciences, social sciences, humanities, and men of affairs. The first woman was elected in 1788, and three women were elected on the same night Charles Darwin became a member.

Election to the society is not easy. Whitfield Bell, the society's historian, tells the story of the young man who had recently won the Nobel Prize. He was being considered for membership, but it was decided that he was too young and would have to wait until he proved himself. George Washington, John Adams, Thomas Jefferson (who also was the society's president in 1797), John Madison, John Quincy Adams, Ulysses Grant, and Woodrow Wilson were members but were elected before they became president. Herbert Hoover, William Taft, and Theodore Roosevelt were elected while they were president.[16] Clearly, the society is very accomplished in recognizing achievement and ability.

The American Philosophical Society meets twice a year, in the fall and spring, for 2 to 3 days, to hear "papers on every topic of human knowledge from archaeology to zoology, from medieval law to modern genetics."[17] Dr. Rhoads has spent a good deal of his later years involved with this organization. He was instrumental in raising funds to purchase a nearby building for expansion of the library, which requires the largest part of the budget. Whitfield Bell credits Rhoads and former Society President Crawford Greenewalt for the physical expansion and strong financial standing of the society.[18] According to Arlin Adams, the society's current president,

Jonathan's wise leadership and thoughtful guidance have made it possible for this remarkable organization to continue to support and inspire

hundreds of leaders and scholars throughout the world—including scores of young medical students.[19]

Herman Goldstine, a friend and patient of Dr. Rhoads since 1943 and chief executive officer of the society, says that Rhoads, as president, gave him complete freedom to change some of its existing laws and never interfered with his recommendations or decisions. Like so many others, Dr. Goldstine was impressed with Rhoads' uncanny business acumen and his ability to achieve consensus in their many meetings.[20] David Stokes, former treasurer of Haverford College, describes Rhoads in a meeting:

Over the years I must have attended hundreds of meetings at which Jonathan was present. He had a style which was predictable but so effective. His physical dimensions and presence were unique, and these added to his humility and sincerity and made him a force to be reckoned with.

All the boards and meetings that we took part in together were conducted by consensus. Jonathan would wait patiently for the participants to express themselves, sometimes heatedly, and then would quietly, at the appropriate moment, come forward with "I would hope we could proceed along the lines of 'thus and so,'" and nearly always it was "thus and so" that was agreed to.[21]

Rhoads uses humor occasionally to gain consensus. Stokes describes Rhoads' approach:

I recall at one meeting of the Germantown Friends School, the question of accepting funds from the State which were generated by horse racing came before the group. After a lively discussion of why we shouldn't accept them, Jonathan made a comment about not looking a gift horse in the mouth. This settled the matter, as his closing comments usually did.[22]

Rhoads modestly explains his method of gaining consensus:

If you haven't done your homework, it's a good idea to hear what's going on before you open your mouth too much. I think often there are two times when you can speak most effectively in a group. One is when the thing starts off, and sometimes if you then take a strong position, it doesn't solve the controversy but it sort of directs it. The other way is to wait until the discussion is pretty well advanced and see whether you can find a solution that will reconcile enough points of view to prevail.[23]

In the same conversation he noted that he had received a letter from a fellow alumnus and former Haverford College board member. In the letter, the person mentioned that another board member thought that the Quaker way of reaching a decision was a waste of time. He disagreed, saying that it did take longer but the decisions stuck better.

Rhoads adds:

So I think sometimes if you wait until the end of a discussion, you may see something that can be compromised and sometimes you can't. And other times by waiting that long, some forceful proponents will have gotten a decision you really don't agree with, but if that's the case you probably can't do anything about it anyhow. I have failed to gain a consensus many more times than I have succeeded. . . . There's nothing like trying.[24]

Many of his friends have expressed surprise at Rhoads' sense of humor. He loves a good joke or story, and he loves to tell them. Invariably, before the punch line he would break into a grin and chuckle—traits that became infectious regardless of the quality of the humor. In connection with this, Leonard Miller comments on Rhoads' ability to surprise people:

What I have found in my dealings with him is that he has certain principles, not only about money but about everything, virtually. And those principles will not be broken no matter what the circumstances are. . . .

Jonathan has the ability to surprise you. Almost every time you speak to him in any serious way, his responses are not usually like the responses you expect to get. . . . Whenever I went to see him about something, I had no idea what his response was going to be. As a matter of fact, after I left the office on many occasions I didn't know what he said. We could have a very nice chat for 20–30 minutes and I thought was very congenial, and then I left and I would ask myself, "What exactly did he commit himself to, which questions did he answer yes or no." . . . He has an unbelievable breadth of knowledge. He has a very indirect wit and unless you know him you sometimes don't know it's a joke. He has a way of speaking and thinking that is very unusual.[25]

In addition to his activities in the American Philosophical Society, Rhoads continues to be involved in most of the institutions he has attended. He serves on the boards of Germantown Friends School, the Westtown School, and Haverford College.

In 1982 Rhoads was recognized for his 50 years of service and contributions to the University of Pennsylvania. He surprised several members of the audience that night with an unexpected tribute. George Spaeth, an ophthalmologic surgeon and a colleague of Rhoads, describes his reaction:

Brooke Roberts and a variety of others told some brief stories about their relationship with Dr. Rhoads. But the high point of the evening was what Dr. Rhoads himself did. And what did he do? He talked about the people who had been of most help to the development of his professional career. He had invited those people to the celebration. He spoke of them all by name. They were his secretaries![26]

He paid tribute to his secretaries Irene Brown, Marion Carbone, and Jinny Mager. It was they who were able to place him in the right place at the right time during the busiest years of his life and make his complex travel adventures seem effortless. Currently, he is loyally and ably assisted by Ruth Brown and Jeannie Shapin. They all express the view that working for Dr. Rhoads is the equivalent of a wonderful education, not just another job.

In the decade from 1983 to 1993, Dr. Rhoads took 391 trips and traveled to 28 countries. Sadly, his colleagues Harry Vars, William Altemeier, Elliot Stellar, and Crawford Greenewalt and close friend Ted Hetzel passed away.

In 1987, Rhoads announced his retirement from private practice just before his 80th birthday. Jack Mackie and Leonard Miller watched Rhoads operate on his last few patients. Jack Mackie remembers:

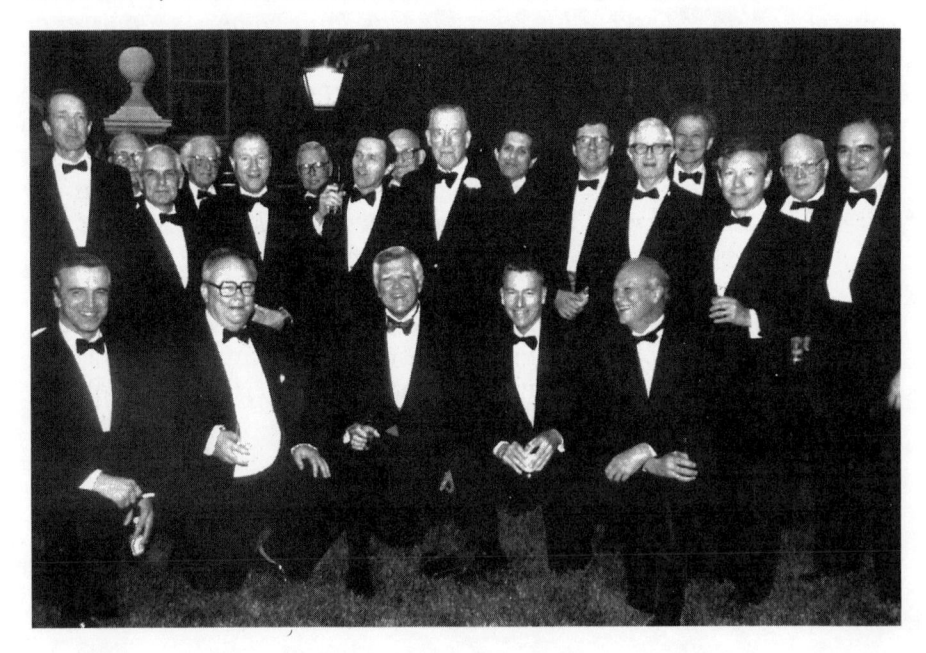

80th Birthday celebration—Dr. Rhoads with his colleagues and former residents.

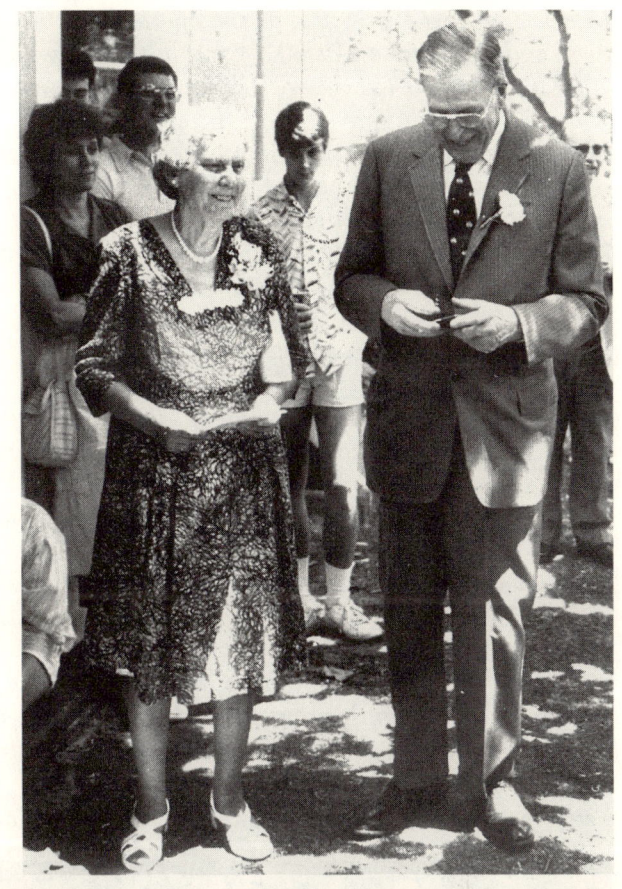

Terry and Jonathan Rhoads (right) at their 50th wedding anniversary in New Hope, Pennsylvania—1986.

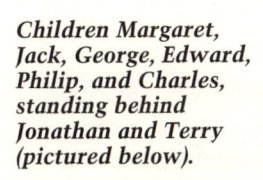

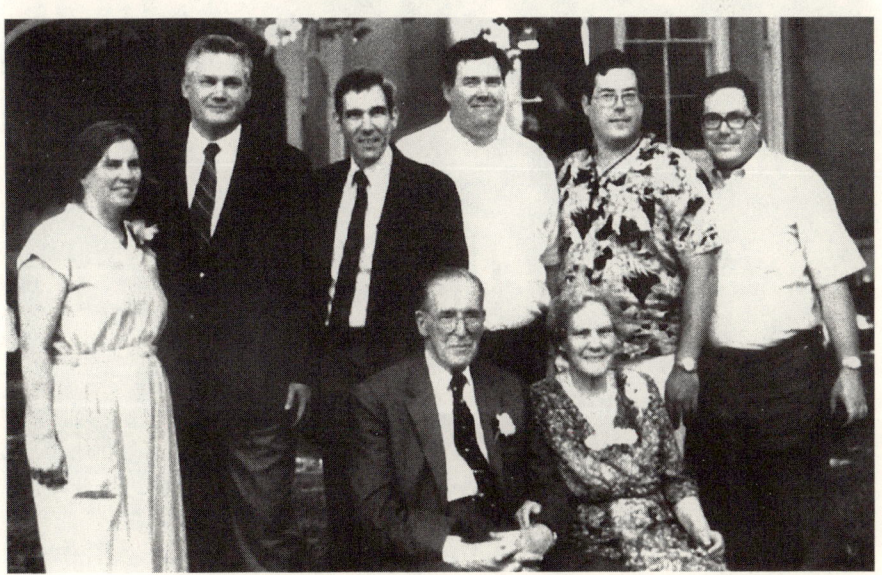

Children Margaret, Jack, George, Edward, Philip, and Charles, standing behind Jonathan and Terry (pictured below).

I think the best I saw him at the operating table was the last operation he ever did when he was 80. I wouldn't say it was the best, but it was as good as anyone I ever saw. He had a woman whom he thought he was going to do a Whipple on, and she turned out to be inoperable. Because he was close to quitting, he wanted me to scrub with him. He went through that case as well as I have ever seen, all of the thought processes, all the things he needed to look at to make judgments on. Then it became apparent she needed shunts. . . . His hand was steady and I could tell no difference at age 80 than when I first started with him.[27]

And Leonard Miller adds:

He was a superb technical surgeon. In the last couple of years he operated I watched him do a Whipple. . . . He was beautiful.[28]

Looking back on his years of practice, Rhoads observes:

Well, even when I started in medicine, cancer was still an important cause of death, though it did not count for as large a proportion of deaths as it does now because the infectious diseases carried so many people off. Dr. Eliason informed me fairly early in life that I would find that my practice would grow old with me. I would start out with fractures and appendicitis and move into middle age, into gallbladder disease

Terry Rhoads (below) in her rose garden at 131 West Walnut Lane.

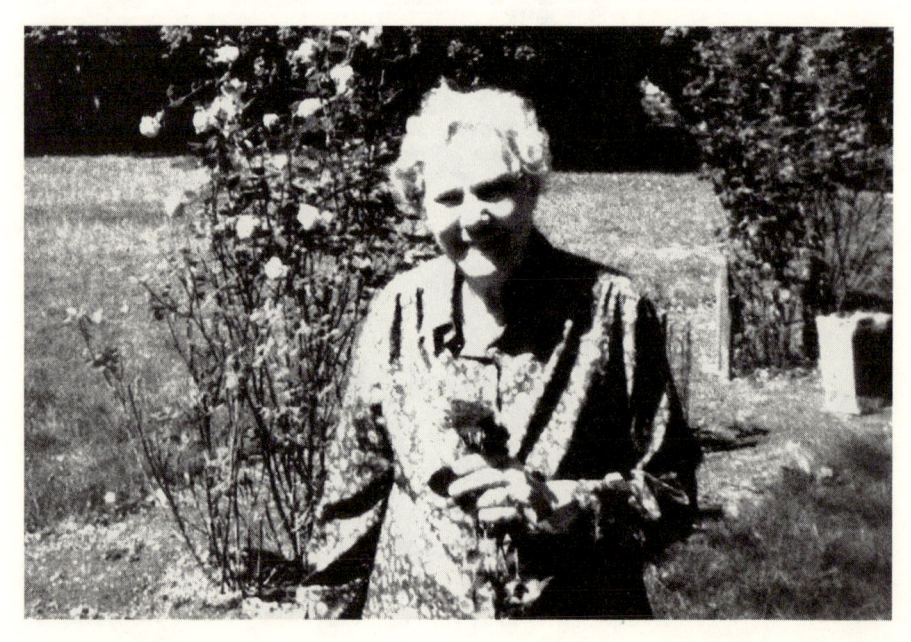

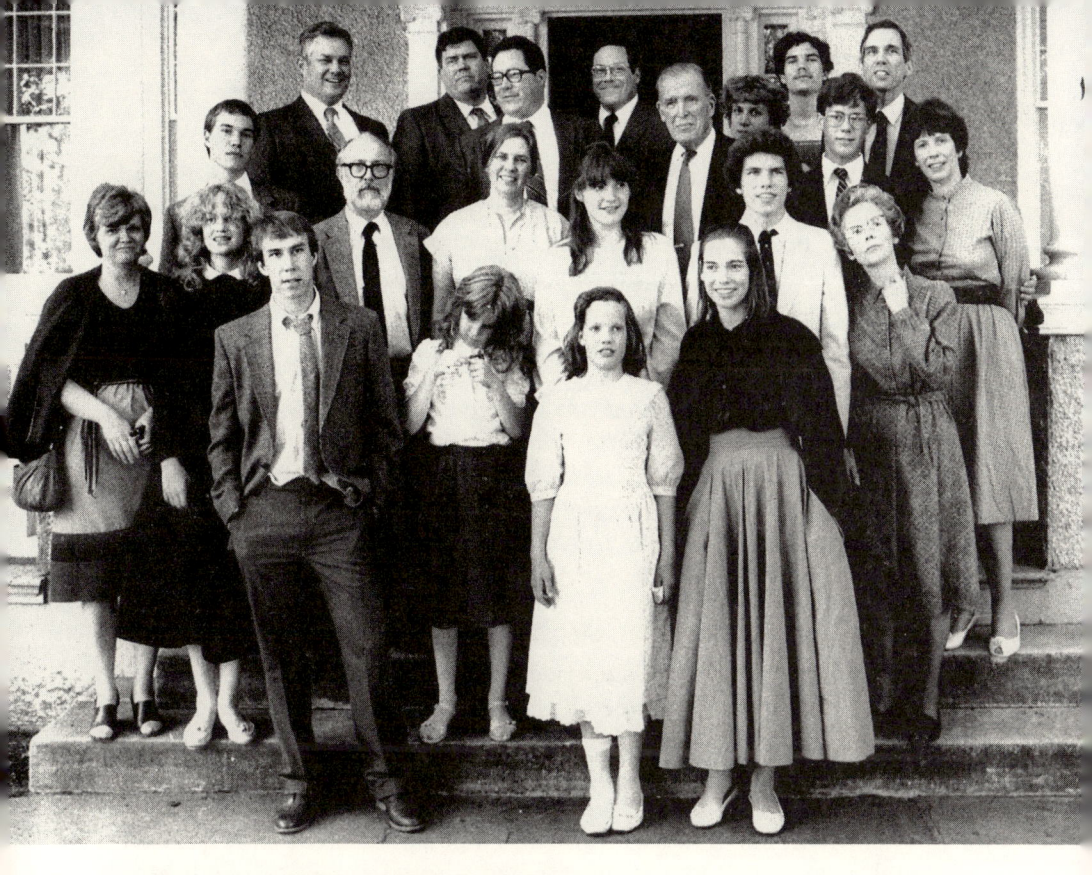

Dr. Jonathan E. Rhoads with his family, May 1987.
Front row (l to r): Barbara Rhoads (Mrs. Philip Rhoads), Deborah (Philip and Barbara's daughter), Benjamin Kendon (Adam and Margaret's son), Johanna (Philip and Barbara's daughter), Margaret and Mary Teresa (Jonathan, Jr. and Julia's daughters).
Middle row (l to r): Angus Kendon (Adam and Margaret's son), Adam Kendon (Margaret's husband), Margaret (Dr. Rhoads' daughter), Ruth Anne (Jonathan, Jr. and Julia's daughter), James (George and Frances' son), Frances (George's wife).
Back row (l to r): Dr. Rhoads' sons, Jonathan, Jr., Edward, Charles, and Philip; Dr. Rhoads; Gudrun (Adam and Margaret's daughter), Thomas (George and Frances' son), Garrett (Philip and Barbara's son), George (Dr. Rhoads' son), and Julia (Jonathan, Jr.'s wife).

and ulcers, and when I got old I'd be taking care of cancer. *In a sense, that turned out to be true.*[29]

As Rhoads' 80th birthday drew near, Clyde Barker prepared a two-day celebration to include a day-long scientific symposium in his honor. His professional colleagues, friends, and former residents paid their respects. Over 400 people attended this celebration. On the first evening, Stan Dudrick concluded his remarks by saying that he hoped they would all be there for his 90th birthday, to which Dr. Rhoads replied, "Well, Stan, you had better start taking care of yourself if you want to be there!"

This gala event was followed by great sadness when, three days later, Terry, his wife of 51 years, passed away suddenly at a luncheon. Although not a Quaker, her funeral service was held in the Germantown Friends Meeting, where she was buried along with other members of the Rhoads family. Many people spoke warmly of her kind acts and love of roses. She was especially loved by her grandchildren. Her daughter-in-law Julia has said of her:

She was a most extraordinary grandmother. And the kids adored her. The children absolutely loved her to pieces. They knew exactly where she was coming from. . . . They thought she hung on the moon. All were devastated when she died. She could let her hair down and have a level of joy and play and excitement with the children. . . . She loved them as teenagers, and she gloried in adolescence and made everybody feel special.[30]

In 1990, Jonathan Rhoads married Katharine "Kitty" Evans Goddard in a Quaker ceremony attended by 40 close relatives and friends at his New Hope home. She is a third cousin, long-time friend, and widow of the University of Pennsylvania Provost David Goddard. Mrs. Rhoads graduated from Vassar College and the University of Pennsylvania School of Medicine. She was trained as a pediatrician at the Children's Hospital and for many years maintained a private practice in Chestnut Hill, Pennsylvania, one of the first group practices in the country. She

At Maple Grove, New Hope, Pennsylvania, wedding of Jonathan Rhoads and Katharine Goddard, with members of the immediate family—1990.

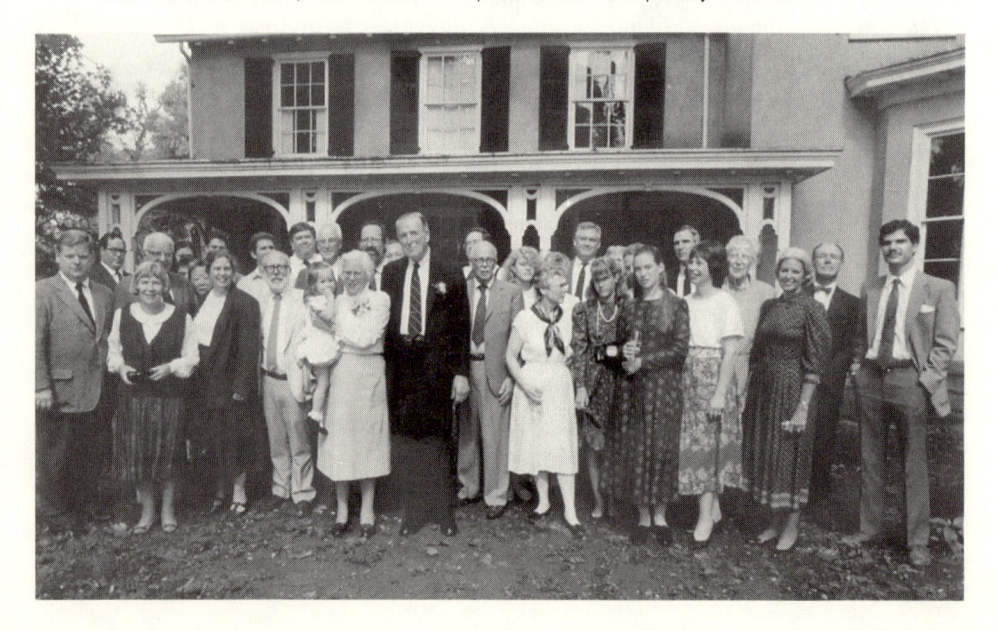

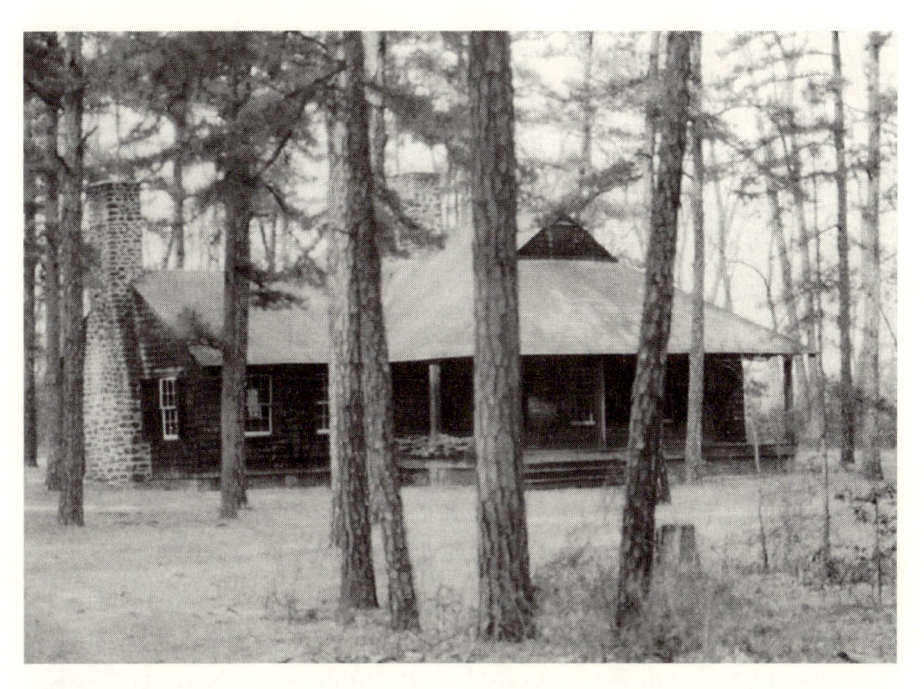

Four Way Lodge.

served on the board of the Children's Seashore House for many years and followed Elizabeth Ravdin for a term as its chairman. Rhoads' son Jack quipped that his father only married pediatricians who graduated from Vassar and were married to provosts.

The couple lives at the Quadrangle, a retirement community near the Haverford College campus. They continue to maintain a busy professional and social life. They travel extensively and according to Kitty have visited, among other places, the "four most beautiful cities in the world—San Francisco, Hong Kong, Cape Town and Rio de Janeiro." "Dr. Rhoads," she says, "never says no to a trip."[31]

The Rhoadses generally spend their summer vacations, or part of them, in New England. They visit the Folin summer home in Kearsarge and then drive to Mt. Desert Island in Maine, where they both have relatives. When they are not attending professional meetings, they enjoy going to the Science and Art Club, where members listen to and discuss a wide variety of intellectual subjects. They also belong to The Friendly Eights, a Quaker group devoted to meeting other members of the Meeting on an informal basis.[32]

In May of every year, Rhoads faithfully drives to the New Jersey Pinelands to attend the annual meeting of "Four Way Lodge," established in the 1920s by a group of Quakers, mostly graduates of Haverford College, for weekend retreats. According to David Stokes,

He loved our annual members meeting at the Four Way Lodge. He would drive in late in the evening, fresh from a meeting somewhere. He would somehow disentangle himself from behind the steering wheel of one of GM's latest creations—I think he was even able to fit into a Corvette—always wearing his huge black shoes, and, of course, a suit and a tie. Although he may not have seen most of the members for many months or a year, he reentered their lives as though he had been talking to them yesterday. He inquired of the children or relatives, what they were doing, or launched off into broad philosophical discussions. Then after dinner, he would silently melt into the darkness and head into Mays Landing to use the phone to check on his patients.

On Sunday, after meeting in front of the fire, he would often drive to the wildlife refuge at Brigantine to observe birds. I remember one time he spotted a peregrine falcon flying over the car. The rest of us would have missed it. Then, after a simple lunch, he would quietly say, "I have to drive to New York to catch a plane for London."[33]

On most Sundays after Meeting, Dr. and Mrs. Rhoads return to 131 West Walnut Lane in Germantown, which remains the site of the family's traditional Sunday dinners. As for his six children, Margaret is married, has 3 children, and is a foreign language teacher in the Philadelphia School System. Jack Rhoads is married, has 3 children, and is chairman of the Department of Surgery at the York Hospital in York, Pennsylvania, and

Traditional Sunday dinner at 131 West Walnut Lane.
Left to right, seated: Jack, Edward, George, Philip, Charles, and Margaret.
Standing: Dr. and Mrs. Rhoads.

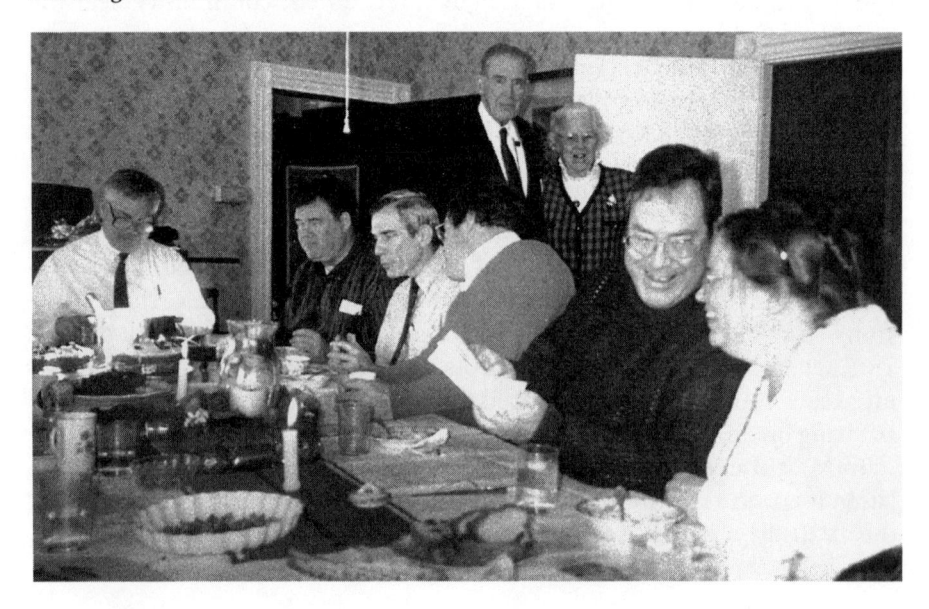

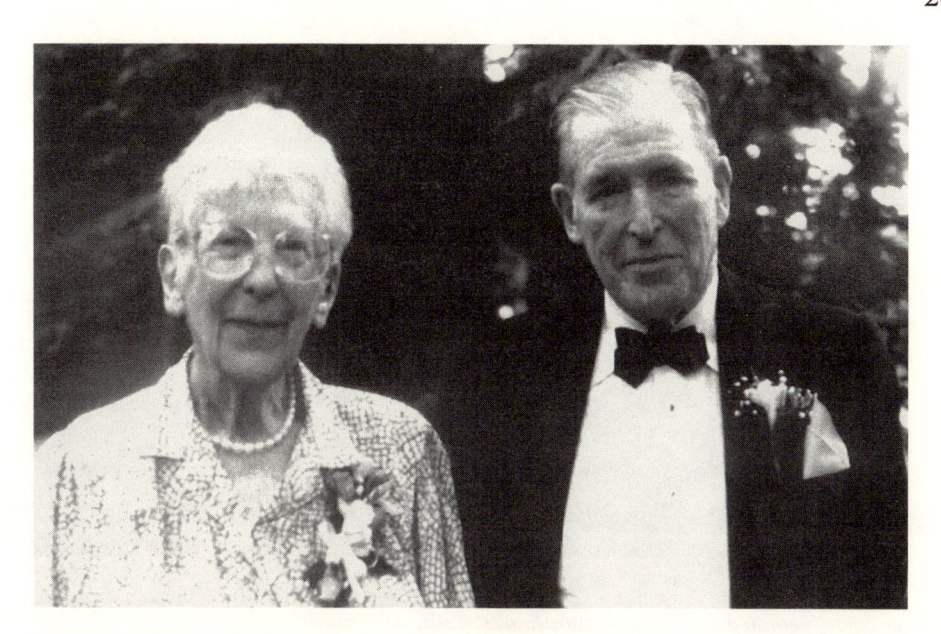

Jonathan Rhoads with his sister Caroline around 1989.

clinical professor of surgery at the University of Pennsylvania and Hershey Medical Center. George is married, has 2 children, and holds an endowed chair in the Department of Epidemiology at the New Jersey School of Medicine and Dentistry in New Brunswick. Edward is an accountant and runs a printing business in Allentown, Pennsylvania, along with his brother Charles. Charles and Philip are married. Philip has his own print shop and is the father of 4 children. According to Dr. Rhoads' daughter-in-law Julia,

Since he and Kitty married and have shared this very rich time together, in some ways he's even more accessible. He has been reaching out to each grandchild in a special way and in an individual way that is new and very heartwarming.[34]

In reviewing his 90 years, Rhoads has been honored with 27 fellowships or memberships in the most prestigious international organizations: the surgical colleges of Canada, Edinburgh, England, Germany, Holland, India, Poland, and South Africa. He belongs to 65 professional societies and has been president of most. He has been the visiting lecturer to the most prestigious academic institutions on 55 occasions. He has sat on the board of 25 organizations. He is the recipient of 27 awards, including the Joseph Goldberger Award of the American Medical Association; the Distinguished Service Award for the American Surgical Association; the Strittmayer Award of the Philadelphia County Medical

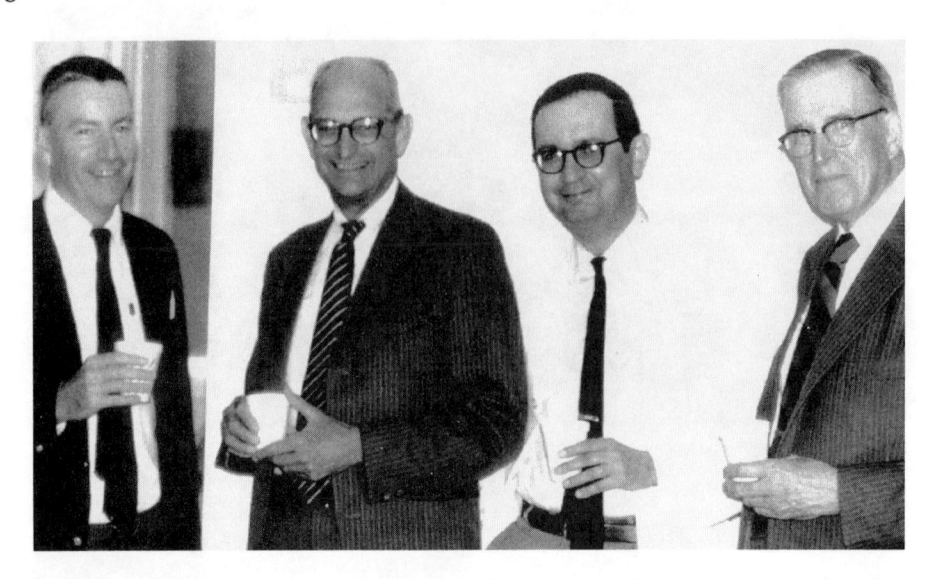

John Rhea Barton Chairmen of Surgery at HUP (left to right): Clyde Barker, Brooke Roberts, Leonard Miller, and Jonathan Rhoads.

Society; the Benjamin Franklin Medal of the American Philosophical Society (its highest honor); and the Distinguished Service Award of the College of Physicians of Philadelphia. In 1979, Dr. Rhoads' colleagues honored him through an endowed professorship in his name, "The Jonathan E. Rhoads Professorship in Surgical Sciences."

He is the founder or founding member of 5 surgical organizations and has served on the editorial boards of 8 professional journals. Rhoads has been the recipient of many honorary degrees from this country's most prestigious institutions: The University of Pennsylvania, Haverford College, Jefferson Medical College, Hahnemann Medical School, the Medical College of Ohio, Duke University, Georgetown University, and Yale University. Clyde Barker tells the story of Rhoads and his honorary degree from Georgetown University:

In 1981, Dr. Rhoads was on his way to Washington from a meeting in Europe, and during the transatlantic flight he realized that he had developed thrombophlebitis. However, he was not deterred from appearing at the commencement by this inconvenience, nor even by his additional self-diagnosis shortly thereafter of a pulmonary embolus. After accepting the degree, he caught the train to Philadelphia, came directly to the Hospital, and gave himself up for heparin treatment over the next several weeks.[35]

In conferring an honorary degree on Dr. Rhoads, President Benno Schmidt of Yale University said:

As physician, scientist, educator, university administrator, editor, civic leader, statesman, and President of the American Philosophical Society, you are considered by Philadelphia colleagues to be a genetic descendant of Ben Franklin, founder of the University of Pennsylvania 250 years ago. In recognition of your singular contributions to shaping the science of surgery and your six decades as the professor who taught future professors, Yale is proud to confer upon you the degree of Doctor of Medical Sciences.[36]

Dr. Rhoads has also been recognized as a great philanthropist by the many institutions with which he has been involved. He has established a prize in chemistry at the Westtown School and, with James Magill, a scholarship program at Haverford College. He has tirelessly raised funds or contributed to his alma maters over the years. He continues to serve on the boards of a number of charitable organizations. In connection with one of them, the Measey Foundation, Rhoads tells the story of his somewhat harrowing initial meeting with William Measey:

I approached Mr. Measey first when I was raising money for the Westtown School. It was suggested that when I meet him, that I should remind him that the wife of our principal was the daughter of a friend of his. I called and he said, "I'd like to meet you. I need to know exactly when you'll be here so we can have the dogs tied and the gates open." He [Measey] had four acres and an old house he had rebuilt. He told me just which entrance to use, so I arrived on time and there were all of these big bushes around and the front of the house was boarded up on the first floor. I kept looking around to see if there were any of those damned dogs lurking behind the bushes ready to take a dive at my throat. They were Dobermans. I pulled up in front of the house, the door swung open, and this well-civilized, well-dressed man came out. He said, "Dr. Rhoads, I presume?" He asked me in and we talked for two hours and he never gave me a nickel.[37]

Dr. Rhoads, along with Mary Johnson, his wife, and two sons, serve on the Board of the Buckingham Mountain Foundation, whose primary benefactor is the University of Pennsylvania. In addition to Buckingham, Rhoads contributes from 3 other sources: his own account, his charitable trust, and with matching money, the Pennwalt Foundation.

In 1992, Jonathan Rhoads was summoned to the office of William Kelley, the chief executive officer of the Medical Center and Health System and dean of the Medical School. Kelley informed Rhoads that the university had decided to name its newest building after him—the

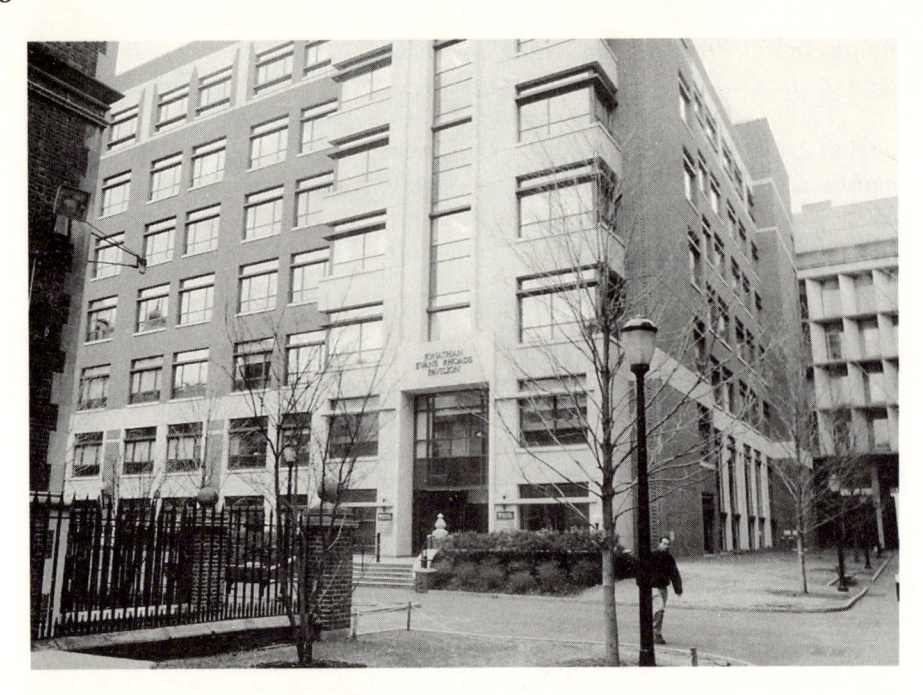

Jonathan Evans Rhoads Pavilion.

Jonathan Evans Rhoads Pavilion. The event was marked by a two-day celebration in the fall of 1994. Located at 36th and Hamilton Walk, the nine-floor, $69 million pavilion was dedicated on October 26 and 27th. William Kelley, in paying tribute to Rhoads, said:

We can only hope to approach the hallmarks of Jonathan's life and career—an overriding commitment to precision, excellence, and fulfillment of long-term goals with the flexibility to accept and meet new challenges as they arise.[38]

Judith Rodin, president of the University of Pennsylvania in representing the entire university community, said:

Penn honors Rhoads by naming the new facility for him, but it is, in truth, Dr. Rhoads who has honored Penn again and again by dedicating his life and his life's work to this University.[39]

Rhoads began his address that evening by saying:

This evening you have heard a great deal about my brighter side, and it is not my intention to balance this with any confessions about my failures, except to say that they have never been scarce.[40]

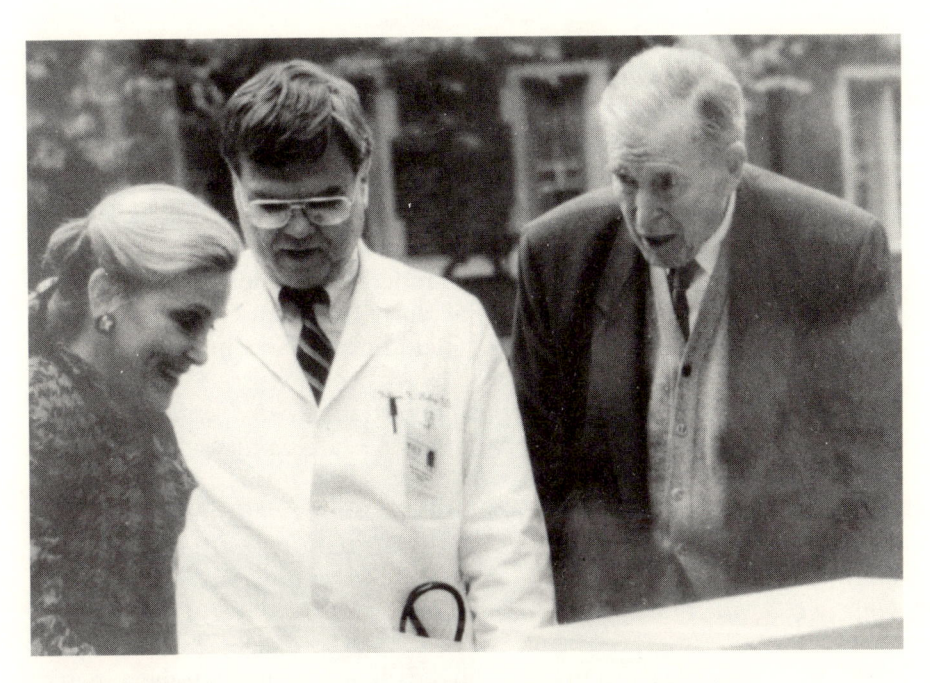

President Judith Rodin, CEO William Kelley, and Jonathan Rhoads—laying of the cornerstone of the Rhoads Pavilion.

Dr. and Mrs. Rhoads on the occasion of the dedication of the Rhoads Pavilion—Dinner, October 1994.

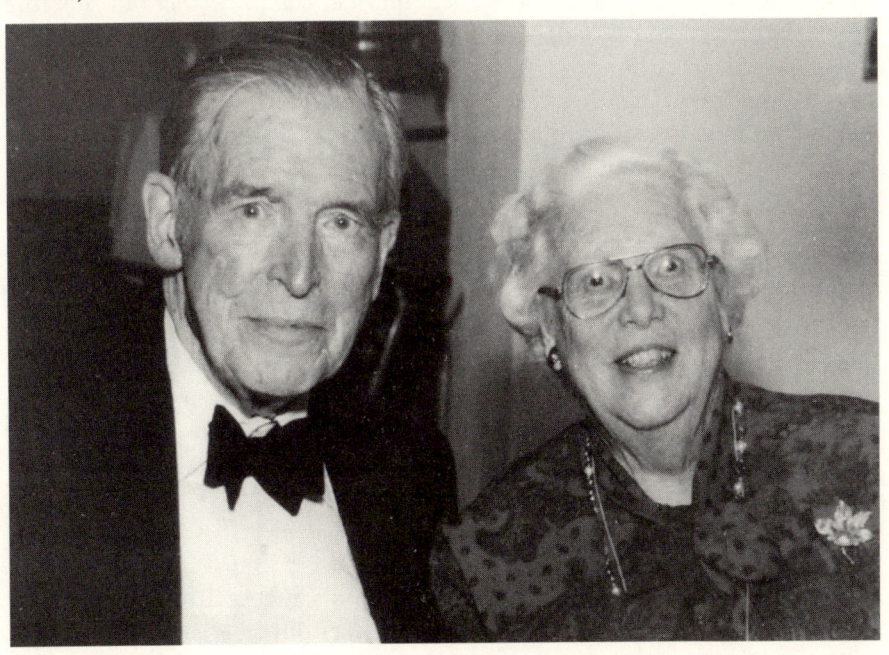

He honored his first wife Teresa and second wife Kitty, his children and grandchildren. He observed that the site of the Rhoads Pavilion was exactly where he had his first contacts with the hospital. He noted that he had gained numerous honors which would not have come to him if he had simply had the traditional three score years and ten: 5 honorary doctorates and 13 other awards had come to him since the age of 70. He paid tribute to William Kelley, Clyde Barker (whom he noted had not dated the blank resignation Rhoads had handed him when Barker became chairman), and the past officers, particularly President Gaylord Harnwell and Provost David Goddard. In his concluding remarks he said:

I suppose it is a human failing to wish to be remembered, and I have often had a special admiration for some of the early Quakers who refused to have their graves marked, believing I suppose that it was a form of vanity, but I am not that good a Quaker and I am simply delighted to have my name perpetuated for a time, at least, by this building. . . . I have come to be grateful to some of my critics as well as to all of my friends, and I thank you ever so much for this wonderful honor and this lovely occasion.[41]

As Rhoads approaches his 90th birthday, he continues to be a man of wide and varied interests, as Jack Mackie observed:

He likes to do everything. There's nothing that the man's not interested in . . . very little that he's ever seen, heard or read, or experienced that he's forgotten. He knows the Bible, finance, business, economics like the back of a hand, as well as he knows surgery.[41]

Sylvan Eisman, a colleague of Rhoads' and, before his retirement, his physician, expresses his amazement at Rhoads' stamina at the age of 89, as he relates in this story:

Do you know what he's done now? This is unbelievable! Have you ever heard of the Penn Reading project? It is now 7 years old. All of the incoming undergraduate freshmen are given a book to read, and on the Sunday before Labor Day, the day of the baccalaureat convocation, they break up these 2200 freshmen into small groups of 12 to 15 and a faculty member discusses a book. The book this year was Hemingway's Moveable Feast. Jonathan Rhoads is a preceptor. Eighty-nine years old and he reads this book and is a preceptor on that afternoon. I asked him if he was going to do this again, and he said, "Well, we'll see what the book is but probably I will."[43]

Keeping up with friends, far and wide, is another Rhoadsian trademark. Dr. Elizabeth Rose, a friend and former colleague, observes:

I don't know if it's his Quaker inheritance, but he has such an awareness of obligation and continuity and helpfulness with a low-key approach.[44]

In paying tribute to Dr. Rhoads on the occasion of his building's dedication, Arlin Adams, stated:

It has been said that there are some individuals who lift the generation they inhabit, so that all whose lives come in contact with theirs walk on higher ground during their own lifetime. Those who have been associated with Dr. Rhoads do indeed walk on higher ground for having known him.[45]

Perhaps with Quaker simplicity in mind, Leonard Miller sums up eloquently those attributes of Dr. Rhoads that are central to his rich legacy:

Master surgeon, devoted scholar, civic leader, wise counselor, firm friend.

ACKNOWLEDGMENTS

The individual and institutionally related sources in our research were many. The authors gratefully acknowledge and extend their thanks to the following (listed alphabetically):

ARCHIVES

College of Physicians of Philadelphia; Columbia University Oral History Project; Enoch Pratt Library-Mencken Curator, Vincent Fitzpatrick; Germantown Historical Society; Johns Hopkins Medical School Archives; Quaker Collection, Haverford College-Betsy Brown and Diana Peterson; University of Pennsylvania Archives-Curtiss Ayers, Mark Frazier Lloyd and Gail Pietrzyk.

INDIVIDUALS

Robert Austrian; A.C. Barger; Whitfield Bell; Harry Bishop; Irene Brown; Ruth Brown; Arthur Brown; Margaret Perry Bruton; Ben Buchwald; Mr. and Mrs. Fred Burgess; Marion Carbone; Robert Cathcart; C. Gene Cayten; Julie Choi, Edward Copeland; Louis Coriell; P. William Curreri; Charles Day; Joseph Diaco; William Dyson; Lydia Edwards; Sylvan Eisman; Barry Ellman; James Finnegan; Archibald Fletcher; Herman Goldstine; Mrs. Phillip Gray; Joseph Green; Marjorie Green; Paul Grotzinger; Dorothy Hallowell; C. Rollins Hanlon; Victor Hanson; James Hardy; Francis Harvey; Becky Hetzel; Richard Hillier; Arthur Holleb; Fairchild Houghton; Dorothy Howorth; Peter Janetta; Mary Johnson; Margaret (Rhoads) Kendon; Fred Kessler; C. Everett Koop; James Long; William Longmire; Barbara Lundy; Dennis Lynch; Jack Mackie; Horace MacVaugh; Dorothy Maxwell; Robert Mayock; Leonard Miller; Sarah Millheim; George Moore; Roland Morgan; S. Burkhart Morrison; William Muller; Henry Murphey; Gerald Murphy; Gary Nicholas; R. Barrett Noone; Martha Jones Oelke; Cynthia Peterson; William Pierce; Eric Renwick; Caroline Rhoads; Charles and Pat Rhoads; Edward Rhoads; George Rhoads; Jonathan E. Rhoads, Jr.; Julia Rhoads; Katharine Rhoads, Philip Rhoads; Eva Martin Rich; Ingram Richardson; Brooke Roberts; Charles Robinson; Francis Rosato; Elizabeth Rose; Henry Royster; Richard Saik; John Sayen; Harris Schumacker; Henry and Edith Schwartz; Cletus Schwegman; Jean Shapin; George Sharpless; Franklin Smith; George Spaeth, Ezra Steiger; George Stephenson; David Stokes; Harvey Sugerman; E. Armistead Talman; R. Carmichael Tilghman; Hilary Timmis; Paul Tschetter; G. Frank Tyers; Anne and Sylvain Van Gobes; Marc Wallack; John and Doris Webster; Jack Wehner; Claude Welch; Raleigh White; Douglas Wilmore; Willis Winn; Leonard Yoder; Jane Ziegler; Mrs. Harold Zintel.

ENDNOTES

INTRODUCTION

1. Robert Austrian, letter to the authors, 11 May 1994.
2. Margaret Bacon, *The Quiet Rebels* (Philadelphia: New Society Publishers, 1985) 13.
3. Philip Benjamin, *Philadelphia Quakers in the Industrial Age* (Philadelphia: Temple University Press, 1976) 141.
4. Howard Brinton, *Quaker Education: Theory and Practice* (Wallingford, Pa.: Pendle Hill Pamphlet #9, 1940) 20.
5. Brinton, 20.
6. Brinton, 24.
7. Julia Rhoads, personal interview, 12 November 1996.
8. Brinton, 24–25.
9. Barbara Lundy, letter to the authors, 7 August 1992.
10. Joan Cassell, "On Control, Certitude and the 'Paranoia' of Surgeons," *Culture, Medicine and Psychiatry* June 1987, Vol. 11 (2), 229.
11. Peter Zeldow and Steven Daugherty, "Personality Profiles and Specialty Choices of Students from Two Medical School Classes," *Academic Medicine* May 1991, Vol. 66 #5, 285.
12. Laura Bleiweiss, "Out of the Depths: A Study in the Sociology of Surgery," diss., University of Pennsylvania, 1974, 18.
13. Jonathan Rhoads, "Quaker Tenets and the Philosophy of the Medical Profession," *Through A Quaker Archway*, ed. Horace Lippincott (New York: Sagamore Press, 1959) 129.
14. Rhoads, 140.
15. Rhoads, 141.
16. William Curreri, *Jonathan E. Rhoads Eightieth Birthday Symposium*, ed. Clyde F. Barker and John Daly (Philadelphia: Lippincott, 1989) 210.
17. Victor Hanson, letter to the authors, 4 July 1992.
18. Michael Sheeran, *Beyond Majority Rule—Voteless Decisions in the Religious Society of Friends* (Philadelphia: Philadelphia Yearly Meeting, 1983) 91.

1 FRIENDS FOR LIFE

1. Liva Baker, *The Justice from Beacon Hill: The Life and Times of Oliver Wendell Holmes*, (New York: Harper Collins, 1991) 66.
2. Jonathan Rhoads, letter to Samuel Morris, 24 November 1891, Quaker Collection, Haverford College, Haverford, Pa.
3. Richard Rhoads, ed. *Jonathan Evans Rhoads and Rebecca Garrett Rhoads and Their Descendents* (Kennett Square, Pa., 1994) 2nd ed., 3.
4. Jonathan Rhoads, personal interview, 12 April 1993.
5. Richard Rhoads, 5.

6. Richard Rhoads, 3.
7. Jonathan Rhoads, personal interview, 12 April 1993.
8. Jonathan Rhoads, personal interview, 12 April 1993.
9. Richard Rhoads, 3.
10. Edward G. Rhoads, letter to Esther Biddle Rhoads, 21 August 1917, Esther Biddle Rhoads Collection, 1153, Quaker Collection, Haverford College, Haverford, Pa.
11. Sharon Kaufman, *The Healer's Tale* (Madison, Wisconsin: Univ. of Wisconsin Press, 1993) 83.
12. Caroline Rhoads, personal interview, 12 August 1992.
13. Jonathan Rhoads, personal interview, 19 April 1993.
14. Philip Benjamin, *Philadelphia Quakers* (Philadelphia: Temple University Press, 1976) 201.
15. Openhouse Brochure, New Hope Historical Society, 9 May 1964, New Hope, Pa.
16. Caroline Rhoads, personal interview, 28 April 1993.
17. John Webster, personal interview, 9 July 1992.
18. Caroline Rhoads, personal interview, 12 August 1992.
19. Caroline Rhoads, personal interview, 28 April 1993.
20. Jonathan Rhoads, personal interview, 12 April 1993.
21. Caroline Rhoads, personal interview, 28 April 1993.
22. Jonathan Rhoads, personal interview, 12 April 1993.
23. Jonathan Rhoads, personal interview, 19 April 1993.
24. Philip Benjamin, *Philadelphia Quakers in the Industrial Age* (Philadelphia: Temple University Press, 1976) 269.
25. Philip Benjamin, *Industrial*, 269.
26. Caroline Rhoads, personal interview, 12 August 1992.
27. Jonathan Rhoads, personal interview, 19 April 1993.
28. Caroline Rhoads, personal interview, 28 April 1992.
29. Margaret Rhoads, letter to Esther B. Rhoads, [c. 1922], Esther B. Rhoads Collection, 1153, Quaker Collection, Haverford College, Haverford, Pa.
30. Margaret Rhoads, letter to Esther B. Rhoads, 8 February 1922, Esther B. Rhoads Collection, 1153.
31. Caroline Rhoads, personal interview, 12 August 1992.
32. Esther B. Rhoads, diary entry, 29 August 1914, Esther B. Rhoads Collection, 1153.
33. Jonathan Rhoads, personal interview, 19 April 1993.
34. Jonathan Rhoads, personal interview, 19 April 1993.
35. Julia Rhoads, personal interview, 12 November 1996.
36. John Moore, ed. *Friends in the Delaware Valley: Philadelphia Yearly Meeting 1681–1981* (Haverford, Pa.: Friends Historical Assoc., 1981) 219.
37. Margaret Rhoads, letter to Esther B. Rhoads, 19 August 1921, Esther B. Rhoads Collection, 1153.
38. Jonathan Rhoads, personal interview, 19 April 1993.
39. Julia Rhoads, personal interview, 12 November 1996.
40. Jonathan Rhoads, personal interview, 4 May 1993.
41. Jonathan Rhoads, personal interview, 4 May 1993.
42. Caroline Rhoads, personal interview, 12 August 1992.
43. Jonathan Rhoads, personal interview, 4 May 1993.
44. Caroline Rhoads, personal interview, 12 August 1992.
45. Margaret Rhoads, letter to Esther B. Rhoads, 9 September 1909, Esther B. Rhoads Collection, 1153.
46. Margaret Rhoads, letter to Esther B. Rhoads, 19 September 1909, Esther B. Rhoads Collection, 1153.
47. Jonathan Rhoads, personal interview, 4 May 1993.
48. Margaret Rhoads, letter to Esther B. Rhoads, 19 September 1909, Esther B. Rhoads Collection, 1153.
49. Margaret Rhoads, letter to Esther B. Rhoads, 10 September 1909, Esther B. Rhoads Collection, 1153.

50. Jonathan Rhoads, personal interview, 13 May 1993.
51. Margaret Rhoads, letter to Esther B. Rhoads, 15 August 1917, Esther B. Rhoads Collection, 1153.
52. Jonathan Rhoads, personal interview, 13 May 1993.
53. Jonathan Rhoads, personal interview, 13 May 1993.
54. Mark S. Hoffman, ed. *The World Almanac and Book of Facts* (New York: Pharos Books, 1992) 521.
55. Jonathan Rhoads, personal interview, 13 May 1993.
56. Jonathan Rhoads, personal interview, 13 May 1993.
57. Jonathan Rhoads, personal interview, 13 May 1993.
58. Margaret Rhoads, letter to Esther B. Rhoads, 19 April 1921, Esther B. Rhoads Collection, 1153.
59. Esther B. Rhoads, letter to Hetty B. Garrett, 3 August 1915, Esther B. Rhoads Collection, 1153.
60. Caroline Rhoads, personal interview, 12 August 1992.
61. Jonathan Rhoads, unpublished memoir, n.d., n.pag.
62. Caroline Rhoads, personal interview, 28 April 1993.
63. Jonathan Rhoads, "Changing Concepts in Breast Surgery," *Sonneborn Memorial Lecture*, Philadelphia, 28 April 1982.
64. Edward G. Rhoads, letter to Esther B. Rhoads, 26 July 1922, Esther B. Rhoads Collection, 1153.
65. Edward G. Rhoads, letter to Esther B. Rhoads, 11 September 1921, Esther B. Rhoads Collection, 1153.
66. Jonathan Rhoads, personal interview, 24 May 1993.
67. E. Digby Baltzell, *Puritan Boston and Quaker Philadelphia* (Boston: Beacon Press, 1979) 279.
68. Susanna Smedley, *Catalog of Westtown Through the Years* (Philadelphia: Lyon and Armor, 1945) 6.
69. Jonathan Rhoads, unpublished chapter for *Lives of the Presidents of the American Cancer Society*, 1983, 3–4.
70. Edward G. Rhoads, letter to Esther B. Rhoads, 9 October 1921, Esther B. Rhoads Collection, 1153.
71. Jonathan Rhoads, letter to Esther B. Rhoads, [c. 1921], Esther B. Rhoads Collection, 1153.
72. Jonathan Rhoads, letter to Esther B. Rhoads, [c. 1921], Esther B. Rhoads Collection, 1153.
73. Margaret Rhoads, letter to Esther B. Rhoads, 30 October 1921, Esther B. Rhoads Collection, 1153.
74. Margaret Rhoads, letter to Esther B. Rhoads, 19 April 1921, Esther B. Rhoads Collection, 1153.
75. Margaret Rhoads, letter to Esther B. Rhoads, 13 November 1921, Esther B. Rhoads Collection, 1153.
76. Jonathan Rhoads, letter to Esther B. Rhoads, 11 December 1921, Esther B. Rhoads Collection, 1153.
77. Jonathan Rhoads, letter to Esther B. Rhoads, 11 December 1921, Esther B. Rhoads Collection, 1153.
78. John Webster, personal interview, 9 July 1992.
79. Jonathan Rhoads, personal interview, 7 June 1993.
80. Jonathan Rhoads, personal interview, 7 June 1993.
81. John Webster, personal interview, 9 July 1992.
82. Margaret Rhoads, letter to Esther B. Rhoads, 17 September 1922, Esther B. Rhoads Collection, 1153.
83. John Webster, personal interview, 9 July 1992.
84. John Webster, personal interview, 9 July 1992.
85. Jonathan Rhoads, personal interview, 1 June 1993.
86. Helen Hole, *Westtown Through the Years* (Philadelphia: Lyon and Armor, 1942) viii.

87. John Webster, personal interview, 9 July 1992.
88. *Year's Record of Westtown School for 1924* (Westtown, Pa.) 14.
89. Hole, viii.
90. Jonathan Rhoads, personal interview, 7 June 1993
91. Jonathan Rhoads, personal interview, 7 June 1993.
92. Becky Hetzel, personal interview, 21 June 1993.
93. John Webster, personal interview, 9 July 1992.
94. Jonathan Rhoads, personal interview, 1 June 1993.
95. Francis Harvey, letter to the authors, 14 May 1992.
96. Perry Bruton, letter to the authors, 13 May 1992.
97. Sarah Millheim, letter to the authors, 12 June 1992.
98. Becky Hetzel, personal interview, 21 June 1993.
99. Margaret Rhoads, letter to Esther B. Rhoads, 11 December 1921, Esther B. Rhoads Collection, 1153.
100. Margaret Rhoads, letter to Esther B. Rhoads, 8 February 1922, Esther B. Rhoads Collection, 1153.
101. *Year's Record*, 112.
102. Ingraham Richardson, letter to the authors, May 1992.
103. Edward G. Rhoads, letter to Esther B. Rhoads, 5 September 1923, Esther B. Rhoads Collection, 1153.
104. Edward G. Rhoads, letter to Esther B. Rhoads, 9 September 1923, Esther B. Rhoads Collection, 1153.
105. Edward G. Rhoads, letter to Esther B. Rhoads, 14 September 1923, Esther B. Rhoads Collection, 1153.
106. John Webster, personal interview, 9 July 1992.
107. Hole, 379.
108. Margaret Rhoads, letter to Esther B. Rhoads, 17 October 1923, Esther B. Rhoads Collection, 1153.
109. Margaret Rhoads, letter to Esther B. Rhoads, 11 November 1923, Esther B. Rhoads Colleciton, 1153.
110. Margaret Rhoads, letter to Esther B. Rhoads, 2 September 1924, Esther B. Rhoads Collection, 1153.

2   SWIMMING THE BOSPORUS

1. Margaret Rhoads, letter to Esther B. Rhoads, 8 September 1925, Esther B. Rhoads Collection, 1153, Quaker Collection, Haverford College, Haverford, Pa.
2. Jonathan Rhoads, personal interview, 7 June 1993.
3. Robert Stevens, "Philadelphia Friends and Higher Education: The Case of Haverford College," published speech to the Newcomen Society, 1 November 1983, n.pag.
4. *Haverford College Bulletin*, Vol. xxvi, No. 3, January 1928, 8.
5. Gregory Kannerstein, ed. *The Spirit and the Intellect: Haverford College, 1833–1983* (Haverford, Pa.: Haverford College, 1983), 56.
6. Kannerstein, 60.
7. *The Haverford Record* (Haverford, Pa.: Haverford College, 1928), 101.
8. Stevens, n.pag.
9. Kannerstein, 119.
10. *Haverford Record*, 87.
11. *Haverford College News*, 11 November 1924.
12. *Haverford College News*, 28 October 1924.
13. Jonathan Rhoads, letter to Esther B. Rhoads, 21 October 1924, Esther B. Rhoads Collection, 1153.
14. Jonathan Rhoads, letter to Esther B. Rhoads, 21 October 1924, Esther B. Rhoads Collection, 1153.

15. Ingram Richardson, letter to the authors, May, 1992.
16. Margaret Rhoads, letter to Esther B. Rhoads, 6 November 1924, Esther B. Rhoads Collection, 1153.
17. Jonathan Rhoads, letter to Esther B. Rhoads, 22 March 1925, Esther B. Rhoads Collection, 1153.
18. Edward G. Rhoads, letter to Esther B. Rhoads, 10 April 1925, Esther B. Rhoads Collection, 1153.
19. Margaret Rhoads, letter to Esther B. Rhoads, 29 November 1924, Esther B. Rhoads Collection, 1153.
20. *Haverford News*, passim, 1924–1928.
21. Jonathan Rhoads, personal interview, 9 June 1993.
22. Jonathan Rhoads, letter to Esther B. Rhoads, 21 October 1924, Esther B. Rhoads Collection, 1153.
23. Edward G. Rhoads, letter to Esther B. Rhoads, 28 July 1924, Esther B. Rhoads Collection, 1153.
24. Margaret Rhoads, letter to Esther B. Rhoads, 2 September 1924, Esther B. Rhoads Collection, 1153.
25. *Haverford Record*, 88.
26. Jonathan Rhoads, personal interview, 6 June 1995.
27. Bellangee, J. "Fairhope The Forerunner," *Twentieth Century Magazine*, Vol. IV, No. 4, September 1911, 483–484.
28. Jonathan Rhoads, letter to Esther B. Rhoads, 8 November 1925, Esther B. Rhoads Collection, 1153.
29. *Haverford News*, 15 February 1926.
30. Margaret Rhoads, letter to Esther B. Rhoads, 6 January 1926, Esther B. Rhoads Collection, 1153.
31. Margaret Rhoads, letter to Esther B. Rhoads, 24 January 1926, Esther B. Rhoads Collection, 1153.
32. Margaret Rhoads, letter to Esther B. Rhoads, 30 January 1926, Esther B. Rhoads Collection, 1153.
33. Caroline Rhoads, personal interview, 28 April 1993.
34. Jonathan Rhoads, personal interview, 25 August 1994.
35. S. Burkhart Morrison, letter to the authors, 14 May 1992.
36. *Haverford News*, 7 March 1927.
37. *Haverford News*, 11 January 1926.
38. Steven Gragert, ed., *Will Rogers Weekly Articles: The Hoover Years—1929–1931* (Stillwater, Oklahoma: Oklahoma University Press, 1981), 44.
39. Jonathan Rhoads, personal interview, 7 June 1993.
40. Jonathan Rhoads, personal interview, 7 June 1993.
41. Jonathan Rhoads, personal interview, 7 June 1993.
42. Ingram Richardson, letter to the authors, May 1992.
43. *Haverford Record*, 75.
44. Kannerstein, 76.
45. Jonathan Rhoads, personal interview, 9 June 1993.
46. Kannerstein, 74.
47. Jonathan Rhoads, personal interview, 9 June 1993.
48. Jonathan Rhoads, personal interview, 9 June 1993.
49. Jonathan Rhoads, personal interview, 7 June 1993.
50. *Haverford Record*, 57.
51. *Haverford Record*, 101.
52. William Meldrum, letter to Lawrence Baker, 2 June 1928, Johns Hopkins Medical School.
53. Henry S. Pratt, letter to Lawrence Baker, 6 June 1928, Johns Hopkins Medical School.
54. Lawrence Baker, memorandum to himself, 19 June 1928, Johns Hopkins Medical School.

3 CAN WE GIVE HIM BACK HIS $18?

1. Jonathan Rhoads, unpublished memoir, n.d., 1.
2. Ingram Richardson, letter to authors, May 1992.
3. Jonathan Rhoads, unpublished chapter for *Lives of the Presidents of the American Cancer Society*, 1983, 6.
4. Jonathan Rhoads, application to Johns Hopkins Medical School, 1928.
5. Thomas B. Turner, *Heritage of Excellence, The Johns Hopkins Medical Institutions—1914–1947* (Baltimore: The Johns Hopkins University Press, 1974) 227.
6. Augusta Tucker, *Miss Suzie Slagle's* (Baltimore: The Johns Hopkins University Press, 1939) xv.
7. Turner, 7.
8. Turner, 173.
9. Turner, 173.
10. Turner, 173.
11. Sharon Kauffman, *The Healer's Tale* (Madison: University of Wisconsin Press, 1993) 105.
12. Joanne Argersinger, *Toward a New Deal in Baltimore* (Chapel Hill: Univ. of North Carolina Press, 1988) 2–3.
13. Argersinger, 12.
14. Argersinger, 13.
15. Turner, 242.
16. Jonathan Rhoads, letter to Royal Davis, 9 November 1928.
17. Jonathan Rhoads, unpublished memoir, n.d., n.pag.
18. Jonathan Rhoads, letter to Royal Davis, 9 November 1928.
19. Jonathan Rhoads, "Biographical Outline for Alpha Omega Alpha Interview," 23 February 1977, 4.
20. Turner, 173.
21. Jonathan Rhoads, letter to Royal Davis, 9 November 1928.
22. Jonathan Rhoads, letter to Royal Davis, 9 November 1928.
23. Becky Hetzel, personal interview, 21 June 1993.
24. Jonathan Rhoads, letter to Royal Davis, 20 March 1929.
25. E. Cowles Andrus, letter to L.H. Weed, 20 March 1929.
26. Paul Tschetter, letter to authors, 15 April 1992.
27. Henry G. Schwartz, letter to authors, [circa 1992].
28. Lydia Edwards, letter to authors, 10 May 1992.
29. R. Carmichael Tilghman, letter to authors, 22 May 1992.
30. Harris Schumacker, letter to authors, 3 June 1992.
31. Harris Schumacker, letter to the authors, 3 June 1992.
32. Jonathan Rhoads, letter to Royal Davis, 9 November 1928.
33. Jonathan Rhoads, letter to Royal Davis, 4 January 1929.
34. Jonathan Rhoads, personal interview, 24 July 1993.
35. Samuel Meites, *Otto Folin: America's First Clinical Biochemist* (Washington, DC: American Association for Clinical Chemistry, 1989), 210–211.
36. Philip Schaeffer, "Otto Folin (1867–1934)," *Journal of Nutrition*, 52, 1954, 8.
37. Meites, 210.
38. Rhoads, AOA, 5.
39. Jonathan E. Rhoads, letter to Esther B. Rhoads, [c. 1934], Esther B. Rhoads Collection, 1153, Haverford College, Haverford, Pa.
40. H. L. Mencken, *Thirty Five Years of Newspaper Work*, ed. F. Hobson, V. Fitzpatrick and B. Jacobs (Baltimore: Johns Hopkins Univ. Press, 1994) 207.
41. Turner, 273.
42. Turner, 279.
43. Turner, 100–101.
44. Jonathan Rhoads, personal interview, 7 July 1994.
45. Jonathan Rhoads, letter to Royal Davis, 27 January 1930.
46. Jonathan Rhoads, personal interview, 7 July 1994.

47. Jonathan Rhoads, letter to Royal Davis, 18 May 1930.
48. Jonathan Rhoads, letter to Royal Davis, 23 April 1930.
49. Jonathan Rhoads, letter to Royal Davis, 31 April 1930.
50. Jonathan Rhoads, letter to Royal Davis, 23 April 1930.
51. Jonathan Rhoads, personal interview, 25 August 1994.
52. Jonathan Rhoads, personal interview, 7 July 1993.
53. Turner, 310.
54. H.L. Mencken, "Johns Hopkins Hospital, I: The Dispensary," *The Evening Sun*, 6 July 1937, 31.
55. Turner, 304.
56. Jonathan Rhoads, personal interview, 25 August 1995.
57. Turner, 244.
58. Kauffman, 97.
59. *Hopkins Medical News*, Vol. 8, No. 2, May–June, 1983, 5.
60. Jonathan Rhoads, letter to Royal Davis, 19 January 1931.
61. Jonathan Rhoads, personal interview, 10 June 1993.
62. Jonathan Rhoads, personal interview, 10 June 1993.
63. Jonathan Rhoads, personal interview, 10 June 1993.
64. E. Cowles Andrus, letter to William Pepper, 5 November 1931.
65. L.H. Thorpe, letter to E. Cowles Andrus, 11 November 1931.
66. Jonathan Rhoads, letter to Royal Davis, 12 December 1931.
67. Jonathan Rhoads, letter to Royal Davis, 12 December 1931.
68. Jonathan Rhoads, letter to Royal Davis, 19 December 1931.
69. Turner, 409.
70. Turner, 406.
71. Turner, 409.
72. Jonathan Rhoads, personal interview, 7 July 1993.
73. Jonathan Rhoads, personal interview, 10 June 1993.
74. Turner, 441.
75. Jonathan Rhoads, personal interview, 7 July 1994.
76. Turner, 442.
77. Turner, 444.
78. Jonathan Rhoads, letter to Walter Menninger, 24 February 1995.
79. Jonathan Rhoads, personal interview, 10 June 1993.
80. Soma Weiss, letter to E. Cowles Andrus, 6 April 1932.
81. Jonathan Rhoads, personal interview, 10 June 1993.
82. Meites, 210.
83. Jonathan Rhoads, AOA, 6.
84. Jonathan Rhoads, personal interview, 10 June 1993.
85. Jonathan Rhoads, letter to Esther B. Rhoads, 9 July 1933, Esther B. Rhoads Collection, 1153.
86. *Board of Managers Report*, Hospital of the University of Pennsylvania, 1932–1933.
87. *Board of Managers Report*, HUP,1932–1933.
88. Jonathan Rhoads, address, University of Pennsylvania Medical School, Class of '39, 14 May 1994.
89. John Webster, personal interview, 9 July 1992.
90. Jonathan Rhoads, letter to Royal Davis, 7 August 1932.
91. Jonathan Rhoads, letter to Royal Davis, 9 September 1932.
92. Jonathan Rhoads, letter to Royal Davis, 7 August 1932.
93. Jonathan Rhoads, letter to Royal Davis, 8 July 1933.
94. John Webster, personal interview, 9 July 1992.
95. Jonathan Rhoads, letter to Esther B. Rhoads, 8 July 1933, Esther B. Rhoads Collection, 1153.
96. Jonathan Rhoads, personal interview, 7 June 1993.
97. Jonathan Rhoads, letter to Esther B. Rhoads, 8 July 1933, Esther B. Rhoads Collection, 1153.

98. Jonathan Rhoads, letter to Esther B. Rhoads, 8 July 1933, Esther B. Rhoads Collection, 1153.
99. John Webster, personal interview, 9 July 1992.
100. Jonathan Rhoads, letter to Esther B. Rhoads, 8 July 1933, Esther B. Rhoads Collection, 1153.
101. Pendleton Tompkins, letter to Jonathan Rhoads, 13 October 1987.
102. Jonathan Rhoads, personal interview, 10 June 1993.
103. Brooke Roberts, personal interview, 2 April 1992.
104. Jonathan Rhoads, personal interview, 10 June 1993.
105. Jonathan Rhoads, personal interview, 10 June 1993.
106. Brooke Roberts, personal interview, 2 April 1992.
107. Jonathan Rhoads, personal interview, 10 June 1993.
108. Pendleton Tompkins, letter to Jonathan Rhoads, 13 October 1987.
109. Jonathan Rhoads, letter to Royal Davis, 7 September 1933.
110. Margaret Rhoads, letter to Esther B. Rhoads, 22 October 1933, Esther B. Rhoads Collection, 1153.
111. Margaret Rhoads, letter to Esther B. Rhoads, 22 October 1933, Esther B. Rhoads Collection, 1153.
112. Clyde Barker and John Daly, ed. *Jonathan E. Rhoads 80th Birthday Symposium* (Philadelphia: Lippincott, 1989), 270.
113. Jonathan Rhoads, AOA, 8.
114. Kauffman, 87.

4 MR. PIM PASSES BY

1. I.S. Ravdin, "The Reminiscences of Isidor Ravdin," (New York: Columbia University Oral History Project, 1963) 68.
2. I.S. Ravdin, 1–15 passim.
3. I.S. Ravdin, 28–30, passim.
4. I.S. Ravdin, 41–42.
5. O.H. Wangensteen, "Isidor Schwaner Ravdin—Versatile Surgeon and Nonpareil Surgical Statesman." *Surgery* 56: 609–610, 1964.
6. I.S. Ravdin, Authorized Translation. *Operative Surgery. General and Special Considerations.* Vol. 1, ed. Martin Kirschner (Philadelphia: J. B. Lippincott) 1931.
7. W.E. Lee, I.S. Ravdin, G. Tucker and E.P. Pendergrass. "Studies on Experimental Pulmonary Atelectasis; Production of Atelectasis." *American Surgery* 88: 15–20, 1928.
8. C.G. Johnston, I.S. Ravdin, C. Riegel, C.L. Allison. "Studies on Gallbladder Function; Anion-Cation Content of Bile from Normal and Infected Gallbladder." *Journal of Clinical Investigation* 12: 67–75, 1933.
9. P.M. Mecray, R.P. Barden, I.S. Ravdin. "Nutritional Edema: Its Effect on Gastric Emptying Time Before and After Gastric Surgery." *Surgery* 1: 53–64, 1937.
10. James Hardy, *The World of Surgery (1945–1985)* (Philadelphia: University of Pennsylvania Press, 1986) 124–125.
11. S. Farber and I.S. Ravdin. "Civilian Activities at the National Level." *Surgery* 56: 611–613, 1964.
12. Farber and Ravdin, 608.
13. Farber and Ravdin, 610.
14. Jonathan Rhoads, unpublished memoir, n.d., n.pag.
15. Jonathan Rhoads, "Surgical Training in Retrospect," speech, Dublin, Ireland, 3 July 1989.
16. Rhoads, "Training," 3 July 1989.
17. Charles Johnston, letter to I.S. Ravdin, 16 August 1934.
18. Jonathan Rhoads, letter to Esther B. Rhoads, December 1934, Esther B. Rhoads Collection, 1153, Quaker Collection, Haverford College, Haverford, Pa.

19. Charles Frazier, letter to I.S. Ravdin, 25 March 1935.
20. Report of the Board of Managers, Hospital of the University of Pennsylvania, 1934–1935.
21. Jonathan Rhoads, "Biographical Outline for AOA Interview," 23 February 1977, 7.
22. Samual Meites, *Otto Folin: America's First Clinical Biochemist* (Washington, DC: American Association for Clinical Chemistry) 221.
23. Jonathan Rhoads, personal interview, 24 July 1993.
24. Jonathan Rhoads, "Academic Pitfalls in America—1907–1982," Roswell Park Memorial Lecture, Buffalo, New York, 17 February 1982.
25. Jonathan Rhoads, personal interview, 21 September 1994.
26. Jonathan Rhoads, "The Importance of Small Molecules in Major Surgery," Mixter Lecture, Montreal, Canada, 1 October 1995.
27. Jonathan Rhoads, personal interview, 21 September 1994.
28. Jonathan Rhoads, "Surgery in the Elderly," speech, Bryn Mawr, Pa., 22 March 1979.
29. Jonathan Rhoads, personal interview, 24 July 1993.
30. Jonathan Rhoads, personal interview, 21 September 1994.
31. Jonathan Rhoads, personal interview, 20 October 1993.
32. Henry Royster, letter to the authors, 14 August 1992.
33. Jonathan Rhoads, personal interview, 23 October 1993.
34. Jonathan Rhoads, personal interview, 23 October 1993.
35. Jonathan Rhoads, personal inteview, 23 October 1993.
36. I.S. Ravdin, letter to Alan O. Whipple, 20 April 1940.
37. Jonathan Rhoads, personal interview, 20 October 1993.
38. Jonathan Rhoads, personal interview, 20 October 1993.
39. Jonathan Rhoads, personal interview, 20 October 1993.
40. Albert Keim and Grant Stoltzfus, *The Politics of Conscience: The Historic Peace Churches and America at War* (Scottsdale, Pa.: Herald Press, 1988) 71.
41. Keim and Stoltzfus, 73.
42. Keim and Stoltzfus, 82.
43. Rhoads, AOA, 10.
44. Robert Stevens, "Philadelphia Friends and Higher Education: The Case of Haverford College," published speech to the Newcomen Society, 1 November 1983.
45. Jonathan Rhoads, personal interview, 20 October 1993.
46. Jonathan Rhoads, "Quaker Tenets and the Philosophy of the Medical Profession," *Through a Quaker Archway*, ed. Horace Lippincott (New York: Sagamore Press, 1959) 134.
47. Rhoads, AOA, 12.
48. Jonathan Rhoads, letter to the Procurement and Assignment Office, 2 May 1942.

5 THE BATTLE OF SPRUCE STREET

1. C. Everett Koop, personal interview, 19 August 1994.
2. Edward D. Churchill, *Surgeon to Soldier* (Philadelphia: J.B. Lippincott, 1972) 61.
3. Churchill, 62.
4. I.S. Ravdin, letter to the Dean of the School of Medicine, 10 December 1941, The Papers of I.S. Ravdin, 1917–1972, University of Pennsylvania Archives, Philadelphia, Pa.
5. Jonathan Rhoads, personal interview, 18 November 1994.
6. Churchill, 27.
7. Robert Mayock, personal interview, 5 April 1995.

8. Board of Managers Report, June, 1941–May 31, 1942, Hospital of the University of Pennsylvania, Philadelphia.
9. Richard R. Lingeman, *Don't You Know There's A War Going On?: The American Home Front—1941–1945* (New York: G. P. Putnam's Sons, 1970), 243.
10. William Dyson, personal interview, 1 March 1993.
11. William Dyson, personal interview, 1 March 1993.
12. C. Everett Koop, *Koop: The Memoirs of America's Family Doctor* (New York: Random House, 1991), 63.
13. C. Everett Koop, personal interview, 19 August 1994.
14. C. Everett Koop, "Harold Zintel—1912–1993," *Transactions of the American Surgical Association*, ed. Clyde Barker (Philadelphia: J.B. Lippincott, 1993) 387–388.
15. Jonathan Rhoads, personal interview, 18 November 1994.
16. Jonathan Rhoads, personal interview, 23 October 1993.
17. C. Everett Koop, personal interview, 19 August 1994.
18. Robert Mayock, personal interview, 5 April 1995.
19. Robert Mayock, personal interview, 5 April 1995.
20. Jonathan Rhoads, personal interview, 5 June 1995.
21. Jonathan Rhoads, personal interview, 5 June 1995.
22. Jonathan Rhoads, personal interview, 23 October 1993.
23. Jonathan Rhoads, personal interview, 23 October 1993.
24. C. Everett Koop, personal interview, 19 August 1994.
25. C. Everett Koop, personal interview, 19 August 1994.
26. Jonathan Rhoads, personal interview, 18 November 1994.
27. C. Everett Koop, personal interview, 19 August 1994.
28. Jonathan Rhoads, personal interview, 18 November 1994.
29. C. Everett Koop, personal interview, 19 August 1994.
30. Jonathan Rhoads, personal interview, 18 November 1994.
31. C. Everett Koop, personal interview, 19 August 1994.
32. C. Everett Koop, personal interview, 19 August 1994.
33. Jonathan Rhoads, personal interview, 5 June 1995.
34. C. Everett Koop, personal interview, 19 August 1994.
35. Jonathan Rhoads, personal interview, 5 June 1995.
36. Jonathan Rhoads, personal interview, 5 June 1995.
37. C. Everett Koop, personal interview, 19 August 1994.
38. C. Everett Koop, personal interview, 19 August 1994.
39. Dorothy Maxwell, personal interview, 12 December 1995.
40. Jonathan Rhoads, personal interview, 18 November 1994.
41. Signed, "One of your Third Year Students," letter to Jonathan Rhoads, 29 October 1942, University of Pennsylvania Archives.
42. Jonathan Rhoads, "Quaker Tenets and the Philosophy of the Medical Profession," *Through a Quaker Archway*, ed. Horace Lippincott (New York: Sagamore Press, 1959) 135-136.
43. Jonathan Rhoads, personal interview, 5 June 1995.
44. Jonathan Rhoads, personal interview, 5 June 1995.
45. Jonathan Rhoads, personal interview, 5 June 1995.
46. Jonathan Rhoads, personal interview, 23 October 1993.
47. Jonathan Rhoads, personal interview, 23 October 1993.
48. Jonathan Rhoads, personal interview, 23 October 1993.
49. Jonathan Rhoads, personal interview, 23 October 1993.
50. Jonathan Rhoads, personal interview, 23 October 1993.
51. *Archway*, 136.
52. Jonathan Rhoads, "Memoir of a Surgical Nutritionist," *JAMA*, Vol. 272 No. 12, 28 September 1994, 966.
53. Robert Mayock, personal interview, 5 April 1995.
54. Robert Mayock, personal interview, 5 April 1995.
55. C. Everett Koop, interview, 19 August 1994.

6 THE CHIEF, THE COW, AND THE CORTISONE

1. *The Scope*, the yearbook of the University of Pennsylvania Medical School, 1941.
2. Cletus Schwegman, personal interview, 30 October 1996.
3. Leonard Miller, "William T. Fitts, 1915–1980," *Transactions of the American Surgical Association*, ed. Lloyd Nyhus (Philadelphia: J.B. Lippincott, 1980) 63–66.
4. Mary Johnson, personal interview, 13 August 1993.
5. Mary Johnson, personal interview, 13 August 1993.
6. Leonard Miller, personal interview, 10 July 1994.
7. Jonathan Rhoads, personal interview, 27 October 1993.
8. Jonathan Rhoads, personal interview, 27 October 1993.
9. Jonathan Rhoads, personal interview, 27 October 1993.
10. Jonathan Rhoads, personal interview, 27 October 1993.
11. Jonathan Rhoads, personal interview, 27 October 1993.
12. Jonathan Rhoads, personal interview, 27 October 1993.
13. Caroline Rhoads, letter to Esther B. Rhoads, 23 September 1946, Esther B. Rhoads Collection, 1153, Quaker Collection, Haverford College, Haverford, Pa.
14. Jonathan Rhoads, "Biographical Outline for AOA Interview," 23 February 1977.
15. Caroline Rhoads, letter to Esther B. Rhoads, 8 October 1946, Esther B. Rhoads Collection, 1153.
16. Jonathan Rhoads, AOA, 20.
17. Rhoads, AOA, 22.
18. Rhoads, AOA, 20.
19. Rhoads, AOA, 22.
20. Jonathan Rhoads, personal interview, 27 October 1993.
21. Jonathan Rhoads, letter to Esther B. Rhoads, 14 January 1947, Esther B. Rhoads Collection, 1153.
22. Jonathan Rhoads, personal interview, 27 October 1993.
23. Jonathan Rhoads, letter to I.S. Ravdin, 21 January 1947, University of Pennsylvania Archives.
24. Jonathan Rhoads, letter to Esther B. Rhoads, 14 January 1947, Esther B. Rhoads Collection, 1153.
25. Jonathan Rhoads, letter to Esther B. Rhoads, 14 January 1947, Esther B. Rhoads Collection, 1153.
26. Jonathan Rhoads, letter to I.S. Ravdin, 2 February 1947, University of Pennsylvania Archives.
27. I.S. Ravdin, letter to Jonathan Rhoads, 27 February 1947, University of Pennsylvania Archives.
28. Cletus Schwegman, personal interview, 30 October 1996.
29. I.S. Ravdin, letter to Jonathan Rhoads, 27 February 1947, University of Pennsylvania Archives.
30. I.S. Ravdin, letter to Jonathan Rhoads, 27 February 1947, University of Pennsylvania Archives.
31. Rhoads, AOA, 22.
32. Jonathan Rhoads, letter to Esther B. Rhoads, 30 May 1947, Esther B. Rhoads Collection, 1153.
33. Jonathan Rhoads, letter to I.S. Ravdin, 3 August 1947, University of Pennsylvania Archives.
34. I.S. Ravdin, letter to local physicians, 10 September 1947, University of Pennsylvania Archives.
35. Jack Mackie, personal interview, 31 December 1994.
36. Jack Mackie, personal interview, 31 December 1994.
37. Brooke Roberts, personal interview, 2 April 1992.
38. Rhoads, unpublished memoir, n.d., n.pag.
39. Jonathan Rhoads, personal interview, 27 October 1993.

40. Jonathan Rhoads, letter to the Esther B. Rhoads, 23 April 1948, Esther B. Rhoads Collection, 1153.
41. Archibald Fletcher, letter to the authors, 26 February 1994.
42. William Dyson, personal interview, 1 March 1993.
43. Jonathan Rhoads, personal interview, 9 November 1993.
44. I.S. Ravdin, letter to Jonathan Rhoads, 15 July 1948, University of Pennsylvania Archives.
45. Caroline Rhoads, letter to Esther B. Rhoads, 11 February 1951, Esther B. Rhoads Collection, 1153.
46. Jonathan Rhoads, letter to Esther B. Rhoads, 3 March 1951, Esther B. Rhoads Collection, 1153.
47. Margaret Rhoads, personal interview, 16 April 1994.
48. Edward O.F. Rhoads, personal interview, 6 June 1994.
49. David Stokes, letter to the authors, 11 March 1994.
50. Edward Rhoads, personal interview, 6 June 1994.
51. George Rhoads, personal interview, 24 June 1994.
52. Margaret Rhoads, personal interview, 16 April 1994.
53. George Rhoads, personal interview, 24 June 1994.
54. Charles Rhoads, personal interview, 26 May 1994.
55. Margaret Rhoads, personal interview, 16 April 1994.
56. Anne Van Gobes, personal interview, 8 August 1993.
57. Margaret Rhoads, personal interview, 16 April 1994.
58. Margaret Rhoads, personal interview, 16 April 1994.
59. Charles Rhoads, personal interview, 26 May 1994.
60. Jonathan Rhoads, Jr., personal interview, 15 April 1994.
61. Charles Rhoads, personal interview, 26 May 1994.
62. Margaret Rhoads, personal interview, 16 April 1994.
63. George Rhoads, personal interview, 24 June 1994.
64. Margaret Rhoads, personal interview, 16 April 1994.
65. George Rhoads, personal interview, 24 June 1994.
66. Charles Rhoads, personal interview, 26 May 1994.
67. Edward Rhoads, personal interview, 6 June 1994.
68. Jonathan Rhoads, personal interview, 27 October 1993.
69. Jonathan Rhoads, personal interview, 27 October 1993.
70. J.E. Rhoads, J.G. Allen, H.N. Harkins and C.A. Moyer, *Surgery: Principles and Practice*, 1st ed. (Philadelphia: J.B. Lippincott, 1957) 5.

7 THOUGHT FOR FOOD

1. Francis D. Moore, *Jonathan E. Rhoads Eightieth Birthday Symposium*, ed. Clyde Barker and John Daly. (Philadelphia: J.B. Lippincott, 1989) 250.
2. I.S. Ravdin, J.E. Rhoads, "Certain problems illustrating the importance of knowledge of biochemistry by the surgeon," *Surgical Clinics of North America* 15:85–100, 1935.
3. Jonathan Rhoads, personal interview, 20 December 1993.
4. Jonathan Rhoads, personal interview, 20 December 1993.
5. I.S. Ravdin, M. A. Casberg, "A second look at surgical care in major catastrophes," *American Journal of Surgery* 89:721–724, 1955.
6. David Cooper, personal interview, 11 August 1993.
7. G.P. Mueller, I.S. Ravdin, E. G. Ravdin, "Alterations of bile pigment metabolism in biliary tract disease," *JAMA* 85: 86–88, 1925.
8. Jonathan Rhoads, remarks, Memorial Service for Harry Vars, 1 December 1983.
9. Jonathan Rhoads, remarks, Memorial Service for Harry Vars, 1 December 1983.
10. Jonathan Rhoads, remarks, Memorial Service for Harry Vars, 1 December 1983.
11. David Cooper, personal interview of Harry Vars, 25 April 1983.

12. S. Goldschmidt, H.M. Vars, I.S. Ravdin, "Influence of foodstuffs upon susceptibility of liver to injury by chloroform and probable mechanism of their action," *J Clinical Investigations* 18: 277–289, 1939.
13. R.P. Barden, I.S. Ravdin, W.D. Frazier, "Hypoproteinemia as a factor in retardation of gastric emptying after operations of the Billroth I or II types," *American Journal Roentgenology* 38: 196–202, 1937.
14. Barden, 196–202.
15. Jonathan Rhoads, personal interview, 14 December 1993.
16. W.D. Thompson, I.S. Ravdin, I.L. Frank, "Effect of hypoproteinemia on wound disruption," *Archives of Surgery* 36: 500–508, 1938.
17. J.E. Rhoads, H.F. Hottenstein, I.F. Hudson, "The decline in the strength of catgut after exposure to living tissues," *Archives of Surgery* 34: 377–397, 1937.
18. J.E. Rhoads, W. Kasinkas, "The influence of hypoproteinemia on the formation of callus in experimental fracture," *Surgery* 11: 38–44, 1942.
19. Jonathan Rhoads, personal interview, 14 December 1993.
20. F.N. Gurd, H.M. Vars, I.S. Ravdin, "Composition of the regenerating liver after partial hepatectomy in normal and protein-depleted rats," *Am J Physiology* 152: 11–21, 1948.
21. I.S. Ravdin, E. Thoroughgood, C. Riegel, R. Peters, J.E. Rhoads, "The prevention of liver damage and the facilitation of repair in the liver by diet," *JAMA* 121: 322–324, 1943.
22. Jonathan Rhoads, remarks, Memorial Service for Harry Vars, 1 December 1983.
23. Douglas Waugh, ed. *The Gurds—The Montreal General and McGill—A Family Saga*, (Burnstown, Ontario: General Store Publishing House, 1996) 233.
24. Jonathan Rhoads, personal interview, 14 December 1993.
25. J.E. Rhoads, A. Stengel, Jr., C. Riegel, F.A. Caori, W.D. Frazier, "The absorption of protein split products from chronic isolated colon loops," *Am J Physiology* 125: 707-712, 1939.
26. Jonathan Rhoads, personal interview, 14 December 1993.
27. V. Henriques, A.C. Anderson, "Ueber Parenterale Ernahrung durch Intravenose Injektion," *Ztschr F Physiol Chem Strassb* lxxxviii: 357–369, 1913.
28. Janet Weinberg, "Nutrition Through A Needle: Closing Pandora's Box," *Science News*, 106: 90, 1974.
29. W.M Parkins, C.E. Koop, C. Riegel, H.M. Vars, J.S. Lockwood, "Gelatin as plasma substitute, with particular reference to experimental hemorrhage and burn shock," *Ann Surg* 118: 193–214, 1943.
30. Jonathan Rhoads, personal interview, 22 December 1993.
31. Jonathan Rhoads, personal interview, 22 December 1993.
32. John Lockwood, letter to Jonathan Rhoads, 10 December 1943.
33. A.G. Fletcher, N.S. GImbel, C. Riegel, "Parenteral nutrition with human serum albumin as source of protein in early postoperative period," *Surgery, Gynecology and Obstetrics* 90: 151–154, 1950.
34. Jonathan Rhoads, personal interview, 22 December 1993.
35. C.E. Koop, J.H. Drew, C. Riegel, J.E. Rhoads, "The effect of preoperative forcefeeding on surgical patients," *Ann Surg* 124: 1165–1174, 1946.
36. Jonathan Rhoads, personal interview, 14 December 1993.
37. Jonathan Rhoads, personal interview, 14 December 1993.
38. P. Nemir, H.R. Hawthorne, B.L. Lecrone, "Simple intestinal obstruction; prolongation of life for 45 days with parenteral alimentation," *Proc Soc Exper Biol and Med* 69: 14–16, 1948.
39. B.J. Duffy, "Clinical use of polyethylene tubing for intravenous therapy, Report on 72 cases," *Ann Surg* 130:929–936, 1949.
40. Jonathan Rhoads, personal interview, 15 December 1993.
41. H.C. Meng, D.W. Wilmore, eds., *Proceedings of the International Conference on Fat Emulsions* (Chicago: American Medical Association, 1970).
42. H.C. Meng, D.W. Wilmore, eds., *Proceedings of the International Conference on Fat Emulsions* (Chicago: American Medical Association, 1970).

43. Jonathan Rhoads, personal interview, 15 December 1993.
44. Jonathan Rhoads, personal interview, 15 December 1993.
45. Jonathan Rhoads, personal interview, 15 December 1993.
46. Jonathan Rhoads, personal interview, 15 December 1993.
47. Jonathan Rhoads, personal interview, 20 December 1993.
48. Jonathan Rhoads, remarks, Memorial Service for Harry Vars, 1 December 1983.
49. David Cooper, personal interview, 11 August 1993.
50. J.E. Rhoads, S.J. Dudrick, H.M. Vars, "History of intravenous nutrition." In *Clinical Nutrition*, Vol. II, eds. J.L. Rombeau, M.D. Caldwell (Philadelphia: W.B. Saunders, 1986) 5.
51. S.J. Dudrick, D.W. Wilmore, H.M. Vars, J.E. Rhoads, "Long-term parenteral nutrition with growth development and positive nitrogen," *Surgery* 64: 134–142, 1968.
52. Dudrick, 137.
53. Douglas Wilmore, personal interview, 20 August 1993.
54. R. Aubaniac, "L'injection intraveineuse sous-claviculaire: advantages et technique," *Press Medicale* 60: 1456, 1947.
55. R.A. Mogil, D.A. DeLaurentis, G.P. Rosemond, "The infraclavicular venipuncture," *Arch Surg* 95: 320, 1967.
56. Douglas Wilmore, personal interview, 20 August 1993.
57. Jonathan Rhoads, personal interview, 20 December 1993.
58. Harry Bishop, personal interview, 12 August 1993.
59. Harry Bishop, personal interview, 12 August 1993.
60. D.W. Wilmore, S.J. Dudrick, "Growth and development of an infant receiving all nutrients exclusively by vein," *JAMA* 203: 140–144, 1968.
61. Douglas Wilmore, personal interview, 20 August 1993.
62. Wilmore and Dudrick, 142.
63. Wilmore and Dudrick, 142.
64. Douglas Wilmore, personal interview, 20 August 1993.
65. Douglas Wilmore, personal interview, 20 August 1993.
66. Autopsy report. Children's Hospital of Philadelphia, 1969.
67. Jonathan Rhoads, personal interview, 20 December 1993.
68. E. Steiger, H.M. Vars, S.J. Dudrick, "A technique for long-term intravenous feeding in unrestrained rats," *Archives of Surgery* 104 (3): 330–332, 1972.
69. S.J. Dudrick, J.E. Rhoads, "New Horizons for intravenous feeding," *JAMA* 215(6): 939–949, 1971.
70. Janet Weinberg, "Nutrition through a needle: Closing Pandora's Box," *Science News*, 106: 90–91, 1974.
71. Jonathan Rhoads, personal interview, 22 December 1993.
72. Jonathan Rhoads, personal interview, 20 December 1993.
73. Jonathan Rhoads, personal interview, 20 December 1993.
74. Jonathan Rhoads, "Academic Pitfalls in America—1907–1982," Roswell Park Memorial Lecture, Buffalo, New York, 17 February 1982.

8 A HAPPY FACULTY

1. *Annual Report of the Provost to President Gaylord Harnwell, 1958–1959*, 29. University of Pennsylvania Archives, Philadelphia, Pa.
2. *Press Release*, University of Pennsylvania New Bureau, 30 April 1959. University of Pennsylvania Archives.
3. *Daily Pennsylvanian*, "Rare Combination," 30 April 1959, No. 123, 2.
4. Howard Brinton, *Quaker Education: Theory and Practice* (Wallingford, Pa.: Pendle Hill Press, 1940) Pamphlet #9, 24.
5. Margaret Rhoads, letter to Esther B. Rhoads, [1924?], Esther B. Rhoads Collection, 1153, Quaker Collection, Haverford College, Haverford, Pa.
6. Jonathan Rhoads, personal interview, 12 November 1993.

7. Jonathan Rhoads, personal interview, 12 November 1993.
8. Jonathan Rhoads, personal interview, 12 November 1993.
9. Marion Carbone, personal interview, 10 December 1994.
10. Jonathan Rhoads, personal interview, 12 November 1993.
11. Jonathan Rhoads, personal interview, 12 November 1993.
12. Jonathan Rhoads, "The State of the University," *Founder's Day Address*, University of Pennsylvania, Philadelphia, Pa., 12 January 1957, 2. University of Pennsylvania Archives.
13. Jonathan Rhoads, letter to C. Canby Balderson, 3 January 1957.
14. Willis Winn, personal interview, 11 December 1996.
15. Jonathan Rhoads, personal interview, 12 November 1993.
16. Jonathan Rhoads, personal interview, 12 November 1993.
17. Jonathan Rhoads, personal interview, 12 November 1993.
18. Jonathan Rhoads, personal interview, 12 November 1993.
19. Loren Eiseley, letter to Jonathan Rhoads, 2 August 1956. University of Pennsylvania Archives.
20. Jonathan Rhoads, *Founder's Day*, 1–3. University of Pennsylvania Archives.
21. Rhoads, *Founders Day*, 3. University of Pennsylvania Archives.
22. Rhoads, *Founder's Day*, 5. University of Pennsylvania Archives.
23. Isaac Roberts, letter to Jonathan Rhoads, 12 June 1957. University of Pennsylvania Archives.
24. *Daily Pennsylvanian*, 4 May 1956, No. 179, 1.
25. Jonathan Rhoads, letter to Stewart Marshall, 6 July 1956. University of Pennsylvania Archives.
26. *Daily Pennslyvanian*, 5 February 1957, No. 180., 1.
27. Jonathan Rhoads, letter to Gaylord Harnwell, 11 February 1957. University of Pennsylvania Archives.
28. Willis Winn, personal interview, 11 December 1996.
29. Clifford Backstrand, letter to Jonathan Rhoads, 16 July 1959. University of Pennsylvania Archives.
30. Jonathan Rhoads, letter to Clifford Backstrand, 20 August 1959. University of Pennsylvania Archives.
31. Unidentified patient, letter to Jonathan Rhoads, n.d. University of Pennsylvania Archives.
32. Jonathan Rhoads, letter to Louis Stein, 23 July 1959. University of Pennsylvania Archives.
33. Lewis Johnson, letter to Jonathan Rhoads, 8 June 1956. University of Pennsylvania Archives.
34. Willis Winn, personal interview, 11 December 1996.
35. Clifford Backstrand, letter to Jonathan Rhoads, 16 July 1959. University of Pennsylvania Archives.

9 I WONDER WHERE THAT PLANE IS GOING?

1. Hilary Timmis, letter to the authors, 22 October 1992.
2. Leonard Miller, personal interview, 10 July 1994.
3. Jack Mackie, personal interview, 31 December 1992.
4. Jack Mackie, personal interview, 31 December 1992.
5. Barry Ellman, letter to the authors, 12 August 1992.
6. Arthur Brown, letter to the authors, 20 August 1992.
7. Marc Wallack, letter to the authors, 18 September 1992.
8. Jonathan Rhoads, "Changing Concepts of Breast Cancer," Hahneman Hospital, Philadelphia, Pa., 12 June 1982.
9. Jonathan Rhoads, personal interview, 27 January 1994.
10. Hilary Timmis, letter to the authors, 22 October 1992.

11. Jonathan Rhoads, "Surgery of the Pancreas," Temple University, Philadelphia, Pa., 11 May 1982.
12. Jonathan Rhoads, personal interview, 27 January 1994.
13. Harvey Sugerman, letter to the authors, 5 March 1993.
14. William Pierce, letter to the authors, 23 June 1992.
15. Armistead Talman, letter to the authors, 2 July 1992.
16. Irene Brown, personal interview, 12 May 1994.
17. Marion Carbone, personal interview, 10 December 1994.
18. Irene Brown, personal interview, 12 May 1994.
19. Irene Brown, personal interview, 12 May 1994.
20. R. Barrett Noone, letter to the authors, 8 December 1992.
21. William Pierce, letter to the authors, 23 June 1992.
22. Jonathan Rhoads, personal interview, 8 February 1994.
23. *Philadelphia Bulletin*, 23 June 1965, 1.
24. Jonathan Rhoads, personal interview, 8 February 1994.
25. Jonathan Rhoads, personal interview, 8 February 1994.
26. Jonathan Rhoads, personal interview, 8 February 1994.
27. Jonathan Rhoads, personal interview, 8 February 1994.
28. Jack Mackie, personal interview, 31 December 1992.
29. Horace MacVaugh, letter to authors, 18 June 1992.
30. Jonathan Rhoads, personal interview, 5 July 1994.
31. American Friends Service Committee, Philadelphia Yearly Meeting, June 3, 1969.
32. Jonathan Rhoads, personal interview, 5 July 1994.
33. Jonathan Rhoads, personal interview, 5 July 1994.
34. Jonathan Rhoads, personal interview, 5 July 1994.
35. Jonathan Rhoads, personal interview, 5 July 1994.
36. Jonathan Rhoads, personal interview, 5 July 1994.
37. Jonathan Rhoads, personal interview, 5 July 1994.
38. Lady Borton, letter to Jonathan Rhoads, 8 December 1989.
39. James Finnegan, letter to the authors, 17 July 1992.
40. Gary Nicholas, letter to the authors, 18 June 1992.
41. Francis Rosato, letter to the authors, 7 July 1992.
42. Raleigh White, letter to the authors, 11 August 1992.
43. Joseph Diaco, letter to the authors, 17 July 1992.
44. C. Gene Cayten, letter to the authors, 4 September 1992.
45. R. Barrett Noone, letter to the authors, 8 December 1992.
46. Francis Rosato, letter to the authors, 7 July 1992.
47. William Curreri, letter to the authors, 26 June 1992.
48. Francis Rosato, letter to the authors, 7 July 1992.
49. Edward Copeland, letter to the authors, 6 August 1992.
50. Barbara Lundy, letter to the authors, 5 August 1992.
51. Hilary Timmis, letter to the authors, 22 October 1992.

10 WISE COUNSELOR, FIRM FRIEND

1. Leonard Miller, personal interview, 10 July 1994.
2. Clyde Barker, *Jonathan Rhoads—Eightieth Birthday Symposium*, ed. Clyde Barker, John Daly (Philadelphia: J.B. Lippincott, 1989) 254.
3. Leonard Miller, personal interview, 10 July 1994.
4. Arthur Holleb, letter to the authors, 25 June 1994.
5. Jonathan Rhoads, personal interview, 27 January 1994.
6. Jonathan Rhoads, personal interview, 27 January 1994.
7. Jonathan Rhoads, personal interview, 27 January 1994.
8. Jonathan Rhoads, personal interview, 27 January 1994.

9. Charles Rhoads, personal interview, 26 May 1994.
10. *Philadelphia Evening Bulletin*, 1 April 1977, 1.
11. Jonathan Rhoads, address, Philadelphia Award, Philadelphia, Pa., 31 March 1977.
12. Jonathan Rhoads, Philadelphia Award, 31 March 1977.
13. Robert Austrian, letter to the authors, 11 May 1994.
14. Robert Cathcart, letter to the authors, 19 March 1994.
15. Jack Mackie and Leonard Miller, personal interviews, 31 December 1992, 10 July 1994.
16. Whitfield Bell, personal interview, 18 November 1996.
17. Jonathan Rhoads, unpublished memoir, n.d., n.pag.
18. Whitfield Bell, personal interview, 18 November 1996.
19. Arlin Adams, address, Rhoads Pavilion Dedication, 26 October 1994.
20. Herman Goldstine, personal interview, 17 November 1996.
21. David Stokes, letter to the authors, 11 March 1994.
22. David Stokes, letter to the authors, 11 March 1994.
23. Jonathan Rhoads, personal interview, 29 April 1994.
24. Jonathan Rhoads, personal interview, 29 April 1994.
25. Leonard Miller, personal interview, 10 July 1994.
26. George Spaeth, letter to the authors, 21 February 1994.
27. Jack Mackie, personal interview, 31 December 1994.
28. Leonard Miller, personal interview, 10 July 1994.
29. Jonathan Rhoads, personal interview, 27 January 1994.
30. Julia Rhoads, personal interview, 12 November 1996.
31. Katharine Rhoads, personal interview, 14 May 1996.
32. Katharine Rhoads, personal interview, 14 May 1996.
33. David Stokes, letter to the authors, 11 March 1994.
34. Julia Rhoads, personal interview, 12 November 1996.
35. Clyde Barker, *Eightieth Birthday*, 254.
36. Benno Schmidt, address, Yale University, New Haven, Conn., 28 May 1990.
37. Jonathan Rhoads, personal interview, 31 March 1994.
38. William Kelley, address, Rhoads Pavilion Dedication, Philadelphia, Pa., 26 October 1994.
39. Judith Rodin, address, Rhoads Pavilion Dedication, Philadelphia, Pa., 26 October 1994.
40. Jonathan Rhoads, address, Rhoads Pavilion Dedication, Philadelphia, Pa., 26 October 1994.
41. Jonathan Rhoads, Dedication, 26 October 1994.
42. Jack Mackie, personal interview, 31 December 1994.
43. Sylvan Eisman, personal interview, 18 December 1996.
44. Elizabeth Rose, personal interview, 13 November 1992.
45. Arlin Adams, address, Rhoads Pavilion Dedication, Philadelphia, Pa., 26 October 1994.

SELECTED BIBLIOGRAPHY

Argersinger, Joanne. *Toward A New Deal in Baltimore*. Chapel Hill: The University of North Carolina Press, 1988.
Aubaniac, R. "L'injection Intraveineuse Sous-Claviculaire Venipuncture." *Press Medicale*. 60, 1947, 1456.
Bacon, Margaret. *The Quiet Rebels*. Philadelphia: New Society Publishers, 1985.
Baker, Liva. *The Justice from Beacon Hill: The Life and Times of Oliver Wendell Holmes*. New York: Harper Collins, 1991.
Baltzell, E. Digby. *Puritan Boston and Quaker Philadelphia*. Boston: Beacon Press, 1979.
Barden, R.P., Ravdin, I.S. and Frazier, W.D. "Hypoproteinemia as a Factor in Retardation of Gastric Emptying after Operations of the Billroth I or II Types." *American Journal of Roentgenology*. 38, 1937, 196–202.
Bellangee, J. "Fairhope The Forerunner." *Twentieth Century Magazine*. 4 (4), September 11, 1911, 483–488.
Benjamin, Philip. *Philadelphia Quakers*. Philadelphia: Temple University Press, 1976.
Benjamin, Philip. *Philadelphia Quakers in the Industrial Age*. Philadelphia: Temple University Press, 1976.
Bleiweiss, Laura. "Out of the Depths: A Study in the Sociology of Surgery." diss., University of Pennsylvania, 1974.
Brinton, Howard. *Quaker Education: Theory and Practice*. Wallingford, Pa.: Pendle Hill Press, 1940.
Cassell, Joan. "On Control, Certitude and 'Paranoia' of Surgeons." *Culture, Medicine and Psychiatry*. 11 (2), June 1987, 229–249.
Churchill, Edward D. *Surgeon to Soldier*. Philadelphia: J.B. Lippincott, 1972.
Dudrick, S. J. and Rhoads, J.E. "New Horizons for Intravenous Feeding." *JAMA*. 215 (6), 1971, 939–949.
Dudrick, S.J., Wilmore, D.W., Vars, H.M. and Rhoads, J.E. "Long-Term Parenteral Nutrition with Growth Development and Positive Nitrogen." *Surgery*. 64, 1968, 134–142.
Duffy, B.L. "Clinical Use of Polyethylene Tubing for Intravenous Therapy—Report of 72 Cases." *Annals of Surgery*. 130, 1949, 929–936.
_____. *Esther B. Rhoads Collection, 1153*. Quaker Collection, Haverford College. Haverford, Pa.
Farber, Sidney and Ravdin, I.S. "Civilian Activities at the National Level." *Surgery* 56, 1964, 611–613.
Fletcher, A. G., Gimbel, N.S. and Riegel, C. "Parenteral Nutrition with Human Serum Albumin as Source of Protein in Early Postoperative Period." *Surgery, Gynecology and Obstetrics*. 90, 1950, 151–154.
_____. *Friends in the Delaware Valley: Philadelphia Yearly Meeting 1681–1981*. Ed. John Moore. Haverford, Pa: Friends Historical Association, 1981.
Goldschmidt, S., Vars, H., and Ravdin, I.S. "Influence of Foodstuffs Upon Susceptibility of Liver to Injury by Choloroform and Probable Mechanism of Their Action." *Journal of Clinical Investigation*. 18, 1939, 277–289.
Gurd, F.N., Vars, H.M. and Ravdin, I.S. "Composition of the Regenerating Liver after Partial Hepatectomy in Normal and Protein-Depleted Rats." *American Journal of Physiology*. 152, 1948, 11–21.

SELECTED BIBLIOGRAPHY

———. *The Gurds—The Montreal General and McGill—A Family Saga*. Ed. Douglas Waugh. Burnstown, Ontario: General Store Publishing House, 1996.
Hardy, James. *The World of Surgery (1945–1985)*. Philadelphia: The University of Pennsylvania Press, 1986.
Henriques, V. and Anderson, A.C. "Ueber Parenterale Ernahrung durch Intravenose Injektion." *Ztschr F. Physiol Chem Strassb* lxxxviii, 1913, 357–369.
Hole, Helen. *Westtown Through the Years*. Philadelphia: Lyon and Armor, 1942.
———. *I.S. Ravdin, Collected Papers 1917–1972*. Philadelphia: The University of Pennsylvania Archives.
Johnston, C.G., Ravdin, I.S., Riegel, C., Allison, C.L. "Studies on Gallbladder Function: Anion-Cation Content of Bile from Normal and Infected Gallbladder." *Journal of Clinical Investigation*. 12, 1933, 67–75.
———. *Jonathan E. Rhoads Eightieth Birthday Symposium*. Ed. Clyde F. Barker and John Daly. Philadelphia: J.B. Lippincott, 1989.
———. *Jonathan Evans Rhoads and Rebecca Garrett Rhoads and Their Descendents*. Ed. Richard Rhoads, 2nd ed. Kennett Square, Pa., 1994.
Kaufman, Sharon. *The Healer's Tale*. Madison, Wisc.: University of Wisconsin Press, 1993.
Keim, Albert and Stoltzfus, Grant. *The Politics of Conscience: The Historic Peace Churches and America at War*. Scottsdale, Pa.: Herald Press, 1988.
Koop, C.E. *Koop: The Memoirs of America's Family Doctor*. New York: Random House, 1991.
Lee, W.E., Ravdin, I.S., Tucker, G. and Pendergrass, E.P. "Studies on Experimental Pulmonary Atelectasis; Production of Atelectasis." *American Surgery*. 88, 1928.
Lingeman, Richard R. *Don't You Know There's A War Going On?: The American Home Front—1941–1945*. New York: G. P. Putnam's Sons, 1970.
Mecray, P.M., Barden, R.P., Ravdin, I.S. "Nutritional Edema: Its Effect on Gastric Emptying Time Before and After Gastric Surgery." *Surgery* 1, 1937, 53–64.
Meites, Samuel. *Otto Folin: America's First Clinical Biochemist*. Washington, D.C.: American Association for Clnical Chemistry, 1989.
Mencken, H. L. *Thirty Five Years of Newspaper Work*. Ed. F. Hobson, V. Fitzpatrick and B. Jacobs. Baltimore: The Johns Hopkins University Press, 1994.
Miller, Leonard. "William T. Fitts, 1915–1980." *Transactions of the American Surgical Association*. Ed. Lloyd Nyhus. Philadelphia: J.B. Lippincott, 1980, 63–66.
Mogil, R.A., DeLaurentis, D.A. and Rosemond, G.P. "The Infraclavicular Venipuncture." *Archives of Surgery*. 95, 1967, 320.
Mueller, G.P., Ravdin, I.S. and Ravdin, E.G. "Alterations of Bile Pigment Metabolism in Biliary Tract Disease." *JAMA*. 85, 1925, 86–88.
Nemir, P., Hawthorne, H.R. and Lecrone, B.L. "Simple Intestinal Obstruction: Prolongation of Life for 45 Days with Parenteral Alimentation." *Proceedings of the Society for Experimental Biology and Medicine*. 69, 1948, 14–16.
Parkins, W.M., Koop, C.E., Riegel, C., Vars, H.M. and Lockwood, J. "Gelatin as Plasma Substitute, with Particular Reference to Experimental Hemorrhage and Burn Shock." *Annals of Surgery*. 118, 1943, 193–214.
———. *Proceedings of the International Conference on Fat Emulsions*. Eds. H.C. Meng and D.W. Wilmore. Chicago: American Medical Association, 1976.
Ravdin, I.S. *Operative Surgery. General and Special Considerations*. Vol. 1 (Authorized Translation) Ed. Martin Kirschner. Philadelphia: J.B. Lippincott, 1931.
Ravdin, I.S. and Casberg, M.A. "A Second Look at Surgical Care in Major Catastrophes." *American Journal of Surgery*. 89, 1955, 721–724.
Ravdin, I.S., and Rhoads, J.E. "Certain Problems Illustrating the Importance of Knowledge of Biochemistry by the Surgeon." *Surgical Clinics of North America*. 15, 1935, 85–100.
Ravdin, I.S., Thoroughgood, E., Riegel, C., Peter, R. and Rhoads, J.E. "The Prevention of Liver Damage and the Facilitation of Repair in the Liver by Diet." *JAMA*. 121, 1942, 322–321.

Rhoads, J.E. "Memoirs of a Surgical Nutritionist." *JAMA.* 272 (12), 1994, 963–966.
Rhoads, J.E., Allen, J.G., Harkins, H.N. and Moyer, C.A. *Surgery: Principles and Practice.* Philadelphia: J.B. Lippincott, 1957.
Rhoads, J.E., Dudrick, S.J. and Vars, H.M. *History of Intravenous Nutrition in Clinical Nutrition.* Vol. II Eds. J.L. Rombeau and M.D. Caldwell. Philadelphia: W.B. Saunders, 1986.
Rhoads, J.E., Hottenstein, H.F. and Hudson, I.F. "The Decline in the Strength of Catgut after Exposure to Living Tissues." *Archives of Surgery.* 34, 1937, 377–397.
Rhoads, J.E. and Kasinkas, W. "The Influence of Hypoproteinemia on the Formation of Callus in Experimental Fracture." *Surgery.* 11, 1942, 38–44.
Rhoads, J.E., Stengel, A., Riegel, C., Caori, F.A. and Frazier, W.D. "The Absorption of Protein Split Products from Chronic Isolated Colon Loops."*American Journal of Physiology.* 125, 1939, 707–712.
Rhoads, Jonathan E. "Quaker Tenets and the Philosophy of the Medical Profession." *Through A Quaker Archway,* Ed. Horace M. Lippincott. New York: Sagamore Press, 1959.
Schaeffer, Philip. "Otto Folin (1867–1934)." *Journal of Nutrition,* 52,1954, 1–11.
Sheeran, Michael. *Beyond Majority Rule—Voteless Decisions in the Religious Society of Friends.* Philadelphia: Philadelphia Yearly Meeting, 1983.
Smedley, Susanna. *Catalog of Westtown Through the Years.* Philadelphia: Lyon and Armor, 1945.
_____. *The Spirit and the Intellect: Haverford College, 1883–1983.* Ed. Gregory Kannerstein. Haverford, Pa.: Haverford College, 1983.
Steiger, E., Vars, H.M. and Dudrick, S.J. "A Technique for Long-Term Intravenous Feeding in Unrestrained Rats." *Archives of Surgery.* 104 (3),1972, 330–332.
Thompson, W.D., Ravdin, I.S. and Frank, I.L. "Effect of Hypoproteinemia on Wound Disruption." *Archives of Surgery.* 36, 1938, 500–508.
Tucker, Augusta. *Miss Suzie Slagle's.* Baltimore: The Johns Hopkins University Press, 1939.
Turner, Thomas. *Heritage of Excellence, The Johns Hopkins Medical Institutions—1914–1947.* Baltimore: The Johns Hopkins University Press, 1974.
Wangensteen, O.H. "Isidor Schwaner Ravdin—Versatile Surgeon and Nonpareil Surgical Statesman." *Surgery* 56, 1964, 609–610.
Weinberg, Janet. "Nutrition Through A Needle: Closing Pandora's Box." *Science News.* 106, August 10, 1974, 90–91.
_____. *Will Rogers Weekly Articles: The Hoover Years—1929–1931.* Ed. Steven Gragert. Stillwater, Okla.: Oklahoma University Press, 1981.
Wilmore, D. W., and Dudrick, S.J. "Growth and Development of an Infant Receiving All Nutrients Exclusively By Vein." *JAMA.* 203, 1968, 140–144.
Zeldow, Peter and Daugherty, Steven. "Personality Profiles and Specialty Choices of Students from Two Medical School Classes." *Academic Medicine.* 66 (5), 1991, 283–287.

INDEX

Abbott, William, 110, 143
Abbott Laboratories, 198, 202
Abbotts Company, 53
Abdominal surgery, 103
Abington Hospital, 141
Academi Nazionale dei Lincei, 1
Acta Chirurgia Scandinavia, 234
Adams, Arlin, 255, 271
Adams, John, 255
Adams, John Quincy, 255
Aequanimitas (Osler), 90
Albumin, intravenous, 189–190, 196
Allen, J. Garrott, 173, 196, 197, 228
Allen, Woody, 249
Altemeier, William, 258
Ambulation, postoperative, 137–139
American Academy, 101
American Association for the Surgery of Trauma, 149
American Board of Surgery, 105
American Cancer Society, 104
 Rhoads' presidency of, 228, 249–250, 252
American College of Surgeons, 187, 228
American Cyanamid, 36
American Friends Service Committee, 19, 21, 60, 117, 239, 240–243
American Indian rights movement, 38
American Institute of Nutrition, 180
American Medical Association, Joseph Goldberger Award of, 210, 265
American Philosophical Society, 1, 228, 255–257, 265
American Red Cross, 189
American Society for Parenteral and Enteral Nutrition, 180, 211
American Surgical Association, 144, 265
Amigen, 186, 188, 189, 191
Amputations, 110
 during Vietnam War, 240–241
Andersen, 186
M.D. Anderson Hospital, 251, 252
Andrus, E. Cowles, 86

Anesthetic agents, injurious effects of, 104
Annals of Surgery, 129–130, 159, 252
Annenberg School of Communications, 220
Anthrax, 144
Antibiotics, 144
Anti-semitism, 117
Appendicitis, 106, 110, 114, 133–134
Armstrong Cork Company, 225–226
Army Ambulance Corps, 102
Army Chemical Warfare School, 147
Army Liver Commission, 198
Army Medical Corps, 140
Army Reserve, 118
Astaire, Fred, 70
Atelectasis, postoperative, 104
Athens, Greece, Rhoads' visit to, 59–60
Aubaniac, R., 203
Australia, Jonathan Rhoads' (grandfather) missionary activities in, 7
Austrian, Robert, 1, 253, 254
Autocrat of the Breakfast-Table, The (Holmes), 90
Avertin, 80, 81

Babson, Roger, 115
Backlog Camp, 40–41, 44, 65
Bacteriology, 98
Ballistocardiograph, 191
Balsham, Jinny Mager, 218
Baltimore, Maryland
 during Great Depression, 67, 74–75
 as site of Johns Hopkins Medical School, 66, 67–68
Baltimore City Hospital System, 79
Barden, Robert, 182
Barker, Clyde, 249, 261, 266, 270
Barker, Lewellys, 79
Barness, Lew, 197
Bay View Hospital, 79–80
Bell, Helen, 36–37, 38, 43, 80, 90

293

Bell, Whitfield, 255
Bell, William, 39
Benjamin Franklin Medal, 265
Berrang, Elizabeth, 153
Bile, 160–161, 179
Binfords, Gurney & Elizabeth, 17
Bishop, Harry, 204–205
Blackburn, Doris, 35
Blood clotting, 111–113
Blood estriol measurement, 160
Blood sugar measurement, Folin-Wu method of, 72–73
Blood transfusions, 104, 122
Board of Associated Universities, 194
Bobst, Elmer, 251
Bok, Edward W., 253
Borton, Lady, 243
Bosporus, Rhoads' swim across, 59
Boston Children's Hospital, 85, 209
Boston City Hospital, 85–86
Boston University School of Medicine, 73, 85–86
Bowles, Gilbert & Minnie, 17
Bradley, Sculley, 218–219, 222
Brain, blood flow measurement in, 81
Brancusi, Constantin, 78
Breast cancer, 232–233
Brethren (religious sect), 117–118
Brightonian Literary Society, 32
Brinton, Eileen, 32
Brinton, Howard, 2, 216
Brookhaven Laboratories, 194
Brooks, Dorothy, 26
Brown, Alice, 41
Brown, Arthur, 232
Brown, Carroll, 37
Brown, Irene, 235–236, 258
Brown, Robert, 107
Brown, Ruth, 258
Brown, Sam, 45
Brown, Thomas, 40, 41
Brunner, Dr., 143
Brunschwig, Alex, 188
Bryan, William Jennings, 76
Bryn Mawr College, 4, 9, 12, 14–15, 240
Bryn Mawr Hospital, 113, 129
Buckingham Mountain Foundation, 267
Buerki, Robin, 124
Bulletin of the International Society of Surgery, 202
Bullit, Orville, 107
Burke-Wadsworth Bill, 118
Burn injury research, 129–130, 186–187
Busing, 239
Butt, Hugh, 112
Byrd, Richard, 8

Canada, Rhoads family's trip to, 27
Cancer, 232–234, 260–261
Cancer, 252
Cancer Chemotherapy Program, 104
Cape Town, South Africa, Rhoads' trip to, 263
Carbone, Marion, 220, 235–236, 258
Carey, Ben, 86
Carnegie Foundation, 62, 62
Carr, John Dixon, 50
Carter, Jimmy, 252
Castle, William B., 72, 86
Catalina Island, Rhoads family's trip to, 28
Catgut, tensile strength of, 107
Cathcart, Robert, 254
Cattel, Richard, 111
Cayten, C. Gene, 246
Chamberlain, Neville, 60
Chapple, Charlie, 143
Chase, Dean, 108
Chen, K.K., 81
Chestnut Hill, Pennsylvania, Katharine Rhoads' medical practice in, 262
Chicago, Rhoads' trips to, 236
Chicago, University of, 84, 108, 173, 213
Children's Hospital of Philadelphia, 110, 113, 128, 129, 130, 133, 165, 197, 262
first intravenous hyperalimentation use at, 204–209
Children's Seashore House, 262
China, Rhoads' trip to, 77–79
Chloroform, injurious effects of, 104
Cholecystectomy, 111, 114–117, 130–132
Churchill, Edward, 121, 123
Cincinnati, University of, 147
Clark, Joseph, 253
Clark, R. Lee, 251
Cleveland Clinic, 210
Clinical trials, of cancer chemotherapy, 104
College of Physicians and Surgeons, 228
College of Physicians of Philadelphia, 265
College of Surgeons, 165
Coller, Frederick, 104
Colorado, University of, 180
Colorectal cancer, 233
Columbia University, 22
  Medical School, 65, 66, 69
  Teachers College, 19
Comfort, William Wistar, 254
Committee on Medical Research, 121–122
Communism, 224–226
Comroe, Bernard, 134
Conscientious objection, 117–119, 123
Consensus, as Quaker ethic, 216–217, 256–257

INDEX

Constantinople, Rhoads' trip to, 58–59
Conway Lake, New Hampshire, 171–172
Coolidge, Calvin, 47, 52, 52
Cooper, David A. Sr, 151, 152, 153, 154, 155, 157
Cooper, Hewlings, 41, 48
Cope, Oliver, 138
Cope, Ralph, 32
Copeland, Edward III, 247
Cordotomy, 94
Cornell University, 48–49, 195
Cortisone, 160–161
Cox, Reavis, 217
Cox Foundation, 198
Critchlow, Robert, 202
Crohn's disease, 111, 162
Crosslands (retirement community), 38
Curreri, William, 4–5, 246–247
Cushing, Harvey, 101
Cutdown, 136–137
Cuthbertson, David, 184
Cyst
 congenital, 136
 sebaceous, 114

Daily Worker, 224
Dam, Henrik, 112
Dandy, J. Walter, 84
Darrow, Clarence, 76
Darwin, Charles, 255
Daveron, Solon, 70, 71, 77
Davis, Royal, 69, 70, 71, 76–77, 80, 82, 90, 97
Deaver, John B., 94, 103, 234
DeLaurentis, Dominic, 203
Denmark, Rhoads' trip to, 253
Denver, Colorado, Rhoads family's trip to 28
Dermatitis, exfoliative, 130–131
Detroit Academy of Surgery, 165
Dextran, 187–188
Diaco, Joseph, 245
Dialysis, 141–142
 peritoneal, 110, 141, 145
Dietitians, 211–212
Dilworth, Richardson, 238–239, 253
Diuretics, use in intravenous hyperalimentation, 194–196
Divinyl ether, 179
DNA, James Watson and, 250, 251
Doisy, Edward A., 112
Drabkin, David, 186
Dracula (Stoker), 76
Dreiser Looks at Russia (Dreiser), 76
Dresden, Germany, Rhoads family's trip to, 28

Drexel University, 16, 21
Drinker, Philip, 81
Dripps, Robert, 133, 187
Droll Tales (de Balzac), 90
Dudrick, Stanley, 177, 198, 199, 200, 202–203, 204–205, 209, 210, 211, 254, 261
Duffy, B.J., 191
Duke Foundation, 36
Duke University, 249, 266
Dyson, William, 124–125, 127, 162

Earlham College, 18, 21, 37
Eastern Virginia Medical School, 246
Eberlen, Walter, 185
Edema
 nutritional, 182 183–184
 pulmonary, as intravenous hyperalimentation complication, 193–194
Eiseley, Loren, 222–223
Eisenhower, Dwight D., 103
Eisenhower, Milton, 227
Eisenlohr, Henrietta, 131
Eisenlohr Pavilion, Hospital of the University of Pennsylvania, 152
Eisman, Sylvan, 270
Elder, David, 241, 243
Eliason, Eldridge L., 93–94, 95–96, 98, 99, 105, 110, 114, 116, 124, 133, 139, 186, 213, 260
Elkinton, Joseph P., 14, 19
Ellman, Barry, 231–232
Elman, Robert, 186
Ely, Richard (great-uncle), 12, 14
Ely, Ruth Anna (maternal grandmother), 11, 12
Enteral nutrition, 212. *See also* Intravenous hyperalimentation
Enterline, Ted, 233
Ephedrine, 81
Erb, William, 114
Eschatin, 129
Esophageal cancer, 213
Ether, 110
Europa, 77
Europe, Rhoads' travels in, 58–60
Evans, Katharine. *See* Rhoads, Katharine Evans Goddard (wife)
Evans, Mary (cousin), 72
Evansville, Indiana, 101, 155, 186

Fairhope, Alabama, 54–55, 56
Farber, Sydney, 251
Farrell, Harry, 113
Fathers and Sons (Turgenev), 76

Federation of the American Society of Experimental Biologists, 179
Filler, Robert, 209
Finnegan, James, 243–244
Fishbein, Morris, 173
Fistula, intestinal, 204
Fitts, William, 147, 148–149, 218, 249
Fletcher, Archie, 160–161
Flippin, Harrison, 113, 133, 144
Folin, Axel, 87
Folin, George, 87
Folin, Johanna, 87, 108
Folin, Laura (mother-in-law), 72–73, 74, 86–87, 89, 109, 164, 169
Folin, Otto (father-in-law), 72–73, 74, 86–87, 89, 107–108, 130, 185–186
Folin, Teresa. See Rhoads, Teresa Folin (wife)
Folin-Wu method, of blood sugar measurement, 72–73
Folkman, Judah, 209
Food and Drug Administration, 251
Footprints of a Quaker: Esther Biddle Rhoads, 20–21
Forsythe, David, 16
Forsythe, John, 83
Fort Benjamin Harrison, 102
Fortner, Joseph, 252, 253
Fortune Magazine, 90
Four Way Lodge, 263–264
Fox, George, 2
Fracture healing, 183–184
France, American Friends Service Committee activities in, 240
Franklin, Benjamin, 228, 255, 266–267
Franklin and Marshall College, 198
Franklin Medal, 265
Frazier, Charles Harrison, 93–94, 102, 103, 107, 110, 176
Frazier, William, 107, 185
Frazier Club, 94
"Frazier's men", 103
Freud, Sigmund, 84–85, 222
Friedman, Milton, 213
Friendly Eights, 263
Friends Free Library, Germantown, Pennsylvania, 15, 25
Friends Girls School, Tokyo, 17, 20, 21, 76
Friends Hospital, Philadelphia, 85
Fry, Alex, 217
Furnas, John, 45, 53, 89

Gallbladder research, 104
Gallbladder surgery, 117, 130–132. See also Cholecystectomy
Gammon, George, 107
Garrett, Philip (paternal great-grandfather), 8–9
Gastroenterostomy, 182
Gastrostomy, in esophageal cancer patients, 213
Gates, John Henry, 224–225
Gelatin, intravenous, 187–188, 189
Gemmill, Kenneth, 70, 77
General Motors Cancer Research Assembly, 252
General practice, Rhoads' interest in, 66
George, Henry, 54
George Harrison Professor of Surgery. See Harrison Professor of Surgery
Georgetown University, 249, 266
Germantown, Pennsylvania, 11
  Edward Rhoads' medical practice in, 10
  James Rhoads' medical practice in, 9, 10
  Quaker community of, 14
  Rhoads family's homes in, 10, 14, 24, 29–30, 57, 97, 106, 162
  during World War I, 26–27
Germantown Friends Meeting, 10, 12, 21, 25, 261–262
Germantown Friends Meeting House, 166
Germantown Friends School, 1–2, 30, 256
  Caroline Rhoads as student at, 22
  Esther Rhoads as student at, 16
  Jonathan Rhoads as student at, 25–26, 30, 31
  Jonathan Rhoads as board member of, 4, 257
  principal of, 45
  Ruth Rhoads as student at, 14–15
Germantown Hospital, 113, 129
Germany
  anti-semitism in, 117
  Rhoads' trips to, 28, 58, 253
Gestapo, 117
Geyer, Robert, 191–192
Gibbon, John, 143, 159
Gibbon, Mary, 143
Gimbel, Nicholas, 148, 189
Girard College, 22
Glucose, intravenous, 176–177, 191, 193, 194, 210
Goddard, David, 262, 270
Goddard, Katharine Evans. See Rhoads, Katharine Evans Goddard (wife)
Goldberger Award, 210, 265
Goldschmidt, Samuel, 104, 179, 181
Goldstine, Herman, 256

INDEX

297

Gottingen, University of, 61
Graduate Hospital, 113–114, 129, 136–137, 197
Graham, Evarts, 104
Grant, Ulysses S., 255
Great Depression, 74–75, 89, 91, 110, 124
Greaves, 112
Green, John, 160
Greenewalt, Crawford, 255, 258
Group practice, of Katharine Evans Goddard Rhoads, 262
Gurd, Frazier, 184–185
Gyorgy, Paul, 197

Hahnemann Medical School, 266
Halsted, William S., 83
Hanoi, Vietnam, 242–243
Hanson, Victor, 5
Hardy, James, 104, 148, 174, 187
Harkins, Henry, 173, 228
Harnwell, Gaylord, 217, 218, 221, 224, 227, 270
Harper's, 52
Harrison, Timothy, 138
Harrison Professor of Surgery, 103, 110, 125, 126
Hartmann's solution, 177–178
Harvard infusion pump, 206
Harvard University
  Medical School
    Folin's professorship at, 72–73, 87
    Ravdin's acceptance by, 102
    Rhoads' application to, 65, 66
    Rhoads as student at, 67, 80–81
    during World War I, 123
  School of Fine Arts, 108
  School of Public Health, 191–192
  Vanderbilt Hall, 86, 87
Harvey, Francis, 39, 41
Haverford College, 1–2, 256
  Board of Managers of, 163
  Esther Rhoads honored by, 21
  Quaker origins of, 45, 46
  Rhoads as student at, 44, 45–64
    academic coursework, 48, 57, 60, 65
    academic performance, 70–71
    classmates and roommates, 38, 47, 50, 60
    European trip during, 57–60
    extracurricular activities, 48–50, 51, 52–53, 54, 56, 57, 62, 63
    graduation, 63
    professors, 60–62, 63
    scholarship, 45, 54
  Rhoads as board member of, 4, 163, 217, 228, 240, 257

Haverford College *(cont.)*
  Rhoads honored by, 266
  Rhoads' opinion of, 47–48, 50, 57, 69
  scholarship fund established by Rhoads, 267
  Stokes Hall, 163
  William Penn Lectures, 154
Haverfordian, 50
Haverford News, 47, 50, 54, 57
Hawthorne, Herbert, 191
Healer's Tale, The (Kauffman), 67
Heart-lung machine, 159
Heess, Rogers, 53
Hemorrhage, postoperative, 111
Henrietta Cigar Factory, 131
Henriques, V., 186
Henry Ford Hospital, 79
Hepatitis, 173
Herrick, Dr., 102
Hershey Medical Center, 264
Hetzel, Becky, 48, 70, 71
Hetzel, Theodore, 36, 37–39, 43, 45, 48, 57–60, 70, 71, 258
  father of, 37–39
Hickam Field, Honolulu, 121
"Hicks operation", 235
Hilbert, David, 61
Hippocrates, 4
Hirohito, Emperor, 20
Hiss, Alger, 224
Hitler, Adolf, 117, 118
Hodes, Philip, 151, 162
Hole, Alan, 37
Hole (Bell), Helen, 36–37, 38, 43, 80, 90
Holland, Rhoads' trip to, 58
Holland American Steamship Company, 57
Hollander, Edward, 57
Holleb, Art, 250
Holmes, Oliver Wendell, 7
Holt, Emmett, 191
Hong Kong, Rhoads' trip to, 263
Honolulu County Medical Society, 121
Hoover, Herbert, 71, 74, 255
Hopkins, Johns, 66
Horn, Robert, 233
Hospital of the University of Pennsylvania, 1, 81, 197
  Dulles wing, 104–105
  Eisenlohr Pavilion, 152
  faculty wives at, 134
  Gates Building and Pavilion, 104–105, 158
  Harrison Department of Surgical Research, 113
    Ravdin's directorship of, 110

Hospital of the University of
  Pennsylvania *(cont.)*
 Harrison Department of Surgical
  Research *(cont.)*
  Rhoads' as acting director of,
   142–143
  during World War II, 119, 121, 122,
   123, 124–132, 136–146
 Harrison Professor of Surgery, 103,
  110, 125, 126
 John Rhea Barton Chairman of Surgery,
  94, 103, 110, 149, 229–231, 261,
  266
 Medical Board Meetings at, 163
 Naval medical unit, 118
 Ravdin Building, 232
 Ravdin Institute, 105
 residency program, 105–106
 Rhoads' internship at, 81–82, 88–99
  1st year, 88–91
  2nd year, 91–99
  nose and throat rotation, 92
  obstetrics rotation, 89–90
  surgical rotation, 93–97
 Rhoads Pavilion, 267–270
 Rhoads' residency at, 99, 105–113
 Surgical Clinic, 94
 surgical statistics of, 107
 White Building, 158
 during World War II, 121, 122, 123,
  124–132, 136–146
 William T. Fitts Surgical Education
  Center, 149
Howard, John, 148
Hull, J. Parker, 32
Huntington Museum, 172
Hyperthyroidism, intravenous hyper-
 alimentation in, 176
Hypoproteinemia, 181–184
Hypoxia, 104
 fetal, 160

Iceland, 236
Illinois, University of, 83
Imitation of Christ, The, 52
"Importance of the Knowledge of
 Biochemistry to the Surgeon"
 (Rhoads and Ravdin), 107, 175
In Defense of Women (Mencken), 76
India, 20th General Hospital in, 123,
 126, 148, 149
Indiana University, 101, 102, 155
Infant Nutrition (Marriott), 90
Infections, postoperative, 110
Influenza epidemic (1918), 26
Informed consent, 110

Interallie Club, 228
International Fat Emulsion Conference,
 192–193
International Surgical Group, 228
International Surgical Society, 201, 243
Intestinal obstruction, 143
Intravenous hyperalimentation, 4,
 175–213
 acceptance by medical community,
  204
 applications of, 176, 209–210
 complications of, 193–194, 202, 213
 definition of, 175
 diuretics use in, 194–196
 fat-containing emulsions use in,
  191–193
 first recognized use of, 204–209
 infusion systems for, 188–189, 191,
  194–195, 197–202, 203–204,
  206
 military research contracts in,
  186–187
 as total parenteral nutrition, 175, 191,
  209, 210–213
Isabella Polk (maid), 164, 170
Islet cell adenoma, pancreatic, 111
Italy, Rhoads' trip to, 253

J.E. Rhoads and Sons, 8
Japan
 Crown Prince and Princess of, 17, 20
 Esther Rhoads' missionary activities
  in, 17–20, 41–42
 Jonathan Rhoads' (grandfather)
  missionary activities in, 7
 Jonathan Rhoads' trip to, 79
 Margaret Rhoads' trip to, 41–42
Japanese-Americans, internment during
 World War II, 240
Japanese Language School, 18
Jaundice, 75
 hemorrhagic tendency in, 111–113
Jefferson, Thomas, 255
Jefferson Medical College, 29, 244, 246,
 249, 266
Jesus Christ, 117
Jews, Hitler's persecution of, 117
Johns Hopkins Medical School, 1–2
 admission practices of, 68
 Baltimore location of, 67–68
 historical background of, 66–67
 outpatient services of, 79
 preclinical faculty of, 69
 Quaker origins of, 66
 revised curriculum of, 67, 69
 Rhoads' application to, 63–64, 65–66

INDEX

Johns Hopkins Medical School *(cont.)*
  Rhoads' attendance at, 65–99
    1st year, 67–72
    2nd year, 74–79
    3rd year, 79–81
    4th year, 81–88
    academic grades, 87
    coursework, 76
    graduation, 87
    health and physical condition, 80, 81
    national boards, 76
  tuberculosis rate at, 80
Johnson, Andrew, 180
Johnson, Dale, 206, 207
Johnson, Julian, 99, 107, 137, 147, 148, 149, 150–151, 237–238
Johnson, Mary, 150, 267
Johnston, Charles, 104, 106, 179
Jonathan Evans Rhoads Pavilion, 267–270
Jones, George, 43
Jones, Jim, 197
Jones, Rufus, 240
Joseph Goldberger Award, 210, 265
Journal of the American Medical Association, 112, 144, 173, 209, 210
Journal of Trauma, 149

Kaplan, 114
Kark, Robert, 198
Karolinska Institute, Stockholm, 252
Kasinkas, William, 183
Kearsarge, New Hampshire, Rhoads' summer home in, 108, 132–133, 151–152, 158, 160, 163, 170–171, 263
Keefer, Chester, 85–86
Kelley, William, 267–268, 269, 270
Kendon, Adam (son-in-law), 168, 261
Kendon, Angus (grandson), 261
Kendon, Benjamin (grandson), 261
Kendon, Gudrun (granddaughter), 261
Kendon, Margaret Rhoads (daughter), 110, 115, 128, 165, 168, 169–170, 171, 264
Kentucky, University of, 159–160
Kern, Richard, 118
Kety, Seymour, 81
Kidney transplantation, 231
Kimbrough, Robert, 153
Kind and Knox Gelatin Company, 187, 188
Kirby, Charles, 138, 148
Kolff, W.J., 142
Koop, Betty Flanagan, 132–133

Koop, C. Everett, 99, 121, 125–126, 127, 130–134, 136, 139, 146, 148, 157, 190
Koproski, Hilary, 253
Korea, Rhoads' trip to, 78, 79
Korea Maru, 17
Korean War, 240
Kwashiorkor, 182

La Follette, Robert, 47
Lahey Clinic, 99, 111
Lane, Richard, 45, 48, 49
Lasker, Mary, 250, 251
Leadbetter, Wyland, 138
League of Nations, 52, 60
Leaves of Grass (Whitman), 219
Lee, Walter Estell, 104, 113–114, 119, 129
Lehr, Herndon B., 192, 249
Leopold and Loeb case, 76
Lewis, Dean, 83
Licensed Agencies for Relief in Asia, 20
Life of Christ and the Saints, The, 52
Life of Saint Francis, The, 52
Lindbergh, Charles, 57, 65
Lincolnshire, England, 7
Lipomul, 192
Literary Digest, The, 52
Lockwood, John, 114, 124, 126–127, 142, 144, 188
London, Jack, 52
Long, Perrin, 121–122
Los Angeles, Rhoads family's trip to, 27
Los Angeles Naval Air Station, 172
Lucke, Bauldin, 179

M.D. Anderson Hospital, 251, 252
MacArthur, Douglas, 19–20, 240
MacCallum, William, 75
Mackie, Jack, 158, 230–231, 234, 237, 239, 247, 258, 260, 270
MacVaugh, Horace III, 240
Madison, James, 255
Magee, James C., 121–122
Mager, Jinny, 258
Magill, James, 254, 267
Manhattan Project, 173
Maple Grove, New Hope, Pennsylvania, 11–12, 14, 24–25, 29–30, 44, 53–54, 57, 73, 151, 259, 262
Marple, Delaware County, Pennsylvania, 7
Marsh, Elizabeth, 83
Massachusetts General Hospital, 107, 138
Maxwell, Dorothy Bender, 139–140, 148

Mayock, Robert, 123, 127, 145
Mayo Clinic, 144, 160
McCarthy, Joseph, 221, 224
McCarthy, Miles, 130
McClelland, 217
McLaughlin, Charles, 98
Mead Johnson Company, 186
Measey, William, 267
Measey Foundation, 267
Mecray, Paul, 182
Medical College of Ohio, 266
Medical schools. *See also* specific medical schools
 nutritional education in, 212
Medical Tower Building, Philadelphia, 113
Meigs syndrome, 111
Mein Kampf (Hitler), 117
Melanee, Frank, 127
Meldrum, William, 60–62, 63, 71
Memorial Hospital, New Jersey, 113
Memorial Sloan-Kettering Hospital, 252
Mencken, H.L., 68, 74–75
Mendel, Lafayette, 179, 180
Meng, Ray, 191
Mennonites, 117–118
Merck Chemical Company, 152, 179, 192
Mexican-American War, 102
Meyer, Adolf, 84–85
Milbourne, 234
Military medicine, 118–119
Miller, Leonard, 150–151, 233, 249, 257, 258, 260, 266
Miller-Abbott tube, 110, 235, 237
Millipore filter, 206, 207
Milne, A.A., 108
Minnesota, University of, 87
Minot, George, 72, 182
Mississippi, University of, 187
Mr. Pim (automobile), 108, 109
Mr. Pim Passes By (Milne), 108
Mix, Tom, 70
Mogil, Robert, 203
Moore, Francis, 175, 196
Moore, Stanley, 32
Moorestown Friends School, 22
Morris, Samuel, 7
Morrison, S.B., 56, 104
Mt. Desert Island, Maine, 263
Mt. Holyoke College, 22, 29
Mt. Teresa, New Hampshire, 108
Moveable Feast (Hemingway), 270
Moyer, Carl, 172, 173, 228
Mueller, George P., 94, 103, 113
Murphy, 72, 182
Murphy, Franklin, 144

National Academy of Sciences, 69
National Board of Medical Examiners, 212
National Cancer Act of 1971, 251, 252
National Cancer Advisory Board, 250, 252
National Cancer Institute, 250–252
National Council for the Prevention of War, 52
National Geographic, 52
National Institutes of Health, 104, 251
National Radio Astronomy Laboratory, 194
National Research Council, 121–122, 143, 165, 197
National Selective Service Act, 118, 124
Natural History Club, 39
Nelson, H.M., 202
Nemir, Paul, 191
New England Journal of Medicine, 203
New Hope, Pennsylvania. *See* Maple Grove, New Hope, Pennsylvania
New Jersey School of Medicine and Dentistry, 264
New Mexico, University of, 155
New Republic, The, 87
New York City Hospital, 99
New Yorker, 46
New York Times, 241
New York University, 191
Nicholas, Gary, 244
Nichols, Roy, 219
Nitobe, Inazo, 17
Nixon, Jim, 190
Nixon, Richard M., 250, 251
Nobel Prize, 182, 213, 225, 239, 250, 251, 252, 255
Noguchi, Isamu, 77–78
Noone, R. Barrett, 236, 246
Nurses' Quarterly, 107
Nu Sigma Nu, 68
Nutritional education, in medical schools, 212
Nutritional research. *See also* Intravenous hyperalimentation
 during World War II, 143

Ohio State University, 210
Old, Old Tales from an Old, Old Book (Smith), 25
Olinger, Chester, 47
Operative Surgery (Kirschner), 104
Orient Express, 58–59
Ormandy, Eugene, 253
Osler, William, 4
Oxford University, 50, 219

INDEX

301

Pan-American Chair of Surgery, 248
Pancreatic cancer, 233–234
Pancreatic islet cell adenoma, 111
Park, Richard, 234
Parke-Davis, 129
Parker, Rebecca, 32
Parkins, William, 187, 188, 191
Parliamentary Club, 32, 39
Paulus family, 74
Paxson, Caroline (aunt), 12
Paxson, Margaret Ely. See Rhoads, Margaret Ely Paxton (mother)
Paxson, Oliver (maternal grandfather), 11, 12
Paxson, Thomas (maternal great-grandfather), 11
Pearl Harbor, Japanese attack on, 121, 121–122, 124
Peking Union Medical College, 81
Pendergrass, Eugene, 104, 107, 182, 232–233, 249–250
Penicillin, 127, 140, 144, 241
Pennoch, David, 32
Penn Reading Project, 270
Penn Relays (swimming event), 126
Pennsylvania, University of. See also Hospital of the University of Pennsylvania
  Educational Survey of, 219–220, 228
  faculty senate of, 217–218
  Founder's Day Address, 223
  German-Jewish professors, 117
  Graduate School of Arts and Sciences, 219
  honorary degree conferred on Rhoads by, 266
  Jack Rhoads' professorship at, 264
  Jonathan Evans Rhoads Pavilion, 267–270
  Law School, 220, 222
  Physics Department, 217
  Rhoads as provost of, 4, 215–228
  Rhoads' 50 years of service to, 257–258
  Rhoads' summer job at, 72
  School of Medicine, 148–149, 150
    as Edward Rhoads' alma mater, 9–10
    entrance requirements of, 60
    as James Rhoads' alma mater, 9
    as Katharine Evans Goddard Rhoads' alma mater, 262
    Rhoads' application to, 65
  School of Social Work, 220, 222
  student riots at, 221, 223–224
Pennsylvania Hospital, Philadelphia, 10, 81, 113–114, 129, 154

Pennwalt Foundation, 267
Pepper, D. Sergeant, 66, 82, 107
Pepper, O.H. Perry, 130
Pepper, William, 66, 71, 82, 102, 218
Perioperative care, 235
Peristalsis, 143
Pernicious anemia, 72, 182
Pershing, John, 102
Persian Gulf, 138
Peter Bent Brigham Hospital, 85–86
Pharmacology, nutritional, 212
Phemister, Dallas, 104
Phi Beta Kappa, 63, 68, 217
Philadelphia
  bicentennial celebration in, 253–254
  Rhoads' love for, 254–255
Philadelphia Award, 253–254
Philadelphia Board of Education, 4
Philadelphia County Medical Society, Strittmayer Award of, 265
Philadelphia Eagles (football team), 190
Philadelphia General Hospital, 81
Philadelphia Municipal Hospital, 144
Philadelphia Quakers in the Industrial Age (Benjamin), 14
Philadelphia Quartz Company, 53
Philadelphia School Board, 238–239
Philadelphia Yearly Meeting, 10, 17, 19, 21, 30, 42, 118
Phipps, Levis, 33, 34
Phipps Clinic, 84
Phosgene, 143
Pickett, Clarence, 239
Pierce, William, 229, 235, 237–238
Piersol Building, 139
Pillsbury, Don, 123
Pithotomy Club, 68
Plasma expanders, 187–188
"Plasma Proteins in Relation to Surgical Therapeusis" (Rhoads), 114
Poison gas, 143, 186–187
Poland, 151
Political prisoners, 242
Polk, Isabella, 164, 170
Pope John Paul, 1
Portacaval shunt, 231
Pratt, Henry S., 63
Pre- and Postoperative Treatment (Mason), 126
Presbyterian Hospital, 193
Presbyterian Missionary Hospital, 240
Presbyterian Sanitorium, Albuquerque, New Mexico, 152, 154–155
Princeton University, 179, 180
"Prison edema", 182
Proceedings of the Society of Biology and Experimental Medicine, 111

Proctoclysis, 185, 186
Protein hydrolysates, intravenous, 186, 189, 191
Protein malnutrition, 104
Protein repletion, 143
Prothrombin, 111
Psychiatric hospital, first in United States, 85
Psychiatry, Rhoads' interest in, 84–85
Pulitzer Prize, 219
Puritan Boston and Quaker Philadelphia (Baltzell), 30

Quadrangle (retirement home), 263
Quakers. *See* Society of Friends
Quang Ngai, Vietnam, 240–241, 243
Quick, Armand J., 111
Quick test, 111, 112–113

Randall, Alexander, 94
Randall, Peter, 141
Rank, Otto, 222
Rationing, during World War II, 124, 132
Rauscher, Frank, 250
Ravdin, Elizabeth, 125, 143, 156, 262
Ravdin, Isidor Schwander, 72, 93–94, 111, 113, 127, 148, 218–219
  as American Cancer Society president, 104
  birth of, 101
  Cancer Chemotherapy National Program establishment by, 104
  cancer treatment approach of, 232–233
  comparison with Rhoads, 229–231
  correspondence with Rhoads, 155, 156–157, 163–164
  cortisone research of, 160–161
  death of, 249
  education of, 101–103
  festschrift for, 103–104
  gallbladder surgery performed on, 114–117
  as Harrison Professor of Surgery, 103
  influence on Rhoads, 98–99
  intravenous hyperalimentation research of, 104, 176, 178–179, 181–183, 185–186, 192
  as John Rhea Barton Professor of Surgery, 103
  as magazine salesman, 101
  military titles of, 103
  as *Operative Surgery* translator, 103–104
  personality of, 96–97, 103, 229
  Philadelphia Award received by, 253

Ravdin, Isidor Schwander *(cont.)*
  physical appearance of, 96, 229
  postoperative ambulatory opinion of, 138
  post-World War II career of, 145–146, 150, 151, 153, 156–157, 158, 160
  publications of, 107, 175
  relationship with patients, 96–97
  remarks on Harvey Cushing, 101
  residency of, 102–103
  as Rhoads' mentor, 101, 105
  Rhoads' regard for, 254
  surgical assistants of, 137
  surgical research position of, 103
  as Vice President of Medical Affairs, 103
  in World War II, 103, 118, 119, 121–122, 134, 145–146, 147, 148, 149
Ravdin Institute, 223
Rawnsley, H.M., 202
Reagan, Ronald, 252
Red Cross, 20, 189
Reed College, 169
Rehabilitation services, during Vietnam War, 240–241
Reid, Legh, 61
Rhoads, Alfred (cousin), 29
Rhoads, Barbara (daughter-in-law), 261
Rhoads, Caroline Paxton (sister), 7, 9, 10, 12–13, 15, 21–22, 53, 55, 56, 153, 164, 265
  influence on nieces and nephews, 169
  relationship with Jonathan Rhoads, 26
  teaching career of, 52
Rhoads, Charles (cousin), 153
Rhoads, Charles (son), 153, 154, 168, 172, 253, 259, 261, 264–265
Rhoads, Deborah (granddaughter), 261
Rhoads, Edward Garrett (brother), 7
Rhoads, Edward Garrett (father), 7, 15, 44
  American Friends Service Committee and, 240
  as chairman of Mission Board, 17
  death of, 55–56, 163
  first automobile of, 23
  health of, 45, 53–55
  Hetzel family and, 37
  medical education of, 9–10
  medical practice of, 26, 28–29
  pacifism of, 11
  politics of, 52
  religious faith of, 25
  retirement of, 53–54
  travels of, 28
Rhoads, Edward (son), 128, 172, 259, 261, 264–265

INDEX

303

Rhoads, Esther Biddle (sister), 7, 15, 55, 56, 57, 153
   American Friends Service Committee and, 240
   character of, 16, 19
   death of, 249
   family's correspondence with, 90, 91–92, 93, 97–98, 106, 155, 157–158, 160, 164–165
   missionary career of, 17–18, 19–21, 52, 76
   as tutor to Crown Prince of Japan, 20
Rhoads, Frances (daughter-in-law), 261
Rhoads, George (son), 114, 128, 135, 166–167, 170, 171–172, 259, 264
Rhoads, Jack (son), 115, 128, 169, 171, 172, 195–196, 259, 264
Rhoads, James (grandson), 261
Rhoads, James (great-uncle), 9, 10, 11
Rhoads, Joanna (granddaughter), 261
Rhoads, Jonathan Evans, 14, 125, 128, 148
   American Cancer Society (Philadelphia division) presidency of, 228, 249–250, 252
   American College of Surgeons chairmanship and governorship of, 228, 236
   American Philosophical Society membership and presidency of, 228, 255–257
   American Surgical Association membership of, 144
   AOA membership of, 86
   automobile driving habits of, 70, 168
   automobiles owned by, 48–49, 263–264, 252
   awards and honors received by, 42, 43, 249, 265, 266–270
   birth of, 7
   Board of Associated Universities membership of, 194
   boating hobby of, 70
   burn injury research by, 129–130
   cancer research and funding involvement of, 249–252
   cancer treatment involvement of, 232–234
   childhood of, 23–26
   colleagues' regard for, 3, 4–5
   College of Physicians of Philadelphia presidency of, 228
   College of Surgeons membership of, 236
   community activities of, 238–240
   comparison with I.S. Ravdin, 229–231
   as conscientious objector, 118–119

Rhoads, Jonathan Evans *(cont.)*
   consensus-gaining ability of, 216–217, 256–257
   correspondence coursework of, 155
   at dedication of Jonathan Evans Rhoads Pavilion, 269
   editorial activities of, 159, 247, 252, 266
   80th birthday celebration of, 258, 261–262
   family life of, 128, 166–167, 170–172
   50th wedding anniversary of, 259
   financial interests of, 167, 169
   Friends Hospital and, 85
   frugality of, 169
   Graduate Hospital appointment of, 113
   grandchildren of, 249, 264, 265
   as Harrison Department of Surgery acting director, 142–143
   Haverford College board of managers membership of, 228
   honorary degrees received by, 249, 266–267, 270
   humor of, 166–167, 254, 256, 257
   illnesses and conditions of, 31, 32–33, 50–52, 80, 81, 133–134, 146, 151–158, 253, 266
   International Surgical Group presidency of, 228
   internship of, 81–82, 88–99
      1st year, 88–91
      2nd year, 91–99
      nose and throat rotation, 92
      obstetrics rotation, 89–90
      surgical rotation, 93–97
   intravenous hyperalimentation development by, 192, 193–199, 201–202, 204–213
   as John Rhea Barton Professor and Chairman of Surgery, 229–248, 266
   last operation of, 258, 260
   marital relationship of, 168
   marriage of
      first, 108–110
      second, 262
   on marriage, 108–109
   memory ability of, 232
   medical school education of, 65–99
      academic performance, 70–71
      coursework, 76
      extracurricular activities, 76
      first year, 67–72
      fourth year, 81–88
      national boards, 76
      second year, 74–79

Rhoads, Jonathan Evans *(cont.)*
  medical school education of *(cont.)*
    second-year examinations, 76–77
    surgical experiences during, 83–84
    third year, 79–81
  on mother's character, 13–14
  nickname of, 71
  operating room behavior of, 137
  operation on aunt by, 234–235
  pacifism of, 118–119, 165
  as Pan-American Chairman of Surgery, 248
  on patenting of research discoveries, 212–213
  patients' gratitude towards, 134, 136, 139, 226
  performance of gallbladdder surgery on I.S. Ravdin, 115–117
  personality and character of, 39–40, 139, 159, 170, 171, 172, 229, 230–231, 248, 270–271
  Phi Beta Kappa membership of, 63
  Philadelphia Award received by, 253–254
  Philadelphia School Board membership of, 238–239
  philanthropic activities of, 267
  physical appearance of, 229
  physical stamina of, 246–247
  political views of, 71, 169, 225–226
  postoperative ambulation position of, 137–139
  private practice of, 114, 129–130, 220, 231
    retirement from, 258
  professional memberships of, 265–266
  publications of, 107, 129–130, 144, 161–162
    "Importance of the Knowledge of Biochemistry to the Surgeon," 107, 175
    on intravenous hyperalimentation, 201–202, 209, 210
    Plasma Proteins in Relation to Surgical Therapeusis, 114
    Surgery: Principles and Practice, 172–174, 228
  as "quintessential" surgeon, 3–4
  relationship with children, 166–167, 169–170, 171–172
  relationship with colleagues, 132
  relationship with residents, 231–232, 243–244, 245–248
  religious faith of, 1–5, 165–166
  religious training of, 25
  on research, 144–145

Rhoads, Jonathan Evans *(cont.)*
  research activities
    collaboration in, 143, 144, 159–160
    cortisone research, 160–161
    failures of, 145, 160–161
    intravenous hyperalimentation research, 4, 175–213
    scar tissue research, 159–160
    during World War II, 143–145
  residency of, 99, 105–113
  resignation as Chairman of Department of Surgery, 249
  retirement activities of, 263–264
  retirement home of, 263
  Rittenhouse Club membership of, 228
  secretaries of, 220, 235–236, 258
  social life of, 134–136
  Society of Clinical Surgery membership and presidency of, 144, 159, 228
  Society of University Surgeons membership of, 144
  students' regard for, 140
  Sunday Breakfast Club membership of, 228
  surgical assistants of, 137, 160–161
  surgical fellowship of, 98–99, 105–107
  surgical innovation by, 234–235
  surgical judgement of, 139–140
  surgical rounds by, 158, 232
  surgical schedule of, 158–159, 220
  surgical specialization of, 98–99
  surgical technique of, 137, 245, 260
  teaching activities of, 4–5, 140–141
  teaching philosophy of, 140–141
  thesis of, 114
  travel and vacations, 53, 132–133, 163, 172, 236, 246–247
    on honeymoon, 109–110
    during internship, 92–93
    at Kearsarge, New Hampshire, 108, 132–133, 151–152, 158, 160, 162–163, 170–171, 263
    during medical school, 76–77, 80, 82, 87
    1972–1982, 249, 253
    during surgical chairmanship, 236, 237–238, 240–244, 245–246, 248
    during retirement, 263
    surgical duties during, 236–238
    during Vietnam War, 240–243
  travel style of, 172
  as University of Pennsylvania provost, 215–228, 235–236
  University of Pennsylvania tribute to, 257–258
Rhoads, Jonathan Evans (grandfather), 7–8

INDEX

Rhoads, Jonathan Evans Jr. (son), 65, 114, 261
Rhoads, Joseph (great-grandfather), 31
Rhoads, Julia (daughter-in-law), 2, 19, 261, 262
Rhoads, Katharine Evans Goddard (wife), 144, 262–263, 264, 265, 269
Rhoads, Margaret Ely Paxson (mother), 10–14, 15, 21–22, 44, 45, 55, 56, 151, 153, 169, 216–217, 259
   advice to daughter, 18–19
   correspondence with daughter, 97–98
   death of, 162–163
   on Rhoads' academic career, 43
   on Rhoads' childhood, 23–24
   on Rhoads' health, 32–33
   regard for daughter-in-law, 87
   travels of, 28, 41–42
Rhoads, Margaret (daughter). *See* Kendon, Margaret Rhoads (daughter)
Rhoads, Margaret (granddaughter), 261
Rhoads, Mary Teresa (granddaughter), 261
Rhoads, Philip (cousin), 83, 217
Rhoads, Philip (son), 153, 154, 156, 172, 265
Rhoads, Philip Jr. (grandson), 261
Rhoads, Rebecca Garrett (grandmother), 7, 8–9
Rhoads, Richard (uncle), 91
Rhoads, Ruth Anne (granddaughter), 261
Rhoads, Ruth Ely (sister), 7, 15–16, 22, 52, 55, 56, 261
Rhoads, Teresa Folin (wife), 37, 72–74, 80–81, 84, 128, 135, 253, 254, 260
   automobile driving habits of, 168
   children of, 153
   courtship of, 82–83, 86, 87–88, 90, 107–108
   death of, 261–262
   50th wedding anniversary of, 259
   financial interests of, 167
   illnesses of, 134, 154
   internship of, 87–88
   as Johns Hopkins student, 79
   marital relationship of, 168
   personality of, 167–168
   political views of, 169
   pregnancy of, 153
   relationship with grandchildren, 262
   religious faith of, 165
   residency of, 108
Rhoads, Thomas (grandson), 160, 261
Rhode, C. Martin, 148, 188–189
Richards, A. Newton, 81, 143, 179
Richards, Esther, 84–85, 85
Richardson, Ingram, 41, 45, 48, 49, 60, 65
Rickets, 110
Riegel, Cecelia, 104, 179, 185, 189
Ringer's solution, 177–178
Rio de Janeiro, Rhoads' trip to, 263
Rittenhouse Club, 228
Rittenhouse Square, 114
Roberts, Brooke, 95, 148, 159, 258, 266
Roberts, Isaac, 223
Roberts' Rules of Order, 39
Rockefeller Foundation, 219
Rodgers, Ginger, 70
Rodin, Judith, 268, 269
Roosevelt, Franklin, 91, 117, 122, 127, 153
Roosevelt, Theodore, 255
Roosevelt administration, 122
Roosevelt Boulevard, Philadelphia, 34
Rosato, Francis, 244–245, 246, 247
Rose, Elizabeth, 270
Rose, W.C., 193
Rosemond, George, 203
Rosenthal, Otto, 125, 130
Roswell Park, New York, 108
Roswell Park cancer center, 252
Royal Society of London, 255
Ruberg, Paul, 210
Ruigh, William, 179
Rusk, Howard, 241
Rusk Rehabilitation Center, 241
Russel, Hugh, 32
Russia, 240
   Rhoads' trip to, 76–77
Rustic Club, 32

Saltonstall, Henry, 141–142
San Diego, California, Rhoads family's trip to, 28
San Francisco, California, Rhoads' trips to, 27, 263
Santa Barbara, California, Rhoads family's trip to, 27
Santa Cruz, California, Rhoads family's trip to, 27–28
Saranac, New York, 151, 154
Savoy Operas (Gilbert), 90
Schmidt, Benno, 251, 266
Schmidt, Carl, 81, 81
Schmidt, L.A., 112
Schmidt Richards Lecture, 1
Schultz, Katherine, 87
Schuylkill River, 177
Schwartz, Henry, 76
Schwegman, Cletus, 147, 147–148, 156, 220
Science and Art Club, 263
Scopes trial, 76
Scott, 163

Seibert, Florence, 177
Selective Service Act of 1940, 118, 124
Serlick, Stanley, 202
Shapin, Jeannie, 258
Sharpless, Amy, 32
Sharpless, Isaac, 45
Shenkin, Henry, 187
Shires, Thomas, 173
Shock, 122, 143
　"speed", 177
　surgical, 186–187
Short bowel syndrome, intravenous hyperalimentation in, 176
Sloan-Kettering Hospital, 252
Sloan-Kettering Institute, 191
Smalley, Ruth, 222
Smith, Esther Morton, 56
Smith, H.P., 112
Smith, Roger, 252
Smith Act, 224
Smits, Helen, 203
Societas Latina, 32
Society of Clinical Surgery, 144, 228
Society of Friends, 2. *See also* American Friends Service Committee
　assistance to German refugees by, 117
　attitudes towards education of women, 46
　beliefs and values of, 2, 216
　conscientious objector proposal of, 117–119
　consensus use by, 216–217, 256–257
　influence on Rhoads, 1–5
　medical profession and, 4
　mental health movement involvement of, 85
　pacifism of, during World War I, 27
　Rhoads on, 4
Society of Organized Charity, 15
Society of University Surgeons, 144, 209
South Alabama, University of, 246
Southwestern Medical School, 173
Spaeth, George, 257–258
Spagna, Pascal, 202
Specialization, medical, 67
"Speed shock", 177
Spencer Morris Prize, 149
Spinal anesthesia, 113, 116, 133
Sprong, David, 74, 75, 80, 87
Sprong, Wilbur, 74, 75
Spruce Street, Philadelphia, 121, 158, 159, 220
S.S. Korea Maru, 17
Stanford University, 173
Stare, Frederick, 191–192
Starr, Isaac, 190–191

Stassen, Harold, 217
Stead Resort, Colorado, 173
Steiger, Ezra, 210
Stellar, Elliot, 258
Stengel, Alfred, 181
Sterre, Douglas, 5
Stevens, Lloyd, 133
Stevens, Robert, 60–61
Stevenson, Robert Louis, 7–8
Stewart, Francis, 29
Stokes, David, 256, 263–264
Stokes, Emlen, 102, 103, 163
Stokes, John, 51, 52, 63
Stokes, Joseph, 72, 81, 82, 110
Stokowski, Leopold, 253
Streptomycin, 152
Strittmayer Award, 265
Subspecialization, 231
Sugerman, Harvey, 234–235
Sulfanilamides, 121, 122, 126, 127, 134, 140
Sunday, Billy, 102
Sunday Breakfast Club, 228
Surgeons, characteristics of, 3–4
Surgeon to Soldier (Churchill), 121–122
Surgery
　during 1930s, 110
　physiological basis of, 104
Surgery: Principles and Practice (Rhoads et al), 172–174, 228
Surgery, 103–104
Surgical Clinics of North America, 107
Swingle, W.W., 179

Taft, William, 255
Talc, 110
Talman, Armistead, 235
Temple Medical School, 83
Temple University, 203, 253, 254
Temporomandibular joint disease, 136
Terrell, Alex, 111
Test, Dan, 83
Texas, University of, 229
Textbook of Pathology (MacCallum), 75
"Third phase of medicine," 241
Thompson, James, 229–230
Thoroughgood, Elizabeth, 184
Thrombosis, deep vein, 138, 139
Thymectomy, 145
Thyroid cancer, 233
Tibia, delayed union of, 149
Tic douloureux, 94
Time, 127
Timmis, Hilary, 229, 233, 248
Tompkins, Pendleton, 94, 97
Toronto Sick Children's Hospital, 209

INDEX

307

Total parenteral nutrition, 175, 191, 209, 210–213
Touchstone, Joseph, 160
Tourtelotte, Dee, 187, 188, 191, 198
Toxemia, of pregnancy, 141–142
Traction, 107
Travelers' Club, 228
Triangle honorary society, 42, 43
Tripler General Hospital, Honolulu, 121
Tuberculosis, 80, 151–158
Tucker, 104
Turner, Thomas B., 75, 85
20th General Hospital, 119, 123, 134, 145–146, 147, 148, 149

Ulin, Alex, 111
Union Club, 228
Union College, 57, 148–149
United Nations Relief and Rehabilitation Authority, 151
U.S. Defense Department, 165
U.S. House of Representatives, Appropriation Committee, 250
U.S. Public Health Service, 165
U.S. Surgeon General, 121–122
University of Pennsylvania Hospital. *See* Hospital of the University of Pennsylvania
University of Pennsylvania Press, 223
Upjohn Company, 192
Uremia, peritoneal dialysis for, 110

"Value of Biochemistry in Surgery" (Rhoads), 107, 175
Van Gobes, Anne, 168
Vars, Harry, 104, 125, 177, 179–181, 186, 187, 191, 195–196, 197, 198–200, 202, 211, 254, 258
Vars, Jonathan, 180
Vascular surgery, 231
Vassar College, 72, 73, 262
Viet Cong, 242
Vietnam, French Indochina War in, 203
Vietnam War, 180, 240–244
Vietnam War Memorial, Washington, D.C., 180
Villa, Pancho, 102
Vining, Elizabeth Gray, 17, 18, 20
Vishay Technologies, 1
Vitamin C deficiency, 183
Vitamin K, 112
Vitamin K, intravenous administration of, 192
Vitamin K deficiency, 112
Volk, Herbert, 154

Wachman, Marvin, 253–254, 254
Walker, Gerry, 130, 148
Wallack, Marc, 232
Wangensteen, Owen, 103, 104
Wangensteen suction, 110
Washington, George, 8–9, 11, 255
Washington University, 173, 186
Watson, James, 250, 251
Webster, Doris, 92
Webster, John, 12, 33–35, 42, 48, 49, 89, 90, 92, 108, 239
Weed, 70–71
Weiss, Soma, 85–86
Welch, William, 66–67
Werner, Dr., 155, 156
Westtown Alumni Association, 9
Westtown Boarding School, 9
Westtown School, 1–2
  Backlog Camp of, 40–41, 44, 65
  Caroline Rhoads as student at, 22
  Edward Rhoads' association with, 9
  Joseph Rhoads as student at, 31
  Margaret Paxson Rhoads as student at, 12
  Rhoads as board member of, 4, 257
  Rhoads' chemistry prize, 267
  Rhoads as student at, 30–35
  Ruth Rhoads as student at, 14–15
  sexual equality principle of, 46
Westtown Through the Years (Hole), 37
Wharton School of Business, 220, 221, 219, 225
Whipple, Alan O., 114–115, 116–117, 127, 233
Whipple, George, 182, 183
Whipple operation, 234
White, Raleigh IV, 245
Whittier College, 172
William Penn Lecture, 254
Williams, Edwin, 218
Willits, Joseph, 219–220
Wills, Rebecca, 38
Wilmington Friends School, 22
Wilmore, Douglas, 202, 203–205, 208, 211
Wilson, Woodrow, 255
Winn, Willis, 221, 225, 228
Wisconsin, University of, 241
Wistar, Richard, 45
Woll, John, 60, 71
Womack, Nathan, 183
Women
  as American Philosophical Society members, 255
  as Haverford College employees, 47
  as interns and residents, 139–140
  Quaker attitudes towards, 46

Women's Foreign Missionary Association, 12
Wood, Francis, 145–146, 198
Wooley, Maryanne, 22
World's Fair, 92–93
World War I, 11, 26–27, 102–103, 123, 240
World War II, 117–119, 121–146, 240
Wound healing, in malnutrition, 183–184
Wretlind, Arvid, 193
Wright, Howell, 74

Yale University, 87–88, 142, 180, 266–267
Yarborough, Ralph, 250
Yarnall, Stanley, 45, 163
York Hospital, 264

Zebly, Miss, 26
Zeppelin (dirigible) disaster (1936), 129
Zintel, Harold, 124, 125, 126, 132, 134, 139, 146, 148, 157
Zurich, University of, 84